RNC-MNN Study Guide

All-in-one RNC-MNN Review + 600 Practice questions with Detailed Answer Explanation for the NCC Maternal Newborn Nursing Exam (4 Full-Length Exams)

Lizzie Z. Dawson
Scarlett Medina
© 2024-2025
Printed in USA.

Disclaimer:

© Copyright 2024 by Lizzie Z. Dawson. All rights reserved.

All rights reserved. It is illegal to distribute, reproduce or transmit any part of this book by any means or forms. Every effort has been made by the author and editor to ensure correct information in this book. This book is prepared with extreme care to give the best to its readers. However, the author and editor hereby disclaim any liability to any part for any loss, or damage caused by errors or omission. Recording, photocopying or any other mechanical or electronic transmission of the book without prior permission of the publisher is not permitted, except in the case of critical reviews and certain other non-commercial uses permitted by copyright law.

Printed in the United States of America.
RNC-MNN ®, NCC ® are registered trademarks. They hold no affiliation with this product. We are not affiliated with or endorsed by any official testing organization.

CONTENTS

1. PREGNANCY, BIRTH RISK FACTORS AND COMPLICATIONS:
   1.1 Antenatal Factors:
   1.2 Intrapartum Factors:
2. MATERNAL POSTPARTUM ASSESSMENT, MANAGEMENT AND EDUCATION:
   2.1 Physiologic Changes and Physical Assessment:
   2.2 Nursing Care:
   2.3 Lactation:
   2.4 Psychosocial and Ethical Issues:
   2.5 Newborn feeding and nutrition:
3. NEWBORN ASSESSMENT AND MANAGEMENT:
   3.1 Transition to Extrauterine Life (Birth to 4 Hours):
   3.2 Physical Assessment and Gestational Age Assessment (to Include Laboratory Values), NEWBORN ASSESSMENT AND MANAGEMENT:
   3.3 Newborn Care and Family Education:
   3.4 Resuscitation and Stabilization:
4. MATERNAL POSTPARTUM COMPLICATIONS:
   4.1 Hematologic:
   4.2 Cardiovascular:
   4.3 Infection:
   4.4 Diabetes:
   4.5 Mood and Substance Use Disorders:
5. NEWBORN COMPLICATIONS:
   5.1 Cardiovascular and Respiratory:
   5.2 Neurological and Gastrointestinal:
   5.3 Hematologic:
   5.4 Infectious Disease:

RNC-MNN Practice Test 1
Answers with Explanation for Practice Test 1
RNC-MNN Practice Test 2
Answers with Explanation for Practice Test 2
RNC-MNN Practice Test 3
Answers with Explanation for Practice Test 3
RNC-MNN Practice Test 4
Answers with Explanation for Practice Test 4

Why do you need to be RNC-MNN Certified?

➢ Firstly, being RNC-MNN certified validates your expertise in the domain, enabling you to stand out among your peers and gain professional recognition. It showcases your commitment to continuous learning and staying updated with the latest advancements in the field.

➢ Additionally, the RNC-MNN certification signifies your ability to deliver safe and high-quality care to patients. This can enhance patient trust and satisfaction, and lead to improved patient outcomes.

➢ Furthermore, the RNC-MNN certification sets you apart in the job market, making you a sought-after candidate. Many employers prioritize hiring RNC-MNN certified candidates due to the added confidence in their skills and knowledge.

➢ Lastly, obtaining the RNC-MNN certification can open up opportunities for career advancement and higher salaries. Many healthcare organizations value the expertise and dedication of RNC-MNN certified candidates and may offer increased responsibilities and compensation packages accordingly.

Willing to Join Our Author Panel?

Dear,

We would like to invite you to join our 'Panel of Authors'.

First of all, Thank you for your hard work and dedication to your patients. We know that the hours are long and the workload is demanding, but you do it with grace and dignity. Your compassion is evident in the way you treat your patients, and we are grateful for all that you do.

We believe that your expertise and experience will be a valuable contribution to our books. Our goal is to provide valuable content that helps our readers to step forward in their career development. This is a unique opportunity to share your expertise with others in need and help shape their future.

The requirements for joining our panel of authors are as follows:
- A minimum experience of 8 years
- Proper certification from a renowned organization
- Good writing and teaching skills
- Enthusiasm in sharing knowledge

If you meet these requirements and are interested in joining our panel, please send us your resume along with a writing sample for our review to
propublisher@zohomail.com.

We would be happy to have you on board!
We are happy that our panel of authors can provide the best content because they are experienced and passionate in their own field. We would love for you to join our panel of authors and help us continue to provide quality content for our readers. You will also be able to connect with other experts in your domain from around the world and build a network of support. Undoubtedly, this will be a great opportunity for you to make a difference in your profession.

Thank You

Why is this book the right choice for you to clear the RNC-MNN Exam?

Latest Study Guide:
If you are looking for an up-to-date study guide for the RNC-MNN Exam, then look no further than this book. This book provides everything you need to know to ace the exam with tons of practice questions to help you prepare. This book is also constantly updated to ensure that it always covers the latest information on the exam as per the outline provided by the NCC ®.

RNC-MNN ® TEST CONTENT OUTLINE

1. Pregnancy, Birth Risk Factors and Complications
2. Maternal Postpartum Assessment, Management and Education
3. Newborn Assessment and Management
4. Maternal Postpartum Complications
5. Newborn Complications

Experienced Set of Authors:
There are many reasons to choose this book over others, but one of the most important is that it is written by experienced authors who are RNC-MNN Certified. The authors of this book have a wealth of experience in taking and passing exams, and we have used our knowledge to create a study guide that is comprehensive and easy to follow.
With our experienced authors and comprehensive coverage, our book is the best way to prepare for this important test.

Detailed rationale for the answer:
We provide an in-depth explanation for each question, so you can understand not only the correct answer but also why it is correct. This book also gives you an ample amount of practice to help you feel confident on exam day.

Similar Question Format as that in the actual exam:
One of the most important features of this book is that the questions and answers follow the same pattern as the actual exam. This is extremely important because you need to be familiar with the format of the exam to do well on it.

Fine Tunes your thinking:
Going through the questions, answers and explanations repeatedly will sharpen your thinking and understanding ability. This will help you to understand the root of the question in the RNC-MNN Exam and make the right selection of the answer.

Clear and Concise:

This RNC-MNN Prep is written in simple language and is not overly technical. This sets this book apart from other study materials because when you are studying for the RNC-MNN Exam, you need to be able to understand the material without getting bogged down in details. This book will help you do just that. This combination of easy-to-understand language and practical testing will help you be successful on the RNC-MNN exam.

Magical Steps to Pass the RNC-MNN Exam with Ease:

1. Belief: You must believe that you can pass the RNC-MNN exam with ease. This belief will help you stay focused and motivated throughout your studies. We help build your confidence by giving you the feel of attending virtual exams in our book, making you familiar with the type of questions that will be asked in the exam, and giving you a thorough idea about all the topics as specified by NCC ®.

2. Visualization: Visualize yourself passing the RNC-MNN exam with flying colors. This will help you stay positive and focused on your goal. Taking multiple tests and solving various questions will help improve your positivity and confidence. We try our best to improve your positivity.

3. Study: Make sure to study all the material thoroughly. Quality Learning is more important than Quantity Learning. Time yourself when you take tests and try to complete them within the stipulated time.

4. Practice: The more you practice the more is the chance of passing the exam. By doing this, you will get a feel for the types of questions that will be asked and how to best answer them. We have an abundant number of questions for you to practice.

5. Relax: On the day of the exam, make sure to relax and stay calm. This will help you think more clearly and perform at your best.

Smart Learning with Trust in Yourself will make Success knock at your door! All the

RNC-MNN Guide

1 PREGNANCY, BIRTH RISK FACTORS AND COMPLICATIONS:

Pregnancy, birth risk factors, and complications are crucial aspects for a Maternal Newborn Nurse. Risk factors include age, obesity, and medical conditions. Complications can arise during pregnancy, labor, or delivery. Preterm birth, preeclampsia, and gestational diabetes are common issues. Maternal health, lifestyle, and genetics play a role in pregnancy outcomes. Nurses must monitor mothers and babies closely for signs of distress. Early detection and intervention can prevent serious complications. Education and support for mothers are essential in promoting healthy pregnancies. Nurses play a vital role in providing care, guidance, and advocacy for pregnant women. Understanding risk factors and complications is key to ensuring safe deliveries and healthy outcomes for both mother and baby.

1.1 Antenatal Factors:

Antenatal factors play a crucial role in pregnancy outcomes. Maternal age, pre-existing health conditions, and lifestyle choices are key factors. Adequate prenatal care and nutrition are essential for a healthy pregnancy. Monitoring maternal weight gain and blood pressure is important. Avoiding harmful substances like alcohol and tobacco is crucial. Genetic factors and family history also impact pregnancy. Folic acid intake can prevent birth defects. Screening for infections and managing chronic illnesses are vital. Mental health support is important for maternal well-being. Antenatal education and support help in reducing birth risks. Overall, addressing antenatal factors is essential for a successful pregnancy and childbirth.

1.1.1 Maternal Health Status:
Maternal health status is crucial for maternal newborn nurses to monitor. Antenatal factors play a significant role in determining maternal health during pregnancy. Factors such as age, nutrition, and pre-existing medical conditions can impact maternal well-being. Monitoring these factors is essential for identifying potential risks and complications.

During pregnancy, various birth risk factors and complications can arise, affecting maternal health. Nurses must be vigilant in assessing these risks and providing appropriate care. Complications such as gestational diabetes, preeclampsia, and preterm labor can have serious consequences if not managed effectively.

By staying informed about maternal health status, nurses can ensure the well-being of both mother and baby. Regular monitoring, early intervention, and effective communication are key in promoting positive outcomes for pregnant women.

1.1.2 Age:
Age is a crucial factor in pregnancy and birth risk assessment. Advanced maternal age, typically defined as **35** years and older, is associated with increased complications. Older mothers may face higher risks of gestational diabetes, hypertension, and chromosomal abnormalities in the fetus. On the other hand, teenage pregnancies also pose unique challenges. Adolescents are more likely to experience preterm birth, low birth weight, and inadequate prenatal care. It is essential for maternal newborn nurses to be aware of the specific risks associated with different age groups. Proper education, monitoring, and support can help mitigate these risks and ensure the best possible outcomes for both mother and baby. Understanding the impact of age on pregnancy and birth is crucial for providing comprehensive care to expectant mothers.

1.1.3 Nutrition:
Nutrition plays a crucial role in antenatal factors, pregnancy, birth risk factors, and complications. A balanced diet rich in vitamins, minerals, and nutrients is essential for the health of both the mother and the baby. Adequate intake of folic acid helps prevent neural tube defects. Iron is important for preventing anemia. Omega-3 fatty acids support brain development. Proper hydration is necessary for overall well-being. Avoiding alcohol, caffeine, and certain foods is recommended. Consulting with a healthcare provider for personalized nutrition advice is beneficial. Good nutrition can help reduce the risk of complications during pregnancy and childbirth. It is important for maternal newborn nurses to educate and support pregnant women in making healthy food choices.

1.1.4 Obstetrical history:
Obstetrical history is crucial for assessing antenatal factors, pregnancy, birth risk factors, and complications. It includes information about previous pregnancies, deliveries, and any complications. Maternal age, medical conditions, and previous obstetrical surgeries are also part of the history.

Subtopics like gestational age at delivery, mode of delivery, and any pregnancy-related complications are essential. Understanding the obstetrical history helps in predicting potential risks during the current pregnancy. It guides healthcare providers in developing a personalized care plan for the mother and baby.

By analyzing the obstetrical history, nurses can identify red flags and provide appropriate interventions to ensure a safe pregnancy and delivery. Regular monitoring and communication with the healthcare team are essential for managing any potential complications.

1.1.5 Psychosocial/Cultural Issues:

Psychosocial/cultural issues in the context of antenatal factors, pregnancy, birth risk factors, and complications are crucial for maternal newborn nurses to consider. Understanding the impact of these issues on maternal health is essential.

Subtopics to consider include mental health, social support, socioeconomic status, cultural beliefs, and access to healthcare.

Psychosocial factors such as stress, depression, and anxiety can affect pregnancy outcomes. Cultural beliefs and practices may influence a woman's decision-making during pregnancy and childbirth.

Addressing these issues requires a holistic approach that considers the physical, emotional, and social well-being of the mother.

Effective communication, cultural competence, and sensitivity are key skills for maternal newborn nurses in providing quality care to diverse populations.

By recognizing and addressing psychosocial/cultural issues, nurses can help promote positive maternal and newborn health outcomes.

1.1.6 Infertility:

Infertility is the inability to conceive after a year of trying. It can be caused by various factors such as age, hormonal imbalances, and lifestyle choices. Antenatal factors like obesity and smoking can increase the risk of infertility.

Pregnancy complications related to infertility include higher chances of miscarriage and ectopic pregnancy. Women with infertility may also have a higher risk of preterm birth and low birth weight babies.

Infertility can lead to emotional distress and strain on relationships. Treatment options include medications, surgery, and assisted reproductive technologies like IVF. It's important for maternal newborn nurses to provide support and education to couples dealing with infertility.

1.1.7 Physiologic Changes and Associated Lab Values:

During pregnancy, there are various physiologic changes that occur in a woman's body. These changes include an increase in blood volume, heart rate, and respiratory rate. Lab values such as hemoglobin and hematocrit may decrease due to dilutional effects. Renal function also changes, leading to alterations in creatinine and blood urea nitrogen levels. Hormonal changes can affect glucose metabolism, resulting in changes in blood sugar levels. Additionally, changes in liver function can impact lab values such as alkaline phosphatase and transaminases. It is important for maternal newborn nurses to monitor these changes closely to ensure the health and well-being of both the mother and the baby.

1.1.8 Antepartum Risk Factors and Complications:

Antepartum risk factors can lead to complications during pregnancy. These factors include maternal age, obesity, and medical conditions like diabetes and hypertension. Substance abuse and smoking also increase risks. Infections such as urinary tract infections and sexually transmitted diseases can cause complications. Poor nutrition and inadequate prenatal care are additional risk factors. Complications may include preterm birth, preeclampsia, and gestational diabetes. Fetal growth restriction and birth defects are also possible. Monitoring and managing these risk factors are crucial for a healthy pregnancy outcome. Education and support for pregnant women are essential in preventing complications. Antenatal care plays a vital role in identifying and addressing these risk factors early on. Early intervention can help reduce the chances of adverse outcomes for both the mother and the baby.

1.1.8.1 Diabetes:

Diabetes is a common condition that can affect pregnancy. Antepartum risk factors include obesity and family history. Antenatal factors such as poor glucose control can lead to complications.

During pregnancy, diabetes can increase the risk of birth defects and miscarriage. It can also cause macrosomia, or large birth weight.

Gestational diabetes is a type of diabetes that develops during pregnancy. It can increase the risk of preeclampsia and preterm birth.

Proper management of diabetes during pregnancy is crucial to reduce complications. This includes monitoring blood sugar levels and following a healthy diet.

Maternal newborn nurses play a vital role in educating and supporting pregnant women with diabetes to ensure a safe pregnancy and delivery.

1.1.8.2 Hypertension (Chronic, gestational):

Hypertension during pregnancy can be chronic or gestational. Chronic hypertension predates pregnancy. Gestational hypertension develops after **20** weeks of pregnancy. It can lead to preeclampsia, a serious condition. Antepartum risk factors include obesity, diabetes, and family history. Antenatal factors like age and race can also play a role. Complications of hypertension include preterm birth and low birth weight. Monitoring blood pressure is crucial. Treatment may involve medication and lifestyle changes. Regular prenatal visits are essential for early detection and management. Maternal Newborn Nurses play a vital role in educating and supporting pregnant women with hypertension.

1.1.8.3 Common Bacterial and Viral Infections:

Common bacterial and viral infections can pose risks during pregnancy. Bacterial infections like urinary tract infections can lead to complications. Viral infections such as influenza can also be harmful. Antepartum risk factors include poor hygiene and exposure to infected individuals. Antenatal factors like weakened immune system increase susceptibility. These infections can cause preterm labor and birth complications. It is crucial for maternal newborn nurses to monitor for signs of infection. Early detection and treatment are essential to prevent adverse outcomes. Education on prevention strategies is key in reducing the risk of infections. Proper hand hygiene and vaccination can help protect both mother and baby. Regular prenatal care is vital in managing and preventing infections during pregnancy.

1.1.8.4 Hematologic (Anemias):
Hematologic (Anemias) in the context of Maternal Newborn Nursing involves various antepartum risk factors and complications. Anemias can be caused by iron deficiency, vitamin B12 deficiency, or folic acid deficiency. These deficiencies can lead to maternal fatigue, preterm birth, and low birth weight. Antenatal factors such as poor nutrition, multiple pregnancies, and chronic diseases can increase the risk of anemia during pregnancy. It is essential for maternal newborn nurses to monitor hemoglobin levels, provide iron supplementation, and educate pregnant women on the importance of a healthy diet. Early detection and management of anemia can prevent adverse outcomes for both the mother and the baby.

1.1.8.5 Cardiac Disease:
Cardiac disease in pregnancy poses risks. Antepartum factors include hypertension and diabetes. Antenatal factors like smoking and obesity increase risk. Complications can arise during pregnancy and birth. Maternal mortality rates are higher. Close monitoring and management are crucial. Consultation with a cardiologist is recommended. Medications may need adjustment. Delivery planning is important. Vaginal delivery is preferred over C-section. Postpartum care is essential. Education on warning signs is necessary. Collaboration with healthcare team is key. Supportive care is vital for positive outcomes. Early recognition and intervention are critical. Maternal Newborn Nurses play a crucial role. Their expertise ensures safe outcomes.

1.1.8.6 Substance Abuse, (e.g. Smoking, Drugs, Alcohol, marijuana):
Substance abuse during pregnancy, including smoking, drugs, alcohol, and marijuana, poses significant risks. These substances can harm the developing fetus and lead to various complications. Smoking increases the risk of preterm birth and low birth weight. Drug use, such as opioids or cocaine, can cause birth defects and developmental delays. Alcohol consumption can result in fetal alcohol syndrome, leading to physical and cognitive impairments. Marijuana use may affect the baby's growth and brain development. Antepartum risk factors, such as maternal addiction and lack of prenatal care, contribute to these issues. Maternal newborn nurses play a crucial role in educating and supporting pregnant women to reduce substance abuse and improve maternal and fetal outcomes.

1.1.8.7 Preterm Labor/Post term Pregnancy:
Preterm labor is when a baby is born before 37 weeks. Risk factors include multiple pregnancies, infections, and high blood pressure. Complications can include breathing problems and developmental delays. Post-term pregnancy is when a baby is born after 42 weeks. Antenatal factors like advanced maternal age and obesity can increase the risk. Complications may include macrosomia and meconium aspiration. Maternal Newborn Nurses play a crucial role in monitoring and caring for mothers at risk for preterm labor or post-term pregnancy. They provide education, support, and medical interventions to ensure the best possible outcomes for both mother and baby. It is important for nurses to be knowledgeable about the signs, symptoms, and management of preterm labor and post-term pregnancy to provide optimal care.

1.1.8.8 Multiple Gestation:

Multiple gestation, or carrying more than one fetus, is a common occurrence in pregnancies. Antepartum risk factors include advanced maternal age and assisted reproductive technology. Antenatal factors such as chorionicity and amnionicity play a role in determining the risks associated with multiple gestation. Complications can arise during pregnancy, such as preterm labor, gestational diabetes, and preeclampsia. Monitoring for these complications is crucial to ensure the health of both the mother and the fetuses. Birth risk factors include preterm birth, low birth weight, and the need for cesarean delivery. Close monitoring and specialized care are essential for women with multiple gestation to prevent and manage potential complications. Maternal newborn nurses play a vital role in educating, supporting, and caring for women with multiple gestation throughout their pregnancy journey.

1.1.8.9 Intrauterine Growth Restriction:
Intrauterine Growth Restriction (IUGR) is a condition where a baby doesn't grow well in the womb. Antepartum risk factors include maternal hypertension, smoking, and poor nutrition. Antenatal factors like placental abnormalities and infections can also contribute to IUGR. Monitoring fetal growth through ultrasounds is crucial for early detection. Complications of IUGR include preterm birth, low birth weight, and stillbirth. Maternal conditions such as preeclampsia and diabetes can increase the risk of IUGR. Proper prenatal care and monitoring are essential to manage IUGR effectively. Close collaboration between healthcare providers is necessary to ensure the best outcomes for both the mother and the baby. Early detection and intervention can help reduce the risks associated with IUGR.

1.1.8.10 Oligohydramnios:
Oligohydramnios is a condition characterized by low amniotic fluid levels in the uterus. This can lead to complications during pregnancy and childbirth.
Antepartum Risk Factors and Complications:
- Maternal dehydration

- Fetal abnormalities
- Placental insufficiency

Antenatal Factors:
- Maternal hypertension
- Diabetes
- Post-term pregnancy

Pregnancy, Birth Risk Factors and Complications:
- Preterm labor
- Intrauterine growth restriction
- Cesarean delivery

Monitoring and management of oligohydramnios is crucial to prevent adverse outcomes for both the mother and the baby. It is important for maternal newborn nurses to be aware of the risk factors and complications associated with oligohydramnios to provide appropriate care and support to pregnant women experiencing this condition.

1.1.8.11 Polyhydramnios:

Polyhydramnios is an excess of amniotic fluid during pregnancy. It can lead to complications such as preterm labor, placental abruption, and fetal malpresentation. Antepartum risk factors include maternal diabetes, fetal anomalies, and multiple gestations. Antenatal factors like maternal age and obesity can also contribute to polyhydramnios. Maternal symptoms may include shortness of breath and abdominal discomfort. Diagnosis is made through ultrasound measurements of amniotic fluid levels. Management may involve monitoring, amniocentesis, and delivery planning. Complications for the newborn include respiratory distress and birth injuries. Maternal risks include postpartum hemorrhage and uterine atony. Close monitoring and timely interventions are crucial in managing polyhydramnios to ensure the best outcomes for both mother and baby.

1.1.9 Fetal Assessment:

Fetal assessment is crucial during pregnancy to monitor the baby's well-being. It involves various methods such as ultrasound, fetal heart rate monitoring, and amniocentesis. Antenatal factors like maternal age, medical history, and lifestyle choices can impact fetal development. Regular assessments help identify any potential risks or complications early on. Monitoring fetal growth, movement, and heart rate patterns are essential indicators of fetal health. Abnormal findings may require further evaluation or intervention to ensure the baby's safety. Maternal Newborn Nurses play a vital role in conducting fetal assessments and providing support to expectant mothers. By closely monitoring fetal well-being, nurses can help promote healthy pregnancies and reduce the risk of complications during childbirth.

1.1.9.1 Biophysical Profile:

A biophysical profile is a prenatal test that assesses fetal well-being. It evaluates five key areas: fetal heart rate, fetal breathing movements, fetal movements, fetal muscle tone, and the amount of amniotic fluid. Each area is scored either **0** or **2**, with a total score out of **10**. This test helps in determining the overall health and development of the fetus. It is often recommended for high-risk pregnancies, such as those with maternal diabetes or hypertension. A low score may indicate the need for further testing or early delivery. The biophysical profile is a valuable tool for maternal newborn nurses in monitoring and managing pregnancies with potential complications. It provides important information to ensure the best possible outcomes for both the mother and the baby.

Nonstress Test:
A nonstress test is a common fetal assessment during pregnancy. It helps monitor the baby's heart rate and movement. The test is usually done in the third trimester. It is used to check the baby's well-being and detect any potential problems. During the test, a belt with sensors is placed on the mother's abdomen to record the baby's heart rate. The test is called "nonstress" because it doesn't put stress on the baby. A normal result shows that the baby's heart rate increases with movement. Abnormal results may indicate a need for further testing or intervention. Nonstress tests are important for identifying any potential risks or complications during pregnancy. Maternal Newborn Nurses play a crucial role in administering and interpreting nonstress tests for pregnant women.

1.1.9.2 Diagnostic Ultrasound:

Diagnostic ultrasound is a common tool in fetal assessment during pregnancy. It helps in evaluating antenatal factors such as fetal growth and development. Ultrasound is used to monitor the baby's health and detect any potential complications. It is a non-invasive procedure that poses no risk to the mother or the baby.

Ultrasound can identify birth risk factors like multiple pregnancies or placental abnormalities. It also helps in diagnosing complications such as ectopic pregnancy or fetal anomalies. The procedure is safe and painless, providing valuable information to healthcare providers. Overall, diagnostic ultrasound plays a crucial role in ensuring the well-being of both the mother and the newborn.

1.1.9.3 Amniocentesis:

Amniocentesis is a prenatal test to check for genetic abnormalities. It involves extracting amniotic fluid from the uterus. The procedure helps in diagnosing conditions like Down syndrome. It is usually done between **15-20** weeks of pregnancy. Amniocentesis carries a small risk of miscarriage. It can also detect neural tube defects. The test is recommended for women over **35**. Results take about **2-3** weeks. Counseling is essential before and after the procedure. It is important to discuss risks and benefits. Amniocentesis can provide valuable information for parents. It helps in making informed decisions about the pregnancy. The test is not mandatory but can be beneficial for some women.

1.1.9.4 Quad Screen/Cell Free DNA Testing:
Quad screen and cell-free DNA testing are prenatal screening tests. Quad screen evaluates risk for Down syndrome, trisomy 18, and neural tube defects. It measures levels of certain substances in the mother's blood. Cell-free DNA testing analyzes fetal DNA in the mother's blood. It screens for chromosomal abnormalities like Down syndrome. Quad screen is done between 15-20 weeks of pregnancy. Cell-free DNA testing can be done as early as 10 weeks. Both tests are non-invasive and carry no risk to the fetus. Results can help parents make informed decisions about further testing or interventions. Maternal Newborn Nurses play a crucial role in educating and supporting families through the testing process. Understanding these tests is essential for providing comprehensive care during pregnancy.

1.1.10 Obesity/Bariatric Surgery:
Obesity is a significant risk factor in pregnancy. It can lead to complications. Bariatric surgery is an option for obese women. It can help improve fertility. However, it may also increase the risk of certain complications during pregnancy. These complications include malnutrition and gestational diabetes. Close monitoring is essential for women who have had bariatric surgery. They may require additional supplements. Adequate nutrition is crucial for the health of both the mother and the baby. Maternal Newborn Nurses play a vital role in educating and supporting these women. They help ensure a healthy pregnancy and safe delivery. Understanding the impact of obesity and bariatric surgery is essential for providing quality care.

1.2 Intrapartum Factors:

Intrapartum factors are crucial during childbirth. These factors include maternal health conditions. Maternal health conditions can impact labor progression. Fetal well-being is also important. Monitoring fetal heart rate is essential. Maternal position during labor affects outcomes. Pain management choices can influence labor. Interventions like induction or augmentation may be necessary. Complications like shoulder dystocia can arise. Maternal exhaustion can prolong labor. Infection risk increases with prolonged labor. Maternal dehydration can impact contractions. Maternal age and weight can affect labor. Intrapartum factors play a significant role in birth outcomes. Maternal Newborn Nurses must be aware of these factors. Understanding intrapartum factors is essential for providing optimal care.

1.2.1 Significance of Fetal Heart Rate Patterns and Blood Gases:
Fetal heart rate patterns and blood gases are crucial indicators during labor. Monitoring these helps assess the baby's well-being and response to labor. Abnormal heart rate patterns may indicate fetal distress. Variations in blood gases can affect oxygen delivery to the baby. Hypoxia can lead to brain damage or even death. Understanding these patterns can guide interventions to optimize outcomes. Different patterns like accelerations, decelerations, and variability provide valuable information. Timely recognition and management of abnormal patterns are essential. Close monitoring and prompt action can prevent complications. Maternal Newborn Nurses play a vital role in interpreting these patterns and collaborating with the healthcare team. Continuous assessment and communication are key in ensuring safe delivery for both mother and baby.

1.2.2 Fetal Heart Rate Abnormalities (Tachycardia, Bradycardia, Altered Variability, Decelerations):
Fetal heart rate abnormalities, such as tachycardia, bradycardia, altered variability, and decelerations, are crucial indicators of fetal well-being during labor. Tachycardia is when the fetal heart rate exceeds 160 beats per minute, while bradycardia is when it falls below 110 beats per minute. Altered variability refers to irregular fluctuations in the heart rate pattern, and decelerations are sudden drops in heart rate during contractions. These abnormalities can be caused by various intrapartum factors, such as maternal fever, hypoxia, or umbilical cord compression. Maternal newborn nurses play a vital role in monitoring and interpreting fetal heart rate patterns to identify and address abnormalities promptly, ensuring the safety and well-being of both the mother and the baby.

1.2.3 Cord Gases:
Cord gases are used to assess fetal well-being during labor. They measure oxygen and carbon dioxide levels in the baby's blood. Low oxygen levels can indicate fetal distress. Acidosis, a condition where blood pH is too low, can also be detected. This can be caused by factors like prolonged labor or umbilical cord compression. High levels of carbon dioxide may suggest respiratory problems in the baby. Monitoring cord gases helps healthcare providers make timely decisions about the need for interventions like cesarean sections. It is an important tool in managing labor and ensuring the safety of both the mother and the baby. Understanding cord gases is crucial for maternal newborn nurses to provide optimal care during childbirth.

1.2.4 Medications Used in Labor:
Medications used in labor help manage pain and promote labor progression. Analgesics provide pain relief during early labor. Opioids are used for moderate to severe pain. Epidurals are common for pain management during labor. They provide effective pain relief. Local anesthetics are used for episiotomies or repairs. Pitocin is a synthetic form of oxytocin. It helps induce or augment labor. Magnesium sulfate is used to prevent seizures in preeclampsia. Antibiotics are given for Group B strep or

other infections. Medications in labor require careful monitoring for side effects. Nurses play a crucial role in administering and monitoring these medications. Understanding the different medications used in labor is essential for maternal newborn nurses.

1.2.4.1 Tocolytics:
Tocolytics are medications used to delay preterm labor contractions. They help prevent premature birth. Tocolytics work by relaxing the uterine muscles. Common tocolytics include magnesium sulfate, terbutaline, and nifedipine. These medications are given to pregnant women experiencing preterm labor. Tocolytics can help buy time for other treatments to take effect. They are not a cure for preterm labor but can delay it. Tocolytics may have side effects such as nausea, dizziness, and rapid heartbeat. It is important for maternal newborn nurses to monitor the mother and baby closely while on tocolytics. Proper administration and monitoring of tocolytics can help improve pregnancy outcomes.

1.2.4.2 Analgesics:
Analgesics are medications used during labor to relieve pain. They can be given orally, intravenously, or through an epidural. There are two main types of analgesics used in labor: opioids and non-opioids. Opioids, such as morphine and fentanyl, work by binding to receptors in the brain to reduce pain. Non-opioids, like acetaminophen and ibuprofen, work by blocking pain signals in the body.

Analgesics can help women manage pain during labor, but they can also have side effects. These side effects may include drowsiness, nausea, and slowed breathing.
It is important for maternal newborn nurses to monitor women receiving analgesics closely for any adverse reactions. Nurses should also educate women about the risks and benefits of using analgesics during labor.

1.2.4.3 Anesthesia:
Anesthesia is used during labor to manage pain and discomfort. There are different types of anesthesia available for women giving birth.
Epidural anesthesia is commonly used, which involves injecting medication into the epidural space in the lower back. This numbs the lower half of the body, providing pain relief during labor.
Spinal anesthesia is another option, where medication is injected directly into the spinal fluid. This provides quick pain relief, but only lasts for a few hours.
General anesthesia may be used in emergency situations or for cesarean sections. It puts the woman to sleep, so she is unconscious during the birth.
Anesthesia carries some risks and side effects, so it is important for maternal newborn nurses to monitor the mother closely.

1.2.5 Complications of Labor:
Complications of labor can arise due to various intrapartum factors. These factors include prolonged labor, fetal distress, and abnormal presentation. Maternal health conditions such as hypertension and diabetes can also lead to complications during labor. Infections, such as chorioamnionitis, can increase the risk of complications.
Other risk factors for labor complications include maternal age, obesity, and multiple pregnancies. Complications during labor can result in emergency interventions like cesarean section or vacuum extraction. These interventions may be necessary to ensure the safety of both the mother and the baby. It is essential for maternal newborn nurses to be knowledgeable about the potential complications of labor and be prepared to provide appropriate care and support during childbirth.

1.2.5.1 Breech and Other Malpresentations:
Breech and other malpresentations can complicate labor and delivery. Breech presentation occurs when the baby's buttocks or feet are positioned to come out first instead of the head. This can increase the risk of birth complications. Other malpresentations include transverse lie and face or brow presentation. These malpresentations can lead to prolonged labor, fetal distress, and the need for a cesarean section. Maternal newborn nurses should be aware of the signs and symptoms of breech and other malpresentations. They should monitor the progress of labor closely and be prepared to intervene if necessary. Proper management of breech and other malpresentations is crucial to ensure the safety of both the mother and the baby.

1.2.5.2 Meconium:
Meconium is a baby's first stool passed in the womb. It can be a sign of fetal distress during labor. Meconium-stained amniotic fluid can lead to respiratory issues for the newborn. Meconium aspiration syndrome occurs when the baby inhales meconium into the lungs. This can cause breathing difficulties and require medical intervention. Maternal factors like post-term pregnancy and maternal hypertension can increase the risk of meconium passage. Intrapartum factors such as prolonged labor or fetal distress can also lead to meconium passage. Maternal newborn nurses should monitor for meconium-stained fluid during labor. They should be prepared to provide immediate care to babies at risk for meconium aspiration syndrome. Understanding the complications associated with meconium is crucial for ensuring the well-being of both mother and baby.

1.2.5.3 Shoulder Dystocia:
Shoulder dystocia is a complication during labor where the baby's shoulder gets stuck behind the mother's pubic bone. This can lead to serious complications for both the mother and the baby. Risk factors for shoulder dystocia include maternal diabetes, obesity, and a history of macrosomia. Intrapartum factors such as prolonged labor or the use of forceps can also increase the risk of shoulder dystocia. Maternal newborn nurses play a crucial role in recognizing the signs of shoulder dystocia and providing prompt and effective interventions to prevent further complications. It is important for nurses to be

knowledgeable about shoulder dystocia and be prepared to act quickly in order to ensure the safety of both the mother and the baby.

1.2.5.4 PROM and Chorioamnionitis:
Premature rupture of membranes (PROM) can lead to chorioamnionitis, an infection of the fetal membranes. Chorioamnionitis can cause complications during labor and delivery. Risk factors for PROM include smoking, infections, and multiple pregnancies. Chorioamnionitis can result in fever, uterine tenderness, and foul-smelling amniotic fluid. It can lead to preterm labor, sepsis, and neonatal infection. Prompt diagnosis and treatment are essential to prevent maternal and fetal complications. Treatment may involve antibiotics, monitoring, and possible early delivery. Maternal newborn nurses play a crucial role in recognizing the signs of PROM and chorioamnionitis, providing care, and supporting the mother and baby throughout the labor and delivery process.

1.2.5.5 Prolonged Labor:
Prolonged labor can lead to various complications for both the mother and the baby. It is often caused by factors such as ineffective contractions, malposition of the baby, or a narrow pelvis. In some cases, medical interventions may be necessary to prevent further risks. Complications of prolonged labor can include maternal exhaustion, fetal distress, and an increased risk of infection. Intrapartum factors, such as the use of epidurals or induction methods, can also contribute to prolonged labor. It is essential for maternal newborn nurses to monitor labor progress closely and intervene when necessary to ensure a safe delivery for both the mother and the baby.

1.2.5.6 Abruption:
Abruption is the premature separation of the placenta from the uterus. It can lead to serious complications for both the mother and the baby.
- Symptoms include vaginal bleeding, abdominal pain, and contractions.
- Risk factors include high blood pressure, smoking, and trauma.
- Diagnosis is based on symptoms, physical exam, and ultrasound.
- Treatment may involve monitoring, bed rest, or emergency delivery.
- Complications can include fetal distress, preterm birth, or maternal hemorrhage.
- Nurses play a crucial role in monitoring for signs of abruption and providing support.

Understanding the signs, risk factors, and management of abruption is essential for maternal newborn nurses to ensure the best outcomes for both mother and baby.

1.2.5.7 Placenta Previa:
Placenta Previa is a condition where the placenta partially or completely covers the cervix. It can cause painless bleeding in the third trimester. There are different types of Placenta Previa based on the location of the placenta. Risk factors include previous C-sections, multiple pregnancies, and advanced maternal age. Diagnosis is usually made through ultrasound. Complications can arise during labor, such as excessive bleeding. Treatment may involve bed rest, monitoring, and cesarean delivery. Nurses should educate patients on signs of bleeding and when to seek medical help. It is important to closely monitor both the mother and baby during labor and delivery.

1.2.5.8 Cord Prolapse:
Cord prolapse occurs when the umbilical cord slips through the cervix before the baby. This can lead to compression of the cord, cutting off oxygen and blood flow to the baby. Risk factors include preterm birth, multiple pregnancies, and breech presentation. Symptoms may include sudden fetal heart rate deceleration and visible or palpable cord. Immediate action is crucial to prevent fetal distress and potential complications. Treatment involves relieving pressure on the cord by changing the mother's position, performing a cesarean section, or pushing the baby's head back into the pelvis. Maternal Newborn Nurses must be vigilant in monitoring for signs of cord prolapse during labor to ensure the safety of both mother and baby.

1.2.5.9 Precipitous Delivery:
Precipitous delivery is a rapid labor and birth process. It occurs in less than 3 hours. This can lead to complications for both the mother and the baby. Maternal risks include severe bleeding and tears. Fetal risks include oxygen deprivation and head trauma. Factors contributing to precipitous delivery include multiparity and previous fast labors. Nurses must be prepared to act quickly and efficiently. They should monitor closely for signs of distress. Immediate interventions may be necessary to ensure a safe delivery. Nurses should provide emotional support to the mother. Education on the risks and warning signs is crucial. Proper documentation and communication with the healthcare team are essential. Training in emergency procedures is vital for maternal newborn nurses.

1.2.6 Methods of Delivery:
Methods of delivery during childbirth include vaginal delivery and cesarean section. Vaginal delivery is the most common method, where the baby is born through the birth canal. Cesarean section, or C-section, involves surgical delivery through an incision in the abdomen and uterus. Indications for a C-section include fetal distress, breech presentation, or maternal health concerns. Other methods such as vacuum extraction or forceps delivery may be used in certain situations. The choice of delivery method depends on various factors like the health of the mother and baby, previous childbirth experiences, and any complications during labor. Maternal newborn nurses play a crucial role in assisting with different delivery methods, providing support and care to both mother and baby throughout the birthing process.

1.2.6.1 Vaginal:
Vaginal delivery is a common method of childbirth. It involves the baby passing through the birth canal. Intrapartum factors can affect the progress of vaginal delivery. These factors include the position of the baby, the mother's health, and the strength of contractions. Maternal pushing efforts also play a crucial role in the success of vaginal delivery. Nurses must monitor the progress of labor closely to ensure a safe delivery. Complications during vaginal delivery can arise, such as tears or infections. Proper care and support are essential during this process. Understanding the risks and factors involved in vaginal delivery is crucial for maternal newborn nurses.

1.2.6.2 Operative Delivery (Forceps, Vacuum, Cesarean):
Operative delivery includes forceps, vacuum, and cesarean sections. Forceps and vacuum are used to assist vaginal delivery. Cesarean section is a surgical procedure for delivery. Intrapartum factors like fetal distress may necessitate operative delivery. Maternal exhaustion or prolonged labor can also be indications. Operative delivery carries risks like maternal hemorrhage and infection. Fetal risks include head trauma and respiratory issues. Maternal consent is crucial before proceeding with operative delivery. Proper training and expertise are essential for safe delivery. Operative delivery should be considered when benefits outweigh risks. Close monitoring and follow-up care are necessary post-operatively. Maternal Newborn Nurses play a vital role in supporting women undergoing operative delivery.

1.2.6.3 VBAC:
VBAC, or Vaginal Birth After Cesarean, is a method of delivery for women who have had a previous C-section. Intrapartum factors, such as labor progression and fetal well-being, play a role in determining if a VBAC is safe. Pregnancy, birth risk factors, and complications can impact the success of a VBAC. Maternal age, BMI, and the reason for the previous C-section are important considerations. The risk of uterine rupture is a major concern during a VBAC. Close monitoring during labor is essential to ensure the safety of both the mother and the baby. Overall, VBAC can be a safe option for many women, but it is important to carefully assess each individual case.

1.2.7 Delayed Cord Clamping:
Delayed cord clamping is the practice of waiting to clamp the umbilical cord after birth. This allows more blood to transfer from the placenta to the baby. Benefits include increased iron levels, better immune system development, and improved cardiovascular stability. Delayed cord clamping can be done for **30** seconds to **5** minutes after birth. It is especially beneficial for preterm infants, as it can reduce the risk of complications such as anemia and intraventricular hemorrhage. Factors to consider include the baby's overall health, the presence of meconium, and the need for resuscitation. Maternal Newborn Nurses play a crucial role in advocating for delayed cord clamping and ensuring that the procedure is done safely and effectively.

2 MATERNAL POSTPARTUM ASSESSMENT, MANAGEMENT AND EDUCATION:
Maternal postpartum assessment involves evaluating physical and emotional well-being after childbirth. Nurses monitor vital signs, bleeding, and pain levels. They assess the uterus for firmness and size. Maternal management includes providing pain relief, promoting breastfeeding, and assisting with postpartum care. Education on self-care, newborn care, and warning signs is crucial. Postpartum depression screening and support are essential. Maternal bonding and family adjustment are also addressed. Effective communication and empathy are key in providing holistic care. Ongoing support and follow-up are important for maternal recovery and well-being.

2.1 Physiologic Changes and Physical Assessment:
Physiologic changes postpartum include uterine involution, vaginal discharge, and breast engorgement. Maternal vital signs should be monitored regularly. Assess for signs of hemorrhage, infection, and thromboembolism. Perform fundal height checks to ensure proper uterine contraction. Evaluate lochia color, amount, and odor for any abnormalities. Monitor for signs of postpartum depression and provide emotional support. Educate on proper perineal care, breastfeeding techniques, and contraception options. Encourage ambulation to prevent blood clots. Document findings accurately for continuity of care. Regular physical assessments are crucial for maternal well-being postpartum.

2.1.1 Reproductive:
Reproductive changes postpartum include involution of uterus, vaginal discharge, and breast engorgement. Maternal Newborn Nurse should assess bleeding, fundal height, and perineum. Monitor vital signs, assess for signs of infection, and provide education on self-care. Encourage breastfeeding, promote bonding, and discuss contraception options. Assess emotional well-being, provide support, and refer for further assistance if needed. Educate on postpartum warning signs, pelvic floor exercises, and resuming sexual activity. Monitor for postpartum depression, provide resources, and encourage self-care practices. Support the mother in her reproductive recovery and adjustment to motherhood.

2.1.2 Cardiopulmonary:
Cardiopulmonary changes postpartum are common. Maternal Newborn Nurses should monitor closely. Respiratory rate may increase due to hormonal shifts. Oxygen consumption decreases gradually. Blood volume decreases, leading to increased heart rate. Blood pressure may fluctuate. Nurses should assess for signs of pulmonary embolism. Educate mothers on deep breathing exercises. Encourage early ambulation to prevent complications. Provide education on signs of respiratory distress. Monitor for symptoms of postpartum hemorrhage. Maternal Newborn Nurses play a crucial role in managing cardiopulmonary changes. Regular assessments and education are key.

2.1.3 Genitourinary:
Genitourinary changes postpartum include increased blood flow to kidneys. This can lead to increased urine output. Maternal bladder tone may decrease, causing urinary retention. Assess for signs of urinary tract infection. Monitor for postpartum hemorrhage. Educate on perineal care and proper hygiene. Encourage adequate fluid intake. Discuss warning signs of complications. Provide resources for lactation support. Address any concerns about urinary incontinence. Support pelvic floor exercises. Offer emotional support during this transition. Remember to assess, educate, and manage genitourinary changes effectively.

2.1.4 Gastrointestinal:
Gastrointestinal changes postpartum can affect maternal well-being. Constipation is common. Encourage fiber intake. Monitor for hemorrhoids. Assess for abdominal distention. Educate on proper hydration. Discuss postpartum bowel movements. Watch for signs of infection. Provide comfort measures for discomfort. Support breastfeeding mothers with dietary advice. Encourage small, frequent meals. Monitor for signs of GI complications. Teach =about warning signs. Offer resources for lactation support. Address concerns about gas and bloating. Overall, understanding maternal gastrointestinal changes is crucial for postpartum care.

2.1.5 Hematological:
Hematological changes postpartum are common. Hemoglobin levels decrease after birth. Physiologic anemia is normal. Iron supplementation may be needed. Monitor for signs of anemia. Assess for excessive bleeding. Thromboembolic risk increases postpartum. Monitor for signs of thrombosis. Educate on signs of complications. Provide education on iron supplementation. Encourage a healthy diet. Monitor for postpartum hemorrhage. Assess for signs of infection. Educate on warning signs. Maternal well-being is crucial. Support and monitor closely. Hematological changes are important to monitor postpartum.

2.1.6 Endocrine:
The endocrine system undergoes changes postpartum. Hormone levels fluctuate significantly.

Subtopics:
- Hormones such as estrogen and progesterone decrease rapidly after delivery.
- Prolactin levels rise to stimulate milk production.
- Thyroid hormones may also fluctuate, leading to potential thyroid disorders.
- Adrenal glands produce cortisol to help the body cope with stress.

Maternal newborn nurses should assess for signs of hormonal imbalance.

Subtopics:
- Symptoms may include mood swings, fatigue, and weight changes.
- Physical assessment should include checking for signs of thyroid dysfunction.
- Education on postpartum hormonal changes and self-care is essential for new mothers.

Management may involve hormone replacement therapy or lifestyle modifications.

Subtopics:
- Supportive care and counseling can help women cope with emotional changes.
- Monitoring hormone levels and symptoms is crucial for maternal well-being.

2.2 Nursing Care:
Nursing care in maternal postpartum assessment, management, and education is crucial. Assessment includes vital signs, uterine firmness, and bleeding. Management involves pain relief, breastfeeding support, and emotional support. Education covers newborn care, postpartum warning signs, and contraception options. Nurses play a key role in providing holistic care to new mothers. It is important to monitor for complications such as postpartum hemorrhage and infection. Effective communication with the mother and family members is essential. Providing a safe and comfortable environment is vital for the mother's recovery. Nurses should also promote bonding between the mother and newborn. Continuous assessment and support are essential in ensuring the well-being of both the mother and baby.

2.2.1 Comprehensive Postpartum Health Assessment:

Comprehensive Postpartum Health Assessment is crucial in nursing care. It involves evaluating physical, emotional, and social well-being of the mother after childbirth. The assessment includes checking vital signs, uterine involution, lochia, and perineum healing. Maternal mental health, breastfeeding, and family support are also assessed. Postpartum complications like hemorrhage, infection, and postpartum depression are monitored. Education on self-care, contraception, and warning signs is provided. Maternal bonding and newborn care are emphasized. The assessment helps in early detection and management of any issues. It ensures the mother's smooth transition to motherhood and promotes overall well-being. Regular follow-up assessments are recommended to monitor progress and address any concerns promptly. Maternal Newborn Nurses play a vital role in providing comprehensive postpartum care.

2.2.1.1 Postoperative Care:

Postoperative care is crucial for maternal newborn nurses. It involves monitoring vital signs. Nurses should assess pain levels regularly. Encourage early ambulation to prevent complications. Provide education on wound care. Monitor for signs of infection. Support breastfeeding if applicable. Ensure proper medication administration. Offer emotional support to the mother. Collaborate with other healthcare providers as needed. Postoperative care plays a vital role in the recovery process.

2.2.2 Common Medications (Indications, Administration, Drug Interactions, Patient Teaching):

Common medications used in maternal postpartum care include pain relievers, such as ibuprofen and acetaminophen. These medications are administered orally to manage postpartum pain. It is important to educate patients on the proper dosage and timing of these medications. Additionally, nurses should be aware of potential drug interactions, such as ibuprofen interacting with blood thinners. Patient teaching should include information on possible side effects and when to seek medical help. Other common medications may include stool softeners to prevent constipation and prenatal vitamins to support postpartum recovery. Nurses play a crucial role in educating patients on the indications, administration, and potential drug interactions of these medications to ensure safe and effective postpartum care.

2.2.2.1 Insulin:

Insulin is a hormone that helps regulate blood sugar levels. It is commonly used to treat diabetes. Insulin is administered through injections or an insulin pump. It is important to monitor blood sugar levels regularly while on insulin therapy. Patient Teaching: Educate patients on proper administration techniques and the importance of monitoring blood sugar levels. Drug Interactions: Insulin may interact with certain medications, so it is important to consult with a healthcare provider before starting any new medications. Nursing Care: Nurses play a crucial role in educating patients about insulin therapy and monitoring their response to treatment. Maternal Postpartum Assessment: In the postpartum period, women with gestational diabetes may require insulin to manage their blood sugar levels. Management and Education: Nurses should provide support and education to new mothers on insulin therapy to ensure optimal outcomes for both mother and baby.

2.2.2.2 Analgesics (Tylenol):

Analgesics like Tylenol are commonly used for pain relief. They are indicated for postpartum discomfort. Tylenol can be administered orally. It is important to be aware of potential drug interactions. Patient teaching should include proper dosage and timing. Nursing care involves monitoring for side effects. Maternal postpartum assessment should include pain level evaluation. Management may include adjusting dosage based on pain intensity. Education should emphasize the importance of following prescribed guidelines. Maternal Newborn Nurses play a crucial role in ensuring safe and effective pain management.

2.2.2.3 Antimicrobials:

Antimicrobials are medications that treat infections caused by bacteria, viruses, fungi, or parasites. They are commonly used in maternal postpartum care to prevent or treat infections. Nurses play a crucial role in administering antimicrobials, monitoring for drug interactions, and educating patients on proper medication use. Maternal postpartum assessment involves evaluating the mother's overall health, including checking for signs of infection. Management of antimicrobials includes ensuring the correct dosage and frequency of administration. Patient education is essential to promote adherence to the prescribed treatment regimen and prevent complications. Nurses should also monitor for any adverse reactions to antimicrobials and report them promptly. Effective communication with healthcare providers and patients is key to successful antimicrobial therapy in the postpartum period.

2.2.2.4 Antihypertensives:

Antihypertensives are medications used to lower high blood pressure. They are commonly prescribed postpartum for women with hypertension. These medications help prevent complications such as stroke or heart attack. Nurses play a crucial role in administering antihypertensives and monitoring their effects. It is important to educate patients on the importance of taking their medication as prescribed. Drug interactions should be carefully monitored to avoid adverse effects. Maternal postpartum assessment includes monitoring blood pressure and evaluating for signs of preeclampsia. Management involves timely administration of antihypertensives and close monitoring of the patient's condition. Education should focus on signs of worsening hypertension and when to seek medical help. Overall, proper use of antihypertensives is essential in managing hypertension in the postpartum period.

2.2.2.5 Diuretics:
Diuretics are medications that help the body get rid of excess water and salt. They are commonly used to treat conditions such as high blood pressure, heart failure, and edema. Diuretics work by increasing the production of urine in the kidneys.

When administering diuretics, it is important to monitor the patient's fluid and electrolyte levels closely. Diuretics can interact with other medications, so it is crucial to be aware of potential drug interactions.

In maternal postpartum care, diuretics may be used to treat postpartum edema. Nurses should assess the patient's fluid status and educate them on the importance of taking the medication as prescribed.

Overall, diuretics play a vital role in managing various conditions, but proper monitoring and patient education are essential in ensuring their safe and effective use.

2.2.2.6 Oxytocics:
Oxytocics are medications used to induce or augment labor contractions. They are also given after childbirth to prevent or treat postpartum hemorrhage. Common oxytocics include Pitocin and Methergine.
- Indications: Used to initiate or strengthen labor contractions.
- Administration: Administered intravenously or intramuscularly as directed.
- Drug Interactions: Can interact with other medications, so consult healthcare provider.
- Patient Teaching: Educate on purpose, administration, and potential side effects.
- Nursing Care: Monitor contractions, fetal heart rate, and maternal blood pressure.
- Maternal Postpartum Assessment: Assess for signs of hemorrhage or adverse reactions.
- Management: Administer as prescribed, monitor closely for effectiveness.
- Education: Instruct on signs of complications and when to seek medical help.

Understanding oxytocics is crucial for maternal newborn nurses to provide safe and effective care.

2.2.2.7 GI Motility Drugs:
GI motility drugs help regulate digestion by promoting movement in the gastrointestinal tract. Common medications include metoclopramide and erythromycin. Metoclopramide is used for GERD and diabetic gastroparesis. Erythromycin is used for gastroparesis. These drugs can interact with other medications, so it's important to check for drug interactions. When administering these drugs, monitor for side effects like diarrhea or dizziness. Educate patients on how to take the medication as prescribed. In maternal postpartum care, these drugs may be used to treat gastrointestinal issues after delivery. Nursing care involves assessing for any adverse reactions and providing education on the importance of taking the medication correctly.

2.2.2.8 Vaccines:
Vaccines are crucial for maternal newborn nurses to understand. They prevent diseases in both mothers and babies. Nurses should know the indications for vaccines and how to administer them safely. Drug interactions with vaccines should be considered to ensure effectiveness. Patient teaching is essential to educate mothers about the importance of vaccines. Maternal postpartum assessment includes checking vaccine history and recommending any necessary vaccinations. Proper management involves scheduling vaccines and monitoring for adverse reactions. Education on vaccine safety and benefits is key for new mothers. Stay updated on vaccine recommendations to provide the best care for mothers and newborns.

2.2.2.9 Rh Immune Globulin (RhoGAM) (Rhophillac):
Rh Immune Globulin (RhoGAM) is given to Rh-negative mothers to prevent Rh incompatibility. It is administered within **72** hours after childbirth. RhoGAM works by preventing the mother's immune system from attacking Rh-positive fetal blood cells. It is crucial to administer RhoGAM to prevent hemolytic disease in future pregnancies.

Nursing care involves verifying the mother's blood type and the baby's blood type. Educate the mother about the importance of RhoGAM administration. Monitor for signs of a transfusion reaction after administration.

Maternal postpartum assessment includes monitoring for signs of Rh incompatibility. Management involves providing emotional support and education. Educate the mother about the need for RhoGAM in future pregnancies.

2.2.2.10 Nicotine Patches:
Nicotine patches are used to help individuals quit smoking. They are applied to the skin. The patches release nicotine into the bloodstream. This helps reduce withdrawal symptoms. It is important to follow the instructions for proper administration.

Nursing care involves assessing the patient's smoking history. Monitoring for side effects is crucial. Educate patients on how to use the patches correctly.

In the postpartum period, nicotine patches should be used with caution. They can affect breast milk. Inform new mothers about he risks. Encourage them to seek alternative methods to quit smoking.

Overall, nicotine patches can be an effective tool in smoking cessation. Proper education and monitoring are essential for success.

2.2.2.11 Antiretroviral:
Antiretrovirals are used to treat HIV/AIDS. They prevent viral replication. Common medications include Tenofovir, Emtricitabine, and Ritonavir. They are administered orally. Drug interactions can occur with other medications. Patient teaching is essential for adherence. Nursing care involves monitoring for side effects. Maternal postpartum assessment includes checking viral load. Management may involve adjusting medication doses. Education on breastfeeding and transmission prevention is crucial.

2.2.2.12 Methadone (subutex) SSI's:
Methadone (subutex) SSI's are commonly used in maternal postpartum care. They help manage opioid dependence. Nursing care involves monitoring for withdrawal symptoms. Patient teaching includes medication administration and potential side effects. Drug interactions should be carefully assessed. Maternal postpartum assessment should include monitoring for signs of addiction. Education on the importance of medication compliance is crucial. Proper management of medication dosage is essential. It is important to provide support and resources for mothers struggling with opioid dependence. Collaboration with healthcare providers is key in ensuring the well-being of both mother and baby.

2.2.2.13 Psychotropic Drugs:
Psychotropic drugs are medications used to treat mental health conditions. They are commonly prescribed for postpartum depression. These drugs can have various indications and administration routes. It is important to be aware of potential drug interactions. Patient teaching is crucial for understanding medication effects and side effects. Nursing care involves monitoring the mother's response to the medication. Maternal postpartum assessment includes evaluating mental health status. Management may involve adjusting medication dosage or type. Education is key in helping mothers cope with postpartum depression. It is essential for maternal newborn nurses to have a good understanding of psychotropic drugs.

2.2.3 Common Problems and Complications:
Common problems and complications in maternal postpartum care include issues like postpartum hemorrhage, infection, and breastfeeding difficulties. Postpartum hemorrhage can occur due to uterine atony or retained placental fragments. Infections may arise from episiotomy or cesarean incisions. Breastfeeding problems can range from latch issues to mastitis. Other common complications include postpartum depression, urinary incontinence, and perineal pain. Maternal newborn nurses play a crucial role in assessing, managing, and educating mothers about these potential challenges. They provide support, guidance, and interventions to promote maternal well-being and optimal recovery. By addressing these common problems and complications promptly, nurses can help mothers navigate the postpartum period with confidence and comfort.

2.2.4 Bladder Distention & Urinary Retention:
Bladder distention and urinary retention are common postpartum problems. Bladder distention occurs when the bladder is not emptied completely. It can lead to urinary retention, which is the inability to urinate. This can be caused by trauma during childbirth, medications, or anesthesia. Nursing care for these issues includes monitoring for signs of distention, such as a firm, tender abdomen. Management may involve catheterization to empty the bladder. Education for the mother should include information on the importance of emptying the bladder regularly. Maternal postpartum assessment should include checking for bladder distention and urinary retention. Prompt recognition and treatment are essential to prevent complications such as urinary tract infections. Proper management and education can help mothers recover comfortably after childbirth.

2.2.5 Hemorrhoids:
Hemorrhoids are common postpartum issues. They can cause pain, itching, and discomfort. Nursing care involves educating mothers on prevention and management. Maternal postpartum assessment should include checking for hemorrhoids. Proper education on diet, hydration, and hygiene is essential. Treatment options include topical creams, sitz baths, and stool softeners. Complications such as thrombosis or infection may occur. Nurses should provide support and reassurance to mothers. Encouraging proper self-care practices is crucial. Education on when to seek medical help is important. Hemorrhoids can impact a mother's quality of life. Proper management can help alleviate symptoms and improve comfort.

2.2.6 Afterpains:
Afterpains are common uterine contractions postpartum. They help uterus return to normal size. Afterpains can be more intense for multiparous women. Nursing care involves assessing pain level and providing comfort measures. Encourage frequent breastfeeding to release oxytocin and reduce afterpains. Educate mothers about afterpains and reassure them it's normal. Monitor for excessive bleeding or signs of infection. Administer pain medication as needed. Encourage rest and proper hydration. Document assessment findings and interventions. Provide emotional support and reassurance to new mothers. Afterpains typically subside within a few days postpartum. Monitor closely for any complications or worsening symptoms. Support mothers in managing afterpains during the postpartum period.

2.2.7 Perineal Edema and Pain:
Perineal edema and pain are common postpartum issues. Nursing care involves assessing for swelling and discomfort. Management includes ice packs, sitz baths, and pain medication. Educate mothers on proper perineal care and hygiene. Encourage rest and avoiding strenuous activities. Monitor for signs of infection and provide support. Perineal pain can impact mobility and breastfeeding. Addressing these concerns promptly can improve maternal well-being.

2.2.8 Breast Engorgement:
Breast engorgement is a common issue postpartum. It occurs when breasts become overfilled with milk. This can lead to pain, swelling, and difficulty breastfeeding. Nursing care involves encouraging frequent feeding, proper latch, and warm compresses.
Maternal postpartum assessment includes checking for redness, warmth, and tenderness. Management may include expressing milk, using cold packs, and wearing a supportive bra. Education on proper breastfeeding techniques and hand expression is crucial. Complications of breast engorgement can include mastitis, a breast infection. Signs of mastitis include fever, chills, and flu-like symptoms. Prompt treatment with antibiotics is necessary. Maternal newborn nurses play a vital role in supporting mothers through this challenging time.

2.2.9 Constipation:
Constipation is a common issue postpartum. It can cause discomfort and pain. Nursing care involves monitoring bowel movements. Encourage fiber-rich diet and hydration. Maternal postpartum assessment should include bowel habits. Management may include stool softeners. Education on prevention and treatment is crucial. Encourage physical activity and adequate fluid intake. Constipation can lead to complications like hemorrhoids. Support new mothers in managing constipation.

2.2.10 Spinal Headaches:
Spinal headaches can occur after epidural anesthesia during childbirth. They cause severe head pain. Treatment includes bed rest, hydration, and pain medication. If severe, a blood patch may be needed. Nursing care involves monitoring symptoms, providing comfort measures, and educating the patient on self-care. Maternal postpartum assessment should include evaluating headache severity, location, and duration. Management may involve adjusting medications or recommending further interventions. Education should focus on warning signs, when to seek help, and ways to prevent spinal headaches in the future. It is important for maternal newborn nurses to be knowledgeable about spinal headaches to provide optimal care for postpartum patients.

2.2.11 Vaginal Lacerations:
Vaginal lacerations are common postpartum complications. They can occur during childbirth. Nursing care involves assessing the severity of the laceration. Proper management includes suturing the laceration if necessary. Maternal postpartum assessment should include monitoring for signs of infection. Education on proper perineal care is essential for preventing complications. Types of vaginal lacerations include first, second, third, and fourth-degree tears. First-degree tears involve the vaginal mucosa. Second-degree tears involve the vaginal mucosa and perineal muscles. Third-degree tears extend to the anal sphincter. Fourth-degree tears involve the anal sphincter and rectal mucosa. Maternal newborn nurses play a crucial role in identifying and managing vaginal lacerations to ensure optimal postpartum recovery for their patients.

2.2.12 Patient Education:
Patient education is crucial in maternal postpartum care. It involves providing information on various aspects of postpartum recovery. Topics include breastfeeding techniques, newborn care, and warning signs of complications. Nurses play a key role in educating new mothers about self-care practices. They also provide guidance on emotional well-being and contraception options. Patient education helps mothers make informed decisions and promotes a smooth transition to motherhood. It is essential for promoting maternal and newborn health. By empowering mothers with knowledge, nurses can enhance their confidence and ability to care for themselves and their babies. Effective patient education leads to better outcomes and satisfaction for both mothers and healthcare providers.

2.2.13 Postpartum Self Care:
Postpartum self-care is crucial for new mothers. It involves physical and emotional well-being. Encourage rest and proper nutrition. Promote gentle exercise and hydration. Discuss emotional changes and support systems. Educate on postpartum warning signs. Emphasize the importance of self-care. Provide resources for mental health support. Encourage open communication with healthcare providers. Offer guidance on breastfeeding and infant care. Support bonding with the newborn. Ensure adequate sleep and relaxation. Monitor for postpartum complications. Empower mothers to prioritize their own health. Postpartum self-care is essential for a smooth recovery.

2.2.14 Contraception:
Contraception is essential for postpartum education. Nurses should discuss various contraceptive options. This includes barrier methods, hormonal methods, and long-acting reversible contraceptives. Patient education should cover effectiveness, side effects, and proper usage. It is important to consider the patient's preferences and medical history. Nurses should provide information on emergency contraception as well. Postpartum contraception helps in family planning and spacing pregnancies. It reduces the risk of unintended pregnancies. Nurses play a crucial role in educating and supporting patients in making

informed decisions about contraception. Regular follow-up is necessary to assess the effectiveness and any issues with the chosen method. Patient education on contraception promotes maternal and newborn health.

2.2.15 Nutrition:
Nutrition is crucial for postpartum mothers. A balanced diet is essential. Include fruits, vegetables, whole grains, and lean proteins. Adequate hydration is important. Encourage drinking plenty of water. Breastfeeding mothers need extra calories. Emphasize the importance of healthy fats. Omega-3 fatty acids are beneficial. Iron-rich foods help prevent anemia. Discuss the benefits of vitamin D. Encourage taking prenatal vitamins. Limit caffeine and sugary drinks. Educate on portion control. Offer resources for meal planning. A well-rounded diet promotes healing and energy. Provide support and guidance for healthy eating habits.

2.3 Lactation:
Lactation is the process of producing breast milk after childbirth. It is essential for infant nutrition. Maternal newborn nurses play a crucial role in supporting lactation. They educate mothers on proper breastfeeding techniques. Nurses assess the baby's latch and feeding patterns. They provide guidance on managing common breastfeeding challenges like engorgement or nipple pain. Nurses also monitor the baby's weight gain to ensure adequate milk intake. Encouraging skin-to-skin contact and frequent nursing sessions can help establish a good milk supply. Nurses may also offer resources for lactation consultants or support groups. Overall, lactation support is vital for promoting maternal-infant bonding and optimal infant growth and development.

2.3.1 Lactation:
Lactation is the process of producing breast milk for newborns. It is essential for infant nutrition and bonding between mother and baby. Maternal postpartum assessment involves evaluating the mother's ability to breastfeed effectively. This includes checking for proper latch, milk supply, and signs of mastitis. Management of lactation issues may involve providing support, education, and resources to help mothers overcome challenges. Education on breastfeeding techniques, proper nutrition, and pumping can improve lactation success. Encouraging skin-to-skin contact and frequent feeding sessions can also enhance milk production. Maternal newborn nurses play a crucial role in supporting and guiding mothers through their lactation journey. By promoting breastfeeding and providing assistance, nurses can help mothers establish a strong breastfeeding relationship with their babies.

2.3.2 Anatomy and Physiology of Lactation:
Anatomy and Physiology of Lactation is crucial for Maternal Newborn Nurses. During lactation, mammary glands produce milk. Hormones like prolactin and oxytocin play a role. The process involves milk production, ejection, and let-down. Understanding breast anatomy is essential. Alveoli produce milk, which travels through ducts to the nipple. Nipple stimulation triggers oxytocin release. This causes milk ejection. Proper latch and suckling are important for successful breastfeeding. Nurses should educate mothers on breastfeeding techniques. They should also assess for any breastfeeding difficulties. Knowledge of lactation anatomy and physiology is vital for maternal postpartum care. It helps nurses support breastfeeding mothers effectively.

2.3.3 Composition of Breast Milk:
Breast milk composition varies throughout lactation. It contains water, carbohydrates, proteins, and fats.
- Water is the main component, essential for hydration.
- Carbohydrates provide energy, mainly in the form of lactose.
- Proteins are crucial for growth and development.
- Fats are necessary for brain development and energy.
- Breast milk also contains antibodies, enzymes, and hormones.
- Colostrum, the first milk produced after birth, is rich in antibodies.
- Mature milk changes in composition to meet the baby's needs.
- Foremilk is watery, while hindmilk is higher in fat.
- Breast milk is easily digested and provides optimal nutrition for infants.

2.3.4 Maternal Nutritional Needs:

Maternal nutritional needs during lactation are crucial for both mother and baby. Adequate intake of nutrients like protein, calcium, and iron supports milk production. Hydration is also essential for milk supply. Mothers should consume a balanced diet with plenty of fruits, vegetables, and whole grains. Omega-3 fatty acids are important for infant brain development. Avoiding alcohol and caffeine is recommended, as they can pass into breast milk. Consulting a healthcare provider for personalized dietary advice is beneficial. Proper nutrition helps mothers recover from childbirth and maintain energy levels. Encouraging healthy eating habits sets a positive example for the newborn. Maternal nutritional needs play a significant role in the overall well-being of both mother and baby.

2.3.5 Normal Breastfeeding Process/Hand Expression:
The normal breastfeeding process involves the baby latching onto the mother's breast. This helps stimulate milk production. Hand expression can be used to collect breast milk. It is important to ensure proper positioning for effective breastfeeding. Encourage skin-to-skin contact between mother and baby. This helps establish a strong bond. Educate mothers on the benefits of breastfeeding. Provide guidance on proper latch techniques. Monitor for signs of successful breastfeeding. Offer support and reassurance to new mothers. Hand expression can help relieve engorgement. It is important to promote a comfortable and relaxing environment. Maternal newborn nurses play a crucial role in supporting breastfeeding mothers. Regular assessment and education are key components of successful breastfeeding.

2.3.6 Positioning:
Positioning is crucial for successful breastfeeding. Proper positioning ensures effective milk transfer.

Subtopics:
1. Correct positioning prevents nipple pain and discomfort.
2. Positioning helps baby latch on correctly for efficient feeding.
3. Different positions like cradle hold, football hold, and side-lying position can be used.
4. Maternal comfort is also important during breastfeeding.
5. Hand expression can help with milk supply and relieve engorgement.
6. Lactation consultants can provide guidance on positioning and latching techniques.
7. Maternal postpartum assessment includes checking for signs of mastitis or blocked ducts.
8. Education on proper positioning can prevent breastfeeding complications. Maternal newborn nurses should be knowledgeable about different positions and techniques to support successful breastfeeding.

2.3.7 Latch On:
Latch On is a crucial aspect of breastfeeding. It refers to the baby attaching to the breast. Proper latch ensures effective milk transfer and prevents nipple pain. Maternal Newborn Nurses play a vital role in educating mothers on achieving a good latch. They assess latch quality during breastfeeding sessions. Nurses also teach hand expression techniques to help with milk supply. Lactation consultants may be involved for complex latch issues. Maternal postpartum assessment includes evaluating latch success and addressing any concerns. Nurses provide support and guidance to improve latch if needed. Education on latch techniques is essential for successful breastfeeding. Nurses empower mothers to establish a strong latch for optimal breastfeeding experience.

2.3.8 Suck/Swallow/Sequence:
During breastfeeding, the baby's suck/swallow/sequence is crucial. The baby should suck rhythmically. Swallowing should occur without difficulty. The sequence should be coordinated. Proper latch helps with suckling. Adequate milk transfer is essential. Ineffective suckling can lead to issues. Maternal education on this is important. Hand expression can aid milk flow. Lactation consultants can assist. Maternal postpartum assessment is vital. Management of any breastfeeding problems is necessary. Education on proper positioning is key. Understanding suck/swallow/sequence promotes successful breastfeeding. Regular monitoring ensures baby's well-being. Maternal support is beneficial for breastfeeding success. Overall, mastering suck/swallow/sequence is vital for successful breastfeeding.

2.3.9 Timing (Frequency and Duration):
Timing (Frequency and Duration) is crucial in the normal breastfeeding process. Newborns should breastfeed **8-12** times daily. Each feeding should last **10-20** minutes per breast. Adequate frequency and duration ensure proper milk production and infant nutrition. Maternal postpartum assessment includes monitoring feeding patterns. Educate mothers on recognizing hunger cues and proper latch techniques. Encourage skin-to-skin contact for successful breastfeeding. Assess maternal comfort and infant weight gain to evaluate feeding effectiveness. Support mothers in establishing a breastfeeding routine. Proper timing promotes bonding and milk supply. Monitor frequency and duration to ensure infant growth and maternal well-being. Timely feedings enhance the breastfeeding experience for both mother and baby.

2.3.10 Feeding Cues:
Feeding cues are signals that indicate a baby is hungry or full. Babies show hunger cues by rooting, sucking on hands, or making sucking motions. Crying is a late hunger cue. It's important to feed the baby when they show early hunger cues to prevent excessive crying. Babies also show signs of being full by turning away from the breast or bottle, falling asleep, or becoming less interested in feeding. It's essential for maternal newborn nurses to educate new mothers on recognizing these cues to establish successful breastfeeding. Proper latch and positioning during feeding can also help ensure adequate milk transfer. Understanding feeding cues is crucial for promoting successful breastfeeding and ensuring the baby's nutritional needs are met.

2.3.11 Breast/Nipple Care:
Breast/nipple care is crucial for lactating mothers. Proper care can prevent issues like engorgement, mastitis, and cracked nipples. Encourage frequent breastfeeding to establish milk supply and prevent engorgement. Teach proper latch techniques to prevent nipple pain and damage. Advise on using lanolin cream for cracked nipples. Ensure breasts are supported with a well-fitting bra. Educate on hand expression and pumping if needed. Monitor for signs of mastitis like redness, pain, and fever. Encourage good hygiene practices to prevent infections. Provide emotional support and reassurance during breastfeeding

challenges. Regularly assess breasts for any abnormalities. Proper breast/nipple care can promote successful breastfeeding and maternal well-being.

2.3.12 Use of Supplementary/Complementary Feedings:
Supplementary/complementary feedings can support breastfeeding. Introduce solids around **6** months. Start with iron-rich foods. Offer breast milk before solids. Avoid honey and cow's milk. Monitor baby's cues for hunger. Encourage self-feeding. Gradually increase food variety. Ensure proper nutrition balance. Seek guidance from healthcare provider. Evaluate baby's growth and development. Stay patient and responsive to baby's needs. Remember breast milk is still important. Provide a supportive feeding environment. Keep breastfeeding as the main source of nutrition. Consult with a lactation consultant if needed. Support mother-baby bonding during feedings. Promote healthy eating habits from the start.

2.3.13 Use of Breastfeeding Devices:
Breastfeeding devices like nipple shields can help with latch issues. They can also aid in protecting sore nipples. Breast pumps are useful for expressing milk. They can help maintain milk supply. Hands-free pumping bras can make pumping more convenient. Nursing pillows can provide support during breastfeeding. Nipple protectors can help with inverted nipples. It is important to choose the right size and type of device. Proper education on how to use these devices is crucial. Consultation with a lactation consultant may be beneficial. Regular assessment of the baby's latch is necessary. Overall, breastfeeding devices can be valuable tools in supporting successful breastfeeding.

2.3.14 Expressing and Storing Breast Milk:

Expressing breast milk helps mothers store milk for later use. It can be done manually or with a breast pump. Proper storage is crucial to maintain milk quality. Milk can be stored in clean containers in the refrigerator or freezer. Label containers with date and time of expression. Thaw frozen milk in the refrigerator or under warm water. Avoid microwaving breast milk. Breast milk can be stored for different durations depending on storage method. Follow guidelines for safe handling and storage. Expressing and storing milk can help mothers continue breastfeeding when apart from their baby. It is important for maternal newborn nurses to educate mothers on proper techniques.

2.3.15 Contraindications to Breast Feeding:

Contraindications to Breastfeeding include maternal HIV infection.

Other contraindications are active tuberculosis, herpes simplex virus on the breast, and using illicit drugs.

Maternal chemotherapy, radioactive isotope therapy, and certain medications are also contraindications.

Infants with galactosemia, phenylketonuria, or maple syrup urine disease should not breastfeed.

Maternal alcohol consumption, smoking, and certain medications can also be contraindications.

Consult with healthcare providers for guidance on contraindications to breastfeeding.

2.3.16 Maternal Complications:
Maternal complications can arise postpartum, affecting breastfeeding and lactation. Contraindications to breastfeeding include maternal infections, substance abuse, and certain medications. Maternal postpartum assessment is crucial to identify complications like hemorrhage, infection, and hypertension. Proper management and education are essential for maternal well-being. Nurses play a vital role in monitoring maternal health, providing support, and educating mothers on postpartum care. It is important to address any complications promptly to ensure the health and safety of both the mother and the newborn. By staying informed and proactive, maternal newborn nurses can help prevent and manage complications effectively.

2.3.17 Latch on Problems:
Latch on problems can occur due to improper positioning. Ensure baby's mouth covers nipple. Encourage baby to open wide for proper latch. Seek help from lactation consultant if needed. Pain during feeding may indicate latch issues. Look for signs of poor latch like clicking noises. Engorgement can also affect latch. Address engorgement to improve latch. Consider tongue tie as a possible cause. Tongue tie can hinder proper latch. Address tongue tie with healthcare provider if suspected. Proper latch is crucial for effective breastfeeding. Address latch on problems promptly for successful breastfeeding journey.

2.3.18 Nipple Problems:
Nipple problems can arise during breastfeeding. Common issues include soreness, cracking, and bleeding. These problems can make breastfeeding painful and challenging for new mothers. It is important for maternal newborn nurses to assess nipple

problems promptly. Contraindications to breastfeeding may include severe nipple damage or infection. Nurses should educate mothers on proper latch techniques and nipple care. Lactation consultants can provide additional support and guidance. Management of nipple problems may involve using lanolin cream, breast shields, or adjusting feeding positions. Nurses should monitor for signs of infection, such as redness or pus. Maternal postpartum assessment should include checking for nipple problems and providing appropriate interventions. Education on nipple care and breastfeeding techniques is essential for successful lactation.

2.3.19 Breast Engorgement:

Breast engorgement is a common issue for new mothers. It occurs when the breasts become overfilled with milk. This can lead to pain, swelling, and difficulty breastfeeding. Engorgement can be caused by not breastfeeding frequently enough, improper latch, or an oversupply of milk.

To relieve engorgement, mothers can try warm compresses, gentle massage, and frequent nursing or pumping. It is important to empty the breasts regularly to prevent further discomfort. Severe cases may require medical intervention, such as medication to reduce milk production.

Mothers should be educated on proper breastfeeding techniques and how to recognize the signs of engorgement. Encouraging frequent feedings and seeking help from a lactation consultant can help prevent and manage engorgement effectively.

2.3.20 Insufficient Milk Supply:

Insufficient milk supply can be caused by various factors. Maternal health issues, such as hormonal imbalances, can contribute to low milk production. Poor latch or ineffective sucking by the baby can also lead to inadequate milk transfer. Suboptimal breastfeeding techniques and infrequent feedings may further decrease milk supply. Stress, fatigue, and certain medications can negatively impact lactation. It is important for maternal newborn nurses to assess the mother's breastfeeding experience and provide education on proper positioning, latch, and frequency of feedings. Encouraging skin-to-skin contact and frequent nursing sessions can help stimulate milk production. Referral to a lactation consultant may be necessary for additional support. Monitoring the baby's weight gain and diaper output is essential in evaluating milk supply.

2.3.21 Therapeutic Medications:
Therapeutic medications can have contraindications to breastfeeding. It is important to assess maternal postpartum status. Educate mothers on safe medication use while breastfeeding. Monitor for any adverse effects on the newborn. Consult with healthcare providers for guidance. Consider alternative medications if necessary. Stay informed about the latest research on medication safety during lactation. Provide support and reassurance to new mothers. Encourage open communication about any concerns or questions. Prioritize the well-being of both mother and baby. Remember that each situation is unique and may require individualized care. Stay up-to-date on best practices for medication management in the postpartum period.

2.3.22 Infection/Mastitis:
Infection/Mastitis is a common issue in breastfeeding mothers. It can be caused by bacteria entering the breast tissue through a cracked nipple. Symptoms include redness, swelling, and pain in the affected breast. Treatment involves antibiotics and continued breastfeeding. It is important to ensure proper latch and positioning to prevent further complications. Mastitis can lead to a decrease in milk supply if not addressed promptly. Encouraging frequent nursing or pumping can help clear the infection. In severe cases, a breast abscess may form, requiring drainage. Educating mothers on the importance of early detection and treatment is crucial. Maternal Newborn Nurses play a vital role in supporting and guiding mothers through this challenging experience.

2.3.23 Maternal Illness:
Maternal illness can impact breastfeeding. Certain conditions may contraindicate breastfeeding. Maternal postpartum assessment is crucial. Education on maternal illness is essential. Lactation consultants can provide support. Management of maternal illness is important. Monitoring maternal health postpartum is necessary. Maternal newborn nurses play a key role. Educating mothers on maternal illness is vital. Support systems are beneficial for mothers. Collaboration with healthcare providers is essential. Maternal illness can affect newborn health. Understanding contraindications to breastfeeding is important. Providing proper care for mothers is crucial. Maternal illness requires careful monitoring and management. Regular assessments are needed for maternal well-being. Maternal newborn nurses should be knowledgeable about maternal illness. Communication with healthcare team is essential for maternal care.

2.3.24 Perinatal Substance Abuse:

Perinatal substance abuse can have serious consequences for both the mother and the baby. It is important for maternal newborn nurses to be aware of the contraindications to breastfeeding in these cases. Lactation may not be recommended if the mother is using certain substances. Maternal postpartum assessment should include screening for substance abuse. Management may involve referral to a substance abuse treatment program. Education is key in helping mothers understand the risks of substance abuse during pregnancy. Nurses play a crucial role in supporting these mothers and ensuring the health and safety of both the mother and the newborn. It is important to provide non-judgmental care and support to these mothers during this challenging time.

2.3.25 Maternal/Newborn Separation:

Maternal/Newborn separation can occur due to medical reasons or NICU admission. It can impact breastfeeding initiation and bonding. Skin-to-skin contact is important for newborns. Encourage kangaroo care for bonding. Support mothers emotionally during separation. Provide education on expressing breast milk. Offer resources for maintaining milk supply. Monitor maternal mental health. Facilitate communication between mother and baby. Promote family-centered care. Collaborate with healthcare team for holistic care. Assess maternal coping mechanisms. Provide reassurance and support. Educate on the benefits of early reunification. Encourage involvement in newborn care. Monitor for signs of postpartum depression. Support breastfeeding goals. Offer guidance on transitioning back together. Ensure a smooth transition home.

2.3.26 Newborn Complications:

Newborn complications can arise in various forms. These can include respiratory distress syndrome, jaundice, and hypoglycemia.

Respiratory distress syndrome is caused by immature lungs and can lead to breathing difficulties. Jaundice occurs when the baby's liver is unable to process bilirubin effectively, resulting in yellowing of the skin and eyes.

Hypoglycemia is a condition where the baby's blood sugar levels are too low, which can lead to seizures if not treated promptly.

Maternal newborn nurses play a crucial role in identifying and managing these complications. They provide education to mothers on how to recognize signs of these issues and seek timely medical intervention.

Early detection and appropriate management are essential in ensuring the well-being of newborns.

2.3.27 Hyperbilirubinemia:

Hyperbilirubinemia is a common condition in newborns. It occurs when there is an excess of bilirubin in the blood. This can lead to jaundice, a yellowing of the skin and eyes.

Risk factors for hyperbilirubinemia include prematurity, breastfeeding, and blood type incompatibility.

Monitoring bilirubin levels through blood tests is crucial for early detection and management.

Treatment options may include phototherapy or exchange transfusion in severe cases.

Maternal education on breastfeeding techniques and ensuring adequate intake can help prevent and manage hyperbilirubinemia.

Maternal postpartum assessment should include monitoring the baby's skin color and feeding patterns.

Early recognition and intervention are key in preventing complications associated with hyperbilirubinemia.

2.3.28 Hypoglycemia:

Hypoglycemia in newborns can occur due to various reasons.

Causes include maternal diabetes, prematurity, and intrauterine growth restriction.

Symptoms may include jitteriness, poor feeding, and lethargy.

Early detection through blood glucose monitoring is crucial.

Treatment involves feeding the baby to increase blood sugar levels.

Maternal education on signs of hypoglycemia is essential.

Nurses should monitor newborns closely for any signs of hypoglycemia.

Prompt intervention can prevent long-term complications.

Proper lactation support can help maintain stable blood sugar levels in newborns.

Maternal postpartum assessment should include monitoring for signs of hypoglycemia in the newborn.

2.3.29   Multiple Birth:
Multiple births, such as twins or triplets, present unique challenges for maternal newborn nurses. These babies are at higher risk for complications such as prematurity and low birth weight. Nurses must closely monitor these infants for any signs of distress. Lactation support is crucial for mothers of multiples to establish and maintain breastfeeding. Maternal postpartum assessment should include monitoring for signs of postpartum hemorrhage and infection. Education on caring for multiple newborns is essential for parents to ensure their well-being. Nurses play a vital role in providing guidance and support to families of multiples during this challenging time.

2.4   Psychosocial and Ethical Issues:
Psychosocial and ethical issues in maternal postpartum care are crucial. Maternal newborn nurses must address these issues effectively. Postpartum depression is a common psychosocial concern. Nurses should screen for it and provide support. Educating new mothers about self-care is essential. Addressing cultural beliefs and practices is important for ethical care. Respecting patient autonomy and confidentiality is key. Involving families in decision-making can be beneficial. Nurses must be aware of ethical dilemmas that may arise. Providing emotional support and resources is vital. Collaboration with other healthcare professionals is necessary. Overall, addressing psychosocial and ethical issues in maternal postpartum care is essential for promoting the well-being of both mother and baby.

2.4.1   Normal Characteristics of Parent/Infant Interactions:
Parent/infant interactions are crucial for bonding. Parents respond to infant cues. They engage in eye contact, touch, and soothing techniques. Infants show attachment behaviors. They seek comfort and security from parents. Parents provide a safe environment. They meet the infant's needs promptly. Infants develop trust and security. Parents learn to interpret infant cues. They respond with sensitivity and warmth. This strengthens the parent/infant bond. It promotes emotional development. Positive interactions enhance communication skills. Parents learn to understand their infant's needs. They build a strong foundation for future relationships. Understanding normal characteristics of parent/infant interactions is essential for maternal newborn nurses. It helps them support families effectively during the postpartum period.

2.4.2   Maternal Role Transition:

Maternal role transition is a crucial aspect of maternal postpartum assessment, management, and education. It involves the psychological and social adjustments a woman goes through after becoming a mother. This transition includes changes in identity, responsibilities, and relationships. During this period, new mothers may experience a range of emotions, such as joy, anxiety, and stress. They may also face challenges in adapting to their new role and balancing their own needs with those of their baby. As a maternal newborn nurse, it is important to support women during this transition by providing education, counseling, and resources. By understanding the psychosocial and ethical issues related to maternal role transition, nurses can help new mothers navigate this significant life change with confidence and resilience.

2.4.3   Sibling Response:
Sibling response to a new baby can vary. Some siblings may feel excited and eager to help. Others may feel jealous or left out. It is important to prepare siblings for the new arrival. Encourage them to ask questions and express their feelings. Offer reassurance and involve them in caring for the baby. Monitor for signs of jealousy or resentment. Provide one-on-one time with each child. Help siblings adjust to changes in routine and attention. Offer age-appropriate explanations about the baby. Encourage bonding activities between siblings. Address any concerns or conflicts that arise. Sibling response is an important aspect of maternal postpartum assessment and management. It is essential to support the emotional well-being of all family members during this transition.

2.4.4   Barriers and Alterations to Parent/Infant Interactions:
Barriers to parent/infant interactions include maternal mental health issues. These can affect bonding. Lack of support from family or partner is another barrier. Stress and fatigue can also impact interactions. Substance abuse is a significant barrier. Cultural differences may lead to misunderstandings. Alterations to interactions can occur due to medical conditions in either parent or infant. Premature birth can affect bonding. Developmental delays in the infant can alter interactions. Parental anxiety or depression can also lead to changes. Education and support can help overcome barriers. Encouraging skin-to-skin contact and breastfeeding can improve interactions. Providing resources for mental health support is crucial. Addressing cultural

beliefs and practices is important for effective communication. Overall, understanding and addressing barriers can enhance parent/infant interactions.

2.4.5 Cultural/Life-Style Factors Affecting Family Integration:
Cultural and lifestyle factors play a significant role in family integration postpartum. Different cultural backgrounds can influence how families adjust to the new addition. Language barriers, religious beliefs, and traditions can impact communication and bonding within the family. Socioeconomic status and education level can also affect family dynamics. Support systems, such as extended family or community resources, can either facilitate or hinder the integration process. Understanding and respecting these cultural differences is essential for maternal newborn nurses to provide effective care. Education on cultural competence and sensitivity is crucial in promoting family well-being. By acknowledging and addressing these factors, nurses can help families navigate the challenges of postpartum integration.

2.4.6 Abuse/Intimate Partner Violence:
Abuse/Intimate Partner Violence is a serious issue in maternal postpartum care. Nurses must be aware of signs of abuse, such as physical injuries, anxiety, and depression. Screening for abuse should be a routine part of postpartum assessments. Nurses should provide a safe space for mothers to disclose abuse. Referral to support services is crucial for women experiencing abuse. Education on healthy relationships and resources for help should be provided. Confidentiality and ethical considerations are important when dealing with abuse cases. Nurses should be prepared to offer emotional support and guidance to mothers in abusive situations. Overall, addressing abuse in the postpartum period is essential for the well-being of both mother and baby.

2.4.7 Family Dynamics:
Family dynamics play a crucial role in maternal postpartum assessment, management, and education. Understanding the family structure, roles, and relationships is essential. It is important to assess the support system available to the mother.
Subtopics such as communication patterns, decision-making processes, and cultural influences should be considered. The nurse should assess how the family is coping with the new addition.
Educating the family on postpartum care, newborn care, and breastfeeding is vital. Involving the family in the care of the mother and baby can improve outcomes.
Supporting the family as a unit can promote bonding and overall well-being. Effective communication and collaboration with the family are key in providing holistic care.

2.4.8 Adoption:
Adoption is a complex process involving psychosocial and ethical considerations. It is important for maternal newborn nurses to understand the emotional impact of adoption on birth parents, adoptive parents, and the child. Maternal postpartum assessment should include questions about adoption plans and feelings. Nurses should provide support and education to birth parents considering adoption. They should also be knowledgeable about legal and ethical issues surrounding adoption. It is crucial to respect the privacy and confidentiality of all parties involved in the adoption process. Nurses play a key role in helping families navigate the challenges and emotions associated with adoption. By providing compassionate care and resources, nurses can support families through this life-changing experience.

2.4.9 Perinatal Grief:
Perinatal grief is the emotional distress experienced by parents following the loss of a baby during pregnancy, childbirth, or shortly after birth. It can be caused by a variety of factors, including miscarriage, stillbirth, or neonatal death. Maternal newborn nurses play a crucial role in supporting parents through this difficult time. They provide emotional support, education, and resources to help parents cope with their grief. Nurses must be sensitive to the unique needs of grieving parents and provide compassionate care. It is important for nurses to assess the mental health of parents, offer counseling services, and facilitate support groups. By addressing perinatal grief, nurses can help parents navigate the complex emotions associated with loss and begin the healing process.

2.4.10 Ethical Principles:
Ethical principles in maternal postpartum care are crucial for ensuring patient autonomy. Nurses must uphold confidentiality and respect cultural beliefs. Informed consent is essential before any procedure. Nurses should advocate for patient rights and provide unbiased care. It is important to maintain professional boundaries and avoid conflicts of interest. Ethical dilemmas may arise, requiring careful consideration and ethical decision-making. Nurses must prioritize the well-being of both mother and baby. Continuous education on ethical principles is necessary for providing quality care. Adhering to ethical standards builds trust with patients and promotes positive outcomes.

2.4.11 Autonomy:
Autonomy is a key ethical principle in maternal newborn nursing. It refers to a woman's right to make decisions about her own care. This includes the right to consent or refuse treatment.

Subtopics:
- Informed Consent
- Respect for Patient's Choices

Psychosocial and ethical issues may arise when autonomy is not respected. Nurses must support women in making informed decisions.

Maternal postpartum assessment involves evaluating the mother's physical and emotional well-being. Autonomy plays a role in this process.

Management of postpartum care should involve educating women about their options. This empowers them to make decisions that align with their values and preferences.

2.4.12 Beneficence:
Beneficence is an ethical principle that focuses on doing good for others. In the context of maternal newborn nursing, beneficence plays a crucial role in ensuring the well-being of both the mother and the newborn. Nurses must prioritize the best interests of their patients and provide care that promotes their health and safety. This includes advocating for proper postpartum assessment, management, and education to support the mother's recovery and the newborn's development. By upholding the principle of beneficence, nurses can help create a positive and supportive environment for new mothers and their babies. It is essential for maternal newborn nurses to always act in the best interest of their patients and prioritize their overall well-being.

2.4.13 Non-maleficence:
Non-maleficence is an ethical principle in maternal newborn nursing. It involves avoiding harm to the mother and baby during assessment, management, and education. Nurses must prioritize the well-being of their patients. This principle guides decision-making in providing care. It is essential to consider potential risks and benefits. Nurses should strive to do no harm. This principle also applies to communication and education. Ensuring that information provided is accurate and beneficial. Nurses must be vigilant in monitoring for any signs of harm. This principle is crucial in promoting safe and effective care. Adhering to non-maleficence helps in maintaining trust and confidence in nursing care. It is a fundamental aspect of ethical practice in maternal newborn nursing.

2.4.14 Justice:

Justice in the context of maternal newborn nursing involves ensuring fair and equal treatment for all mothers and their newborns. This includes respecting their rights, autonomy, and dignity. Ethical principles guide nurses in making decisions that are just and equitable. Nurses must consider psychosocial and ethical issues that may impact the well-being of mothers and newborns. This includes addressing disparities in access to care and resources. Maternal postpartum assessment, management, and education should be done in a way that promotes justice for all patients. Nurses play a crucial role in advocating for the rights of mothers and newborns, ensuring that they receive the care and support they need. By upholding principles of justice, nurses can help create a healthcare system that is fair and compassionate for all.

2.5 Newborn feeding and nutrition:
Newborn feeding and nutrition are crucial for infant growth and development. Breastfeeding is recommended. It provides essential nutrients and antibodies. It helps in bonding between mother and baby. Proper latch and positioning are important for successful breastfeeding.

Colostrum, the first milk, is rich in nutrients and helps in building the baby's immune system. Newborns need to feed frequently, around **8-12** times a day.

Formula feeding is an alternative for mothers who cannot breastfeed. It is important to prepare formula correctly.

Burping the baby after feeding helps prevent gas and discomfort.

Monitoring the baby's weight gain and diaper output is essential.

Educating mothers about newborn feeding cues and signs of hunger is important.

Overall, ensuring proper feeding and nutrition is vital for the health and well-being of newborns.

2.5.1 Bottle Feeding:
Bottle feeding is a common method of feeding newborns. It involves using infant formula. Proper preparation and storage of formula are essential. Always follow the manufacturer's instructions. It is important to choose the right type of formula for the baby's needs. Bottle feeding allows others to help with feeding. It is important to hold the baby in an upright position while feeding. Burp the baby frequently during feeding to prevent gas. Make sure the baby is not overfed or underfed. Bottle feeding

can be a bonding experience for parents and caregivers. It is important to clean and sterilize bottles properly. Seek guidance from healthcare providers for any concerns about bottle feeding.

2.5.2 Nutritional Needs:
Nutritional needs for newborns are crucial for their growth and development. Bottle feeding provides essential nutrients for infants. Maternal postpartum assessment is important for identifying any nutritional deficiencies. Education on proper nutrition is key for new mothers. Understanding newborn feeding and nutrition is essential for maternal newborn nurses. Providing guidance on breastfeeding and formula feeding is part of their role. Assessing the mother's diet can help ensure she is meeting her nutritional needs. Managing any postpartum nutritional issues is vital for the health of both mother and baby. Educating mothers on the importance of a balanced diet is essential for their well-being. Maternal newborn nurses play a critical role in promoting healthy nutrition for both mothers and newborns.

2.5.3 Formulas:
Formulas are essential for bottle feeding newborns. They provide necessary nutrition. There are different types of formulas available. It is important to choose the right formula for the baby. Formulas should be prepared according to instructions. Always use clean bottles and nipples. Check the expiration date before using. Maternal newborn nurses should educate parents on formula feeding. They should be aware of signs of intolerance. Monitor baby's weight gain and growth. Maternal postpartum assessment includes checking formula feeding. Nurses should provide support and guidance. Proper formula feeding is crucial for newborn health. Nurses play a key role in educating parents. It is important to follow guidelines for safe formula feeding. Regular monitoring and assessment are necessary.

2.5.4 Techniques and Equipment:
Techniques and equipment for bottle feeding are essential for newborn feeding and nutrition. Proper assessment, management, and education are crucial for maternal postpartum care.

Equipment such as bottles, nipples, and bottle brushes are necessary for bottle feeding. Techniques like holding the baby at an angle and pacing the feeding are important for newborns.

Assessment of the mother's postpartum condition includes checking for signs of infection and monitoring vital signs. Management involves providing pain relief and promoting breastfeeding.

Education on proper feeding techniques, safe sleep practices, and postpartum care is vital for new mothers. Maternal newborn nurses play a key role in providing support and guidance during this critical time.

Overall, understanding the techniques and equipment for bottle feeding, newborn feeding, and maternal postpartum care is essential for the well-being of both mother and baby.

3 NEWBORN ASSESSMENT AND MANAGEMENT:

Newborn assessment and management are crucial for maternal newborn nurses.
Assessment includes vital signs, physical exam, and gestational age evaluation.
Nurses must check for any abnormalities or signs of distress.
Management involves monitoring for feeding, weight gain, and jaundice.
They also provide education to parents on newborn care.
Early detection of issues is key for prompt intervention.
Nurses play a vital role in ensuring the well-being of newborns.

3.1 Transition to Extrauterine Life (Birth to 4 Hours):
During the transition to extrauterine life (birth to **4** hours), several important aspects need to be considered by the maternal newborn nurse.
First, the nurse should assess the newborn's respiratory effort, heart rate, muscle tone, reflexes, and skin color.
Monitoring for signs of respiratory distress, such as grunting or cyanosis, is crucial during this time.
The nurse should also ensure that the newborn is kept warm and initiate skin-to-skin contact with the mother to promote bonding and regulate the baby's temperature.
Additionally, the nurse should assess the newborn's feeding readiness and provide guidance and support to the mother if needed.
Overall, close monitoring and support during the first few hours of life are essential for a smooth transition to extrauterine life.

3.1.1 Initial Physiologic Adaptations:
During the transition to extrauterine life, newborns undergo initial physiologic adaptations. These adaptations include the establishment of breathing, circulation, and temperature regulation.
Breathing is initiated as the newborn takes its first breath, clearing the airways of amniotic fluid. The cardiovascular system undergoes changes to adapt to the new environment, with the closure of fetal shunts and an increase in pulmonary blood flow.
Temperature regulation is crucial during this period, as newborns are at risk of hypothermia. Skin-to-skin contact and warm blankets help maintain body temperature.
Monitoring vital signs such as heart rate, respiratory rate, and oxygen saturation is essential during the first few hours of life.

Understanding these initial physiologic adaptations is vital for maternal newborn nurses to provide appropriate care and support to newborns during this critical period.

3.1.2 Thermoregulation:

During the transition to extrauterine life, newborns are at risk for thermoregulation issues. It is crucial to maintain their body temperature within a narrow range. Skin-to-skin contact with the mother helps regulate the baby's temperature. Warm blankets and hats can also be used to prevent heat loss. Cold stress can lead to hypothermia, while overheating can cause hyperthermia. Monitoring the baby's temperature regularly is essential. In cases of hypothermia, warming techniques such as radiant warmers or incubators may be necessary. On the other hand, cooling techniques like removing excess clothing can help in cases of hyperthermia. Proper thermoregulation is vital for the newborn's well-being and should be closely monitored during the first few hours after birth.

3.1.3 Associated Laboratory Findings:

Associated laboratory findings during the transition to extrauterine life include blood glucose levels, hematocrit, and bilirubin levels.

Blood glucose levels are important to monitor as low levels can indicate hypoglycemia. Hematocrit levels help assess for polycythemia or anemia. Bilirubin levels are crucial in evaluating for jaundice.

Other important laboratory findings include blood gas analysis to assess acid-base balance and oxygenation status.

Additionally, newborn screening tests are typically done during this time to detect metabolic disorders.

It is essential for maternal newborn nurses to closely monitor these laboratory findings to ensure the newborn's health and well-being during the critical transition period.

3.2 Physical Assessment and Gestational Age Assessment (to Include Laboratory Values),NEWBORN ASSESSMENT AND MANAGEMENT:

Physical assessment of newborns includes evaluating vital signs, skin color, reflexes, and overall appearance. Gestational age assessment involves using physical characteristics and neurological development to determine the baby's age. Laboratory values such as blood glucose levels and bilirubin levels are also important indicators of the newborn's health. Newborn assessment and management focus on identifying any abnormalities or complications early on to provide timely interventions. This includes monitoring for signs of respiratory distress, infection, or jaundice. Proper feeding, keeping the baby warm, and promoting bonding between the newborn and parents are essential aspects of newborn care. Regular assessments and monitoring are crucial for ensuring the well-being of both the newborn and the mother.

3.2.1 Gestational Age Assessment:

Gestational Age Assessment is crucial in determining a newborn's maturity level. It involves physical examination, neurological assessment, and laboratory tests. Physical features like skin texture, breast tissue, and ear cartilage are evaluated. Neurological signs such as posture, muscle tone, and reflexes are also assessed. Laboratory values like blood glucose levels and bilirubin levels provide additional information. Accurate gestational age assessment helps in planning appropriate care for the newborn. It aids in identifying any potential complications or developmental delays. Nurses play a vital role in conducting these assessments and collaborating with healthcare providers to ensure the well-being of the newborn. Regular monitoring and reassessment are essential to track the baby's progress and adjust care accordingly.

3.2.2 Neurobehavioral and Sensory Assessment:

Neurobehavioral and sensory assessment is crucial in newborn care. It involves evaluating the baby's responses to stimuli. Assessing reflexes, muscle tone, and sensory responses are key components. Neurobehavioral assessment helps in identifying any neurological issues early on. Sensory assessment focuses on the baby's ability to respond to touch, sound, and light. It helps in understanding the baby's sensory development. Nurses use various tools and techniques to assess neurobehavioral and sensory responses. These assessments aid in determining the baby's overall health and well-being. Early detection of any abnormalities can lead to timely interventions and better outcomes for the newborn. Regular monitoring and assessment are essential in providing optimal care for newborns.

3.2.3 Systems Review (Including Common Variations):

Systems review in newborn assessment includes evaluating various body systems for normal function. Common variations may include respiratory distress, cardiac anomalies, and neurological abnormalities. Respiratory system assessment involves observing breathing patterns and auscultating lung sounds. Cardiac system evaluation includes assessing heart rate, rhythm, and presence of murmurs. Neurological assessment focuses on reflexes, muscle tone, and level of consciousness.

Other systems to review are gastrointestinal, genitourinary, and musculoskeletal. Laboratory values such as blood glucose, bilirubin levels, and complete blood count are essential for gestational age assessment.

Understanding common variations in systems review is crucial for early detection and management of potential health issues in newborns. Maternal newborn nurses play a vital role in ensuring comprehensive assessment and care for newborns.

3.2.4 Cardiac:
Cardiac assessment in newborns is crucial. Common variations may include murmurs. Physical assessment should include heart rate and rhythm. Gestational age assessment is important for proper evaluation. Laboratory values such as electrolytes may be checked. Newborns with cardiac issues require prompt management. Monitoring for signs of distress is essential. Collaboration with a pediatric cardiologist may be necessary. Treatment options may include medications or surgery. Family education on care and follow-up is vital. Regular follow-up appointments are recommended. Early detection and intervention can improve outcomes. Maternal Newborn Nurses play a key role in the care of newborns with cardiac concerns.

3.2.5 Respiratory:
Respiratory system is vital for newborns. It includes lungs, airways, and diaphragm. Common variations like transient tachypnea may occur. Physical assessment involves observing breathing patterns and chest movements. Gestational age assessment considers lung maturity. Laboratory values like oxygen saturation are important. Newborn assessment includes checking respiratory rate and effort. Management may involve oxygen therapy or respiratory support. It is crucial to monitor for signs of respiratory distress. Proper assessment and management are essential for newborn well-being.

3.2.6 Gastrointestinal:
The gastrointestinal system in newborns is crucial for digestion and absorption. It includes the stomach, intestines, and anus. Common variations in newborns include imperforate anus and omphalocele. Physical assessment of the gastrointestinal system involves inspecting for distention, auscultating for bowel sounds, and palpating for tenderness. Gestational age assessment may involve checking laboratory values such as bilirubin levels. Newborn assessment includes examining for any abnormalities in the gastrointestinal system, such as hernias or abdominal masses. Management of gastrointestinal issues in newborns may include monitoring feeding tolerance, providing appropriate nutrition, and addressing any congenital anomalies promptly. It is essential for maternal newborn nurses to be knowledgeable about the gastrointestinal system to provide optimal care for newborns.

3.2.7 Integumentary:
The integumentary system includes skin, hair, nails, and glands. Skin is the largest organ. It protects the body from external factors. Common variations include birthmarks, rashes, and skin discoloration. Physical assessment involves inspecting skin for color, texture, and lesions. Gestational age assessment uses physical characteristics and laboratory values. Newborn assessment includes skin inspection for jaundice, birthmarks, and rashes. Management may involve skin care, monitoring for jaundice, and educating parents. Skin plays a crucial role in protecting newborns. Proper assessment and management are essential for newborn health.

3.2.8 Musculoskeletal:
The musculoskeletal system in newborns is crucial for movement and support. Common variations include clubfoot and polydactyly. During physical assessment, check for symmetry, range of motion, and reflexes. Gestational age assessment involves evaluating physical characteristics and laboratory values. Newborn assessment includes examining muscle tone, posture, and spine alignment. Management may include physical therapy or orthopedic interventions. Understanding musculoskeletal development is essential for providing comprehensive care to newborns.

3.2.9 Head, Ears, Eyes, Nose and Throat:
During a newborn assessment, it is important to examine the head, ears, eyes, nose, and throat. The head should be symmetrical and fontanelles should be soft. Ears should be in alignment with the eyes and have no abnormalities. Eyes should be clear with equal pupils and red reflex present. The nose should be patent with no flaring or discharge. The throat should have a midline uvula and intact palate. Assess for any signs of cleft palate or tongue tie. Check for proper suck and swallow reflexes. Any abnormalities should be documented and reported for further evaluation. It is crucial to ensure the newborn's airway is clear and functioning properly. Regular monitoring and assessment of these areas are essential for the overall health and well-being of the newborn.

3.2.10 Endocrine:
The endocrine system regulates hormones. It includes glands like thyroid and adrenal. Hormones control body functions. Imbalances can cause health issues. Common variations include diabetes and thyroid disorders. Physical assessment includes checking hormone levels. Gestational age assessment involves lab tests. Newborn assessment includes checking for endocrine issues. Management may involve medication or monitoring. Understanding endocrine system is crucial for maternal newborn nurses.

3.2.11 Genitourinary:
Genitourinary system includes kidneys, ureters, bladder, and urethra. Common variations include hypospadias and cryptorchidism. Physical assessment involves inspecting genitalia for anomalies. Gestational age assessment includes evaluating kidney function with serum creatinine levels. Newborn assessment includes checking for proper formation of genitalia. Management of genitourinary issues may involve surgical correction. Monitoring urine output is crucial for assessing renal function. Maternal history can provide insights into potential genitourinary issues in newborns. Understanding genitourinary system variations is essential for providing comprehensive care. Regular assessments help in early detection and intervention for genitourinary abnormalities. Knowledge of laboratory values aids in diagnosing genitourinary disorders in newborns. Familiarity with genitourinary system variations ensures effective management and treatment strategies.

3.2.12 Screening (CHD/Car Seat/NBGS):
Screening for Congenital Heart Disease (CHD) involves pulse oximetry. Car seat screening ensures proper fit. Newborn Hearing Screening (NBGS) identifies hearing loss. It is crucial to assess gestational age accurately. Physical assessment includes vital signs. Laboratory values help determine overall health. Newborn assessment involves thorough head-to-toe examination. Maternal Newborn Nurses play a vital role in screening. Proper screening can lead to early intervention. It is essential for nurses to stay updated on screening guidelines. Effective screening improves outcomes for newborns. Regular training on screening protocols is necessary. Collaboration with healthcare team is key. Continuous monitoring and assessment are essential.

3.3 Newborn Care and Family Education:
Newborn care involves assessing and managing the health of the baby. This includes monitoring vital signs, conducting physical exams, and assessing feeding and elimination. Family education is crucial for parents to understand newborn care. Topics covered may include breastfeeding, safe sleep practices, and recognizing signs of illness. Providing emotional support to families is also important. Nurses play a key role in educating and supporting families during this critical time. By empowering parents with knowledge and skills, they can confidently care for their newborn. Effective communication and collaboration with healthcare providers are essential for the well-being of both the baby and the family.

3.3.1 Cord Care:
Cord care is essential for newborns. Keep the cord clean and dry. Avoid covering it with tight clothing. Monitor for signs of infection. Use clean water and mild soap for cleaning. Allow the cord to air dry. Fold diapers below the cord. Be gentle when handling the cord. Watch for redness, swelling, or discharge. Report any concerns to healthcare provider. Proper cord care helps prevent infection. It is important for overall newborn health. Follow healthcare provider's instructions carefully. Remember to wash hands before and after caring for the cord. Cord care is a simple yet crucial aspect of newborn care.

3.3.2 Elimination:
Elimination is a crucial aspect of newborn care. It includes bowel movements and urination. Newborns should have several wet diapers and bowel movements daily. Constipation and diarrhea are common issues. Breastfed babies may have more frequent bowel movements. Urine should be pale yellow in color. Monitor for signs of dehydration. Encourage breastfeeding to prevent constipation. Teach parents about normal elimination patterns. Address any concerns promptly. Seek medical advice for abnormal changes. Proper elimination is essential for newborn health. Regular monitoring and education are key.

3.3.3 Circumcision:
Circumcision is a common procedure for male newborns. It involves removing the foreskin. The decision to circumcise is often based on cultural or religious beliefs. Some parents choose circumcision for health reasons. It can reduce the risk of certain infections. The procedure is usually done within the first few days of life. Before circumcision, the baby's health should be assessed. Pain management is important during and after the procedure. Parents should be educated on proper care of the circumcision site. Complications are rare but can include bleeding or infection. It is essential to monitor the baby for any signs of complications. Family education on circumcision is crucial for informed decision-making. Maternal Newborn Nurses play a vital role in supporting families through the circumcision process.

3.3.4 Comfort Measures:
Comfort measures for newborns include swaddling, skin-to-skin contact, and gentle rocking. Swaddling helps babies feel secure and calm. Skin-to-skin contact promotes bonding and regulates the baby's temperature. Gentle rocking can soothe a fussy newborn. Additionally, using a pacifier or providing a gentle massage can also help comfort the baby. It is important to create a quiet and calm environment for the newborn to promote relaxation. Ensuring that the baby is well-fed and has a clean diaper is essential for their comfort. Educating parents on these comfort measures can help them feel more confident in caring for their newborn. By implementing these strategies, nurses can support both the physical and emotional well-being of the newborn and their family.

3.3.5 Screening (CHD/Car Seat):
Screening for Congenital Heart Defects (CHD) in newborns is crucial. It involves pulse oximetry. This test checks oxygen levels in the blood. Early detection of CHD is important for prompt treatment. Another important aspect is car seat screening. Nurses educate parents on proper car seat use. Ensuring newborns are safely secured in car seats is vital. Proper positioning can prevent injuries. Nurses play a key role in educating families. They provide guidance on safe transportation practices. Regular screenings and education help promote newborn safety. Maternal Newborn Nurses are instrumental in this process. Their knowledge and support are essential for newborn care.

3.3.6 Skin Care:
Skin care for newborns is crucial for their health and well-being. It involves gentle cleansing and moisturizing. It is important to use mild, fragrance-free products. Avoid harsh chemicals that can irritate the delicate skin. Keep the baby's skin clean and dry to prevent rashes. Pay attention to areas like diaper area, folds, and creases. Use gentle baby wipes or warm water for cleaning. Avoid using talcum powder as it can be harmful if inhaled. Protect the baby's skin from the sun by keeping them in the shade. Dress them in loose, breathable clothing. Monitor for any signs of skin irritation or infection. Seek medical advice if needed. Proper skin care helps maintain the baby's skin health and comfort.

3.3.7 Safety:

Safety is crucial in newborn care. Always ensure a safe environment.
Subtopics:
- Safe sleep practices
- Prevention of falls
- Proper hand hygiene

Keep the baby's crib free of loose bedding. Place the baby on their back to sleep.

Avoid leaving the baby unattended on high surfaces. Wash hands before handling the baby.

Check the temperature of bath water before bathing the baby. Keep small objects out of reach.

Educate family members on safe handling of the newborn. Provide guidance on safe sleep practices.

Safety measures are essential for the well-being of the newborn. Stay vigilant and proactive.

3.3.8 Safe Sleep/Tummy Time:
Safe sleep practices are crucial for newborns to prevent Sudden Infant Death Syndrome (SIDS). Always place babies on their backs to sleep. Avoid soft bedding, pillows, and toys in the crib. Ensure the crib is firm and snug-fitting. Room-sharing without bed-sharing is recommended. Tummy time helps strengthen neck and shoulder muscles. Start tummy time when the baby is awake and supervised. Gradually increase tummy time duration. Encourage tummy time multiple times a day. Use a firm surface for tummy time. Never leave the baby unattended during tummy time. Educate families on safe sleep and tummy time practices. Promote safe sleep environments in hospitals and at home. Regularly assess and monitor newborns for safe sleep practices.

3.3.9 Commonly Used Medications:
Commonly used medications in newborn care include antibiotics, vitamin K, and eye ointment. Antibiotics are given to treat infections, vitamin K is administered to prevent bleeding disorders, and eye ointment is used to prevent eye infections. Other commonly used medications include pain relievers for circumcision, medications for jaundice, and vaccines for diseases like hepatitis B. It is important for maternal newborn nurses to be familiar with these medication
s, their indications, dosages, and potential side effects. Nurses should also educate parents about the purpose of each medication and how to administer them safely.
Proper documentation of medication administration is crucial for continuity of care and monitoring of the newborn's response to treatment. Maternal newborn nurses play a key role in ensuring the safe and effective use of medications in newborns.

3.3.10 Oral Sucrose:
Oral sucrose is commonly used for newborn pain management. It is given before painful procedures. Sucrose can reduce pain response in newborns. It is safe and effective. Sucrose is often used during heel sticks. It can also be used for minor procedures. Sucrose can help calm and soothe newborns. It is important for family education. Nurses should educate families on sucrose use. Proper dosing and administration are crucial. Sucrose should be given orally. It is important to follow hospital protocols. Nurses play a key role in sucrose administration. They should monitor newborns closely. Oral sucrose is a valuable tool in newborn care. It can improve the overall experience for newborns and families.

3.3.11 Vitamin K:
Vitamin K is essential for blood clotting. Newborns are given vitamin K injection at birth. Lack of vitamin K can lead to bleeding disorders. Vitamin K deficiency can be life-threatening. Maternal vitamin K intake affects newborn levels. Educate families on the importance of vitamin K. Discuss risks of not giving vitamin K. Monitor newborns for signs of bleeding. Administer vitamin K as per protocol. Document vitamin K administration accurately. Vitamin K is crucial for newborn health. Maternal Newborn Nurses play a vital role in ensuring newborns receive vitamin K.

3.3.12 Vaccines/Immunoglobulins (HBIG, Hep B):
Vaccines/Immunoglobulins (HBIG, Hep B) are crucial for newborn care. Hepatitis B vaccine is given at birth. HBIG is administered to infants born to HBsAg-positive mothers. This helps prevent hepatitis B transmission. Educate families on the importance of these vaccines. Newborns should receive the first dose before discharge. Monitor for any adverse reactions post-vaccination. Ensure proper documentation of vaccine administration. Follow up with families for subsequent doses. Vaccines play a key role in preventing infectious diseases. Maternal Newborn Nurses play a vital role in vaccine education and administration. Stay updated on current vaccine recommendations. Promote vaccination to protect newborns from preventable diseases.

3.3.13 Eye Prophylaxis:
Eye prophylaxis is a common practice in newborn care. It involves the administration of antibiotic ointment to prevent eye infections. This procedure is usually done shortly after birth. The medication used for eye prophylaxis is typically erythromycin

ointment. It helps prevent neonatal conjunctivitis caused by certain bacteria. Eye prophylaxis is important to protect the baby's eyes from potential infections. It is a routine part of newborn care in many healthcare settings. Family education on the importance of eye prophylaxis is essential. Maternal newborn nurses play a key role in administering eye prophylaxis and educating families about its benefits. This simple procedure can help prevent serious eye infections in newborns.

3.3.14 Analgesics:

Analgesics are commonly used medications for pain relief in newborns. They are essential in newborn care to ensure comfort and well-being. There are different types of analgesics, including acetaminophen and ibuprofen, which are safe for newborns when used appropriately.

It is important for maternal newborn nurses to assess the newborn's pain level accurately before administering analgesics. Proper dosage and administration techniques should be followed to prevent any adverse effects.

Family education is crucial in explaining the importance of analgesics in newborn care. Parents should be informed about the proper use of these medications and when to seek medical help.

Overall, analgesics play a significant role in managing pain in newborns, and proper assessment and education are key in ensuring their safe and effective use.

3.4 Resuscitation and Stabilization:

Resuscitation and stabilization are crucial in newborn assessment and management.

Initial steps include drying, warming, and stimulating the baby.

Assess breathing, heart rate, and color to determine the need for resuscitation.

Ventilation and chest compressions may be necessary for newborns in distress.

Stabilization involves maintaining body temperature, blood sugar, and oxygen levels.

Close monitoring is essential to ensure the baby's condition improves.

Collaboration with the healthcare team is key in providing optimal care.

Regular assessments and interventions help in achieving successful outcomes for newborns.

3.4.1 General assessment of status and need for resuscitation:

General assessment of status and need for resuscitation in newborns is crucial. It involves evaluating vital signs, skin color, muscle tone, and reflexes. Assessing the need for resuscitation is based on these factors. Subtopics include heart rate, respiratory effort, and overall appearance. Prompt recognition of signs requiring resuscitation is essential. Effective resuscitation can prevent complications and improve outcomes. Maternal Newborn Nurses play a vital role in this process. They must be skilled in assessing newborns and initiating resuscitation if needed. Training and practice are key to ensuring readiness in emergency situations. Continuous monitoring and reassessment are important for ongoing care. Maternal Newborn Nurses must be prepared to act quickly and confidently to provide life-saving interventions.

3.4.2 Management of resuscitation:

Management of resuscitation in newborns is crucial for maternal newborn nurses.

Key aspects include recognizing signs of distress, initiating interventions promptly, and monitoring response.

Subtopics may include airway management, chest compressions, and medication administration.

Nurses must be prepared to handle various scenarios, such as meconium aspiration or birth trauma.

Effective communication within the healthcare team is essential during resuscitation efforts.

Regular training and simulation exercises help nurses maintain skills and confidence in managing resuscitation.

Overall, the management of resuscitation in newborns requires quick thinking, teamwork, and a calm demeanor.

3.4.3 Airway:

In the management of resuscitation, ensuring a patent airway is crucial. Airway assessment includes checking for obstructions and proper positioning. Proper airway management is essential for effective resuscitation efforts. In newborn assessment and management, maintaining a clear airway is a top priority. Newborns may require suctioning to clear their airway. Nurses must be prepared to provide interventions to secure the airway if needed. Understanding the importance of airway management in resuscitation and stabilization is key for maternal newborn nurses. Continuous monitoring of the airway is necessary to ensure adequate oxygenation and ventilation. Proper airway management can significantly impact the outcome of resuscitation efforts.

3.4.4 Breathing:

Breathing is crucial for newborns' resuscitation and stabilization. It is essential to assess breathing in newborns. Look for signs of respiratory distress. Monitor respiratory rate, effort, and sounds. Assess oxygen saturation levels. Provide appropriate interventions if needed. Administer oxygen therapy if necessary. Ensure proper positioning to support breathing. Monitor for signs of improvement or deterioration. Document all assessments and interventions accurately. Seek help from a healthcare provider if needed. Remember, effective breathing is vital for newborns' well-being.

3.4.5 Circulation:

Circulation is crucial in resuscitation and stabilization of newborns. It involves assessing heart rate, perfusion, and blood pressure. Monitoring circulation helps in early detection of any issues. Proper circulation ensures oxygen and nutrients reach vital organs. Inadequate circulation can lead to organ damage or failure. Maternal Newborn Nurses play a key role in managing circulation. They assess newborns for signs of poor circulation. Nurses administer interventions to improve circulation if needed. Monitoring vital signs is essential in evaluating circulation. Nurses collaborate with the healthcare team to ensure optimal circulation for newborns. Understanding circulation is vital for providing effective care to newborns.

3.4.6 Drug Therapy:

Drug therapy plays a crucial role in resuscitation and stabilization of newborns. Medications are administered to address specific conditions such as respiratory distress syndrome or hypoglycemia.

Subtopics:
- Common drugs used in newborn resuscitation
- Dosage calculations for newborns
- Monitoring for drug effectiveness and side effects

Newborn assessment guides drug therapy decisions. Medications may be given to manage conditions like jaundice or infections.

Subtopics:
- Importance of accurate assessment
- Tailoring drug therapy to individual newborns
- Collaboration with healthcare team for optimal outcomes

Maternal newborn nurses must be knowledgeable about drug therapy to provide safe and effective care for newborns. Regular education and training are essential to stay updated on best practices in drug therapy for newborns.

3.4.7 Evaluation of effectiveness of interventions:

Evaluation of effectiveness of interventions in resuscitation and stabilization, newborn assessment, and management is crucial for maternal newborn nurses.

In resuscitation and stabilization, assessing the response to interventions like chest compressions and medications is essential.

For newborn assessment, evaluating the impact of interventions such as oxygen therapy and temperature regulation is important.

In newborn management, monitoring the effectiveness of interventions like feeding plans and medication administration is key.

Regularly assessing the outcomes of interventions helps nurses make informed decisions and adjust care plans accordingly.

By evaluating the effectiveness of interventions, maternal newborn nurses can ensure the best possible outcomes for both mothers and newborns.

3.4.8 Apgar scores:

Apgar scores are used to assess newborns' health at birth. They measure appearance, pulse, grimace, activity, and respiration. Each category is scored from **0** to **2**, with a total score ranging from **0** to **10**. A score of **7** or above is considered normal. Scores below **7** may indicate the need for resuscitation. Apgar scores are typically done at one minute and five minutes after birth. They help healthcare providers determine if a newborn needs immediate medical attention. Low scores may prompt interventions like oxygen therapy or chest compressions. Apgar scores are a quick and effective way to evaluate a newborn's well-being and guide appropriate care.

4 MATERNAL POSTPARTUM COMPLICATIONS:

Maternal postpartum complications can occur after childbirth. These complications can include postpartum hemorrhage, infection, and postpartum depression. Postpartum hemorrhage is excessive bleeding after delivery. Infection can occur in the uterus or at the site of a cesarean section incision. Postpartum depression is a mood disorder that can affect new mothers. Other complications may include blood clots, urinary incontinence, and wound complications. It is important for maternal newborn nurses to monitor mothers closely for signs of complications. Prompt recognition and treatment of these complications are essential to prevent serious consequences. Education and support for new mothers can also help in preventing and managing postpartum complications. Maternal newborn nurses play a crucial role in caring for mothers during the postpartum period.

4.1 Hematologic:

Hematologic complications in maternal postpartum period can include anemia and thrombocytopenia. Anemia is common due to blood loss during delivery. Iron supplements may be needed. Thrombocytopenia is low platelet count, which can lead to excessive bleeding. It requires close monitoring. Other issues may arise such as clotting disorders or hemolytic disease. These conditions can impact the mother's health post-delivery. Maternal newborn nurses should be aware of these complications. Monitoring blood counts and providing appropriate interventions are crucial. Prompt recognition and management of hematologic issues are essential for the well-being of the mother. Collaboration with healthcare team is important for optimal care. Education on signs and symptoms is vital for early detection and treatment. Hematologic complications can have serious consequences if not addressed promptly.

4.1.1 Hemorrhage:

Hemorrhage is a common maternal postpartum complication. It refers to excessive bleeding after childbirth. There are two main types of postpartum hemorrhage: early and late. Early hemorrhage occurs within **24** hours of delivery, while late hemorrhage occurs between **24** hours and **6** weeks postpartum. Causes of postpartum hemorrhage include uterine atony, lacerations, retained placental tissue, and coagulation disorders. Symptoms may include heavy bleeding, dizziness, and rapid heart rate. Prompt recognition and treatment are essential to prevent complications such as shock and organ failure. Management strategies include uterine massage, administration of uterotonics, and surgical interventions if necessary. Maternal newborn nurses play a crucial role in assessing, monitoring, and managing postpartum hemorrhage to ensure the well-being of both the mother and baby.

4.1.2 Thrombophlebitis:

Thrombophlebitis is a condition where a blood clot forms in a vein. It can occur in the legs or pelvis. Risk factors include immobility, obesity, and smoking. Symptoms may include pain, redness, and swelling in the affected area. Treatment involves blood thinners and compression stockings. Complications can include pulmonary embolism and post-thrombotic syndrome. Prevention strategies include staying active and avoiding prolonged sitting or standing. In pregnant women, thrombophlebitis can be a concern postpartum due to hormonal changes and increased risk of blood clots. Maternal newborn nurses should be aware of the signs and symptoms of thrombophlebitis to provide timely intervention and prevent complications.

4.1.3 Pulmonary embolus:

Pulmonary embolus is a serious complication in postpartum women. It occurs when a blood clot travels to the lungs, blocking blood flow. Risk factors include immobility, obesity, and cesarean delivery. Symptoms may include chest pain, shortness of breath, and coughing. Diagnosis is done through imaging tests like CT scans. Treatment involves blood thinners and oxygen therapy. Prevention strategies include early ambulation and compression stockings. Nurses play a crucial role in monitoring for signs of pulmonary embolus. Prompt recognition and intervention are essential to prevent complications. Education on risk factors and prevention is important for maternal well-being. Pulmonary embolus can be life-threatening if not managed promptly.

4.1.4 DIC/HELLP:
DIC (Disseminated Intravascular Coagulation) and HELLP (Hemolysis, Elevated Liver enzymes, Low Platelet count) are serious maternal postpartum complications. DIC is a life-threatening condition where blood clotting becomes overactive. HELLP syndrome involves liver and blood issues. Both conditions can occur after childbirth. DIC can lead to excessive bleeding and organ damage. HELLP can cause liver rupture and stroke. Symptoms include bruising, jaundice, and abdominal pain. Prompt diagnosis and treatment are crucial. Treatment may involve blood transfusions and medications. Close monitoring is essential to prevent complications. Maternal Newborn Nurses should be aware of signs and symptoms. Early recognition and intervention can improve outcomes for both mother and baby.

4.1.5 Hematoma:
Hematoma is a common postpartum complication in maternal care. It is a collection of blood outside of blood vessels. Hematomas can occur in the vaginal or perineal area after childbirth. They can cause pain, swelling, and bruising. Treatment may include ice packs, pain medication, and sometimes drainage. In severe cases, surgery may be necessary. It is important to monitor for signs of infection, such as fever or increased pain. Proper wound care and monitoring are essential for healing. Maternal Newborn Nurses should educate patients on signs and symptoms of hematoma and provide support during recovery. Early detection and management can prevent complications and promote healing.

4.2 Cardiovascular:
Cardiovascular complications in maternal postpartum period are crucial to monitor. Hypertension, preeclampsia, and heart failure are common issues. These conditions can lead to serious consequences if not managed properly. Nurses should assess vital signs regularly. Keep an eye on blood pressure, heart rate, and oxygen saturation levels. Educate patients on signs of complications. Promptly report any abnormal findings to healthcare provider. Prompt intervention can prevent adverse outcomes. Maternal postpartum care should include close monitoring of cardiovascular status. Early detection and management are key in ensuring maternal well-being. Collaboration with healthcare team is essential for optimal patient outcomes. Regular follow-up visits are important for ongoing assessment and support.

4.2.1 Chronic Hypertension, gestational/Eclampsia:
Chronic hypertension during pregnancy can lead to gestational hypertension or preeclampsia. Gestational hypertension is high blood pressure that develops after **20** weeks of pregnancy. Preeclampsia is a more severe condition that can affect the mother's organs, such as the kidneys and liver. Eclampsia is a rare but serious complication of preeclampsia, characterized by seizures. These conditions can be dangerous for both the mother and the baby, leading to preterm birth or low birth weight. Maternal newborn nurses play a crucial role in monitoring and managing these complications, ensuring the well-being of both mother and baby. Early detection and proper management are essential in preventing adverse outcomes. Regular blood pressure monitoring and close observation are key in the care of pregnant women with chronic hypertension.

4.2.2 Shock:
Shock in the context of maternal postpartum complications refers to a life-threatening condition. It can occur due to severe blood loss during childbirth. This can lead to inadequate blood flow to vital organs. There are different types of shock, including hypovolemic, cardiogenic, and septic shock. Symptoms of shock may include rapid heart rate, low blood pressure, confusion, and cold, clammy skin. Prompt recognition and treatment are crucial to prevent complications. Treatment may involve fluid resuscitation, blood transfusions, and medications to support blood pressure. Close monitoring of the mother's condition is essential to ensure a positive outcome. Maternal newborn nurses play a vital role in identifying and managing shock in postpartum women to promote recovery and well-being.

4.3 Infection:
Infection is a common postpartum complication for mothers. It can occur due to various factors such as prolonged labor, c-section delivery, or weakened immune system. Infections can affect different parts of the body including the uterus, urinary tract, or incision site. Symptoms may include fever, pain, redness, or discharge. Prompt diagnosis and treatment are essential to prevent complications. Antibiotics are often prescribed to treat infections. Proper hygiene practices and wound care can help prevent infections. Educating mothers about signs of infection is crucial for early detection. In severe cases, hospitalization may be required for intravenous antibiotics. Regular follow-up visits are important to monitor recovery progress. Maternal Newborn Nurses play a vital role in educating, assessing, and supporting mothers with postpartum infections.

4.3.1 Endometritis:
Endometritis is an infection that affects the lining of the uterus. It is a common maternal postpartum complication. The condition can occur after childbirth or a miscarriage. Symptoms include fever, abdominal pain, and abnormal vaginal discharge. Risk factors include prolonged labor, C-section delivery, and internal exams. Prompt diagnosis and treatment are essential to prevent complications. Treatment typically involves antibiotics to clear the infection. Proper hygiene and wound care can help

prevent endometritis. Complications of untreated endometritis can include sepsis and infertility. Maternal Newborn Nurses play a crucial role in educating patients about prevention and early detection of endometritis. They also provide support and care for women experiencing this condition.

4.3.2 Wound infection:
Wound infection is a common postpartum complication for mothers. It occurs when bacteria enter the incision site. Signs include redness, swelling, warmth, and pain at the wound site. Proper wound care and hygiene are essential to prevent infection. In severe cases, fever and pus drainage may occur. Prompt treatment with antibiotics is necessary to prevent complications. Risk factors for wound infection include obesity, diabetes, and prolonged labor. Nurses play a crucial role in assessing and monitoring incision sites for signs of infection. Education on proper wound care is important for preventing complications. Collaboration with healthcare providers is essential for timely intervention and management of wound infections in postpartum mothers.

4.3.3 Septic Pelvic thrombophlebitis:
Septic pelvic thrombophlebitis is a serious postpartum complication. It involves infection and inflammation of pelvic veins. The condition can lead to sepsis if not treated promptly. Risk factors include cesarean section and prolonged labor. Symptoms may include fever, pelvic pain, and chills. Diagnosis is made through imaging studies. Treatment involves antibiotics and anticoagulants. Nursing care includes monitoring vital signs and administering medications. Complications can include septic emboli and abscess formation. Prevention strategies include early ambulation and proper hygiene. Maternal Newborn Nurses play a crucial role in recognizing and managing septic pelvic thrombophlebitis. Early intervention is key to preventing serious complications.

4.3.4 Urinary tract infections:
Urinary tract infections are common postpartum complications. They can occur due to catheterization. Symptoms include frequent urination, burning sensation, and cloudy urine. Untreated UTIs can lead to pyelonephritis. Risk factors include prolonged labor, epidural use, and instrumental delivery. Diagnosis involves urine culture and sensitivity testing. Treatment includes antibiotics and increased fluid intake. Prevention strategies include proper perineal care and frequent voiding. Maternal newborn nurses play a crucial role in educating patients about UTI prevention. They should monitor for signs of infection and provide appropriate care. Timely detection and management of UTIs are essential to prevent complications in postpartum women.

4.4 Diabetes:
Diabetes can lead to maternal postpartum complications. It is important for Maternal Newborn Nurses to understand the impact of diabetes on pregnancy.
Diabetes can increase the risk of gestational diabetes, preeclampsia, and cesarean delivery.

Proper management of blood sugar levels is crucial during pregnancy to prevent complications.

Maternal Newborn Nurses should educate mothers on the importance of diet, exercise, and medication compliance.

Regular monitoring of blood sugar levels and fetal growth is essential for a healthy pregnancy.

Nurses should also be aware of the signs and symptoms of hypoglycemia and hyperglycemia in both the mother and baby.

By providing comprehensive care and support, Maternal Newborn Nurses can help mothers with diabetes have a successful pregnancy and postpartum period.

4.5 Mood and Substance Use Disorders:
Maternal postpartum complications can include mood and substance use disorders. Postpartum mood disorders, such as postpartum depression and anxiety, can affect a mother's ability to care for herself and her newborn. Substance use disorders, including alcohol and drug abuse, can also impact maternal health and the well-being of the baby. It is important for maternal newborn nurses to be aware of the signs and symptoms of these disorders, as early detection and intervention can lead to better outcomes for both mother and baby. Nurses can provide support, education, and referrals to resources for mothers experiencing mood and substance use disorders. By addressing these issues promptly, nurses can help mothers navigate the challenges of the postpartum period and promote a healthy start for the newborn.

4.5.1 Sleep disturbances:
Sleep disturbances are common in Mood and Substance Use Disorders. Lack of sleep can worsen these conditions. Postpartum women often experience sleep disturbances. Factors include hormonal changes, newborn care, and anxiety. Maternal sleep disturbances can lead to postpartum depression. Nurses play a crucial role in assessing and managing sleep disturbances. Educating mothers on sleep hygiene and relaxation techniques is important. Referring to mental health professionals may be necessary for severe cases. Monitoring maternal sleep patterns is essential for early intervention. Adequate sleep is crucial for maternal well-being and infant care. Addressing sleep disturbances can improve overall maternal and newborn health.

4.5.2 Postpartum depression/psychosis:

Postpartum depression/psychosis is a common maternal postpartum complication. Postpartum depression is characterized by feelings of sadness, anxiety, and exhaustion. It can affect a mother's ability to care for her newborn. Postpartum psychosis is a more severe condition that includes hallucinations, delusions, and extreme mood swings. It requires immediate medical attention. Risk factors for postpartum depression/psychosis include a history of mental health disorders, lack of social support, and hormonal changes. Screening for these conditions is essential during prenatal and postpartum visits. Treatment options may include therapy, medication, and support groups. Maternal newborn nurses play a crucial role in identifying and supporting mothers experiencing postpartum depression/psychosis. Early intervention can improve outcomes for both the mother and baby.

4.5.3 Substance abuse:

Substance abuse is a common issue among women with mood and substance use disorders. It can lead to maternal postpartum complications. Substance abuse during pregnancy can have serious consequences for both the mother and the baby. It can increase the risk of preterm birth, low birth weight, and developmental delays in the child.

Women who struggle with substance abuse may also face challenges in caring for their newborns. They may have difficulty bonding with their baby or providing a safe and nurturing environment. It is important for maternal newborn nurses to be aware of the signs of substance abuse and provide support and resources to help these women overcome their addiction. By addressing substance abuse early on, nurses can help improve the health outcomes for both the mother and the baby.

5 NEWBORN COMPLICATIONS:

Newborn complications can arise from various factors such as prematurity, birth trauma, or infections. Respiratory distress syndrome is a common complication in premature babies. Other complications include jaundice, hypoglycemia, and sepsis. Birth injuries like fractures or nerve damage can occur during delivery. Infections such as pneumonia or meningitis can also affect newborns. Maternal factors like diabetes or hypertension can increase the risk of complications. Prompt recognition and treatment are crucial in managing newborn complications. Close monitoring of vital signs, laboratory tests, and imaging studies are essential in assessing the severity of the condition. Collaboration with a multidisciplinary team is important in providing comprehensive care for newborns with complications. Education and support for parents are also vital in promoting the well-being of the newborn.

5.1 Cardiovascular and Respiratory:

Newborn complications related to cardiovascular and respiratory systems are common.

Cardiovascular issues may include congenital heart defects, arrhythmias, and heart murmurs.

Respiratory problems can range from transient tachypnea of the newborn to respiratory distress syndrome.

Early detection and prompt intervention are crucial in managing these complications.

Maternal Newborn Nurses play a vital role in assessing, monitoring, and providing care for newborns with cardiovascular and respiratory issues.

They collaborate with healthcare providers to develop treatment plans and educate parents on how to care for their newborns at home.

By staying informed about the latest research and guidelines, Maternal Newborn Nurses can ensure the best outcomes for newborns with cardiovascular and respiratory complications.

5.1.1 Cyanotic Heart Disease:

Cyanotic Heart Disease is a condition where there is a lack of oxygen in the blood. It is a type of congenital heart defect that causes a bluish discoloration of the skin. This condition can lead to serious complications if not treated promptly.

There are different types of Cyanotic Heart Disease, including Tetralogy of Fallot, Transposition of the Great Arteries, and Tricuspid Atresia. These conditions affect the structure of the heart and how blood flows through it.

Symptoms of Cyanotic Heart Disease include shortness of breath, fatigue, and poor weight gain. Diagnosis is usually made through physical examination, imaging tests, and cardiac catheterization.

Treatment options may include medications, surgery, or other interventions to improve blood flow and oxygen levels. It is important for Maternal Newborn Nurses to be aware of the signs and symptoms of Cyanotic Heart Disease to provide appropriate care for newborns with this condition.

5.1.2 Acyanotic Heart Disease:

Acyanotic heart disease is a common congenital heart condition in newborns. It includes various defects like atrial septal defect, ventricular septal defect, and patent ductus arteriosus. These defects lead to abnormal blood flow in the heart. Symptoms may include rapid breathing, poor feeding, and failure to thrive. Diagnosis is done through physical exams, echocardiograms, and chest X-rays. Treatment options include medications, catheter procedures, and surgery. Complications can arise if left untreated, such as heart failure and pulmonary hypertension. Nurses play a crucial role in monitoring newborns with acyanotic heart disease, educating parents, and providing emotional support. Early detection and intervention are key in managing this condition effectively.

5.1.3 Apnea:

Apnea is a common newborn complication related to the cardiovascular and respiratory system. It is characterized by pauses in breathing that last for more than **20** seconds.

Causes of apnea in newborns can include prematurity, infections, neurological issues, and maternal drug use during pregnancy.

Symptoms of apnea may include a bluish tint to the skin, slow heart rate, and weak sucking reflex.

Diagnosis of apnea is typically done through monitoring the baby's breathing patterns and heart rate.

Treatment options for apnea in newborns may include stimulation, medication, or the use of a continuous positive airway pressure (CPAP) machine.

It is important for maternal newborn nurses to be knowledgeable about apnea in order to provide appropriate care and support to newborns experiencing this complication.

5.1.4 Transient Tachypnea of the Newborn:

Transient Tachypnea of the Newborn is a common respiratory condition in newborns. It is characterized by rapid breathing and is usually mild. The main cause is delayed clearance of fetal lung fluid. Symptoms include grunting, flaring nostrils, and chest retractions. Diagnosis is based on clinical presentation and chest X-ray findings. Treatment involves supportive care, such as oxygen therapy and IV fluids. Most infants recover within **72** hours. Complications are rare but can include pneumonia or respiratory distress syndrome. Prevention strategies include proper monitoring during labor and delivery. Education for parents on recognizing signs of respiratory distress is essential. Maternal Newborn Nurses play a crucial role in early detection and management of Transient Tachypnea of the Newborn.

5.1.5 Pneumothorax:

Pneumothorax is a condition where air collects in the space around the lungs. It can cause breathing difficulties in newborns.

Causes of pneumothorax in newborns include trauma during birth or lung diseases.

Symptoms of pneumothorax in newborns include rapid breathing, chest retractions, and bluish skin.

Diagnosis is done through physical examination and imaging tests like chest X-rays.

Treatment may involve oxygen therapy, chest tube insertion, or surgery in severe cases.

Complications of pneumothorax in newborns can include respiratory distress and lung collapse.

Maternal Newborn Nurses should be aware of the signs and symptoms of pneumothorax in newborns to provide prompt care.

5.1.6 Meconium Aspiration:

Meconium aspiration occurs when a newborn inhales meconium-stained amniotic fluid during delivery. This can lead to respiratory distress and potential complications. Meconium is the baby's first stool, which is thick and sticky. It can block the airways and cause breathing difficulties. Risk factors include post-term pregnancy, fetal distress, and maternal hypertension. Symptoms may include rapid breathing, grunting, and bluish skin color. Treatment involves suctioning the airways, oxygen therapy, and sometimes mechanical ventilation. Complications can include pneumonia, airway obstruction, and respiratory failure. Maternal Newborn Nurses should be vigilant for signs of meconium aspiration and provide prompt intervention to ensure the best outcomes for the newborn.

5.2 Neurological and Gastrointestinal:

Newborns can experience neurological and gastrointestinal complications. Neurological issues may include seizures or developmental delays. Gastrointestinal problems could involve feeding difficulties or reflux. These complications can impact a newborn's overall health and development. It is crucial for maternal newborn nurses to monitor these conditions closely. Early detection and intervention are key in managing these issues effectively. Nurses should be knowledgeable about signs and symptoms of neurological and gastrointestinal problems in newborns. They play a vital role in providing care and support to both the baby and the family. Collaboration with other healthcare professionals is essential in ensuring the best outcomes for newborns with these complications. Regular assessments and communication with the healthcare team are important in managing these challenges.

5.2.1 Seizures:

Seizures in newborns can be caused by various factors. They can be classified as either focal or generalized seizures. Focal seizures affect only one part of the brain, while generalized seizures involve the whole brain. Common causes of seizures in newborns include hypoxic-ischemic encephalopathy, infections, metabolic disorders, and genetic factors. It is crucial for maternal newborn nurses to recognize the signs of seizures in newborns, such as rhythmic jerking movements, staring, or repetitive movements. Immediate medical attention is necessary when a newborn experiences a seizure. Treatment may involve medication to control seizures or addressing the underlying cause. Maternal newborn nurses play a vital role in monitoring and providing care for newborns with seizures to ensure optimal outcomes.

5.2.2 Jitteriness:

Jitteriness in newborns can be a common neurological and gastrointestinal complication. It is characterized by tremors or shaking movements in the baby's body. Jitteriness can be caused by various factors such as low blood sugar levels, drug withdrawal, or neurological issues. It is important for maternal newborn nurses to monitor and assess the baby's jitteriness carefully.

Subtopics:
- Causes of jitteriness
- Symptoms of jitteriness
- Assessment and monitoring
- Treatment options

Maternal newborn nurses should work closely with healthcare providers to determine the underlying cause of jitteriness and provide appropriate care. Early detection and intervention are crucial in managing jitteriness in newborns. Proper education and support for parents are also essential in ensuring the well-being of the baby.

5.2.3 Intracranial Hemorrhage:

Intracranial hemorrhage in newborns is a serious condition. It can be caused by trauma during birth or underlying medical conditions.

Subtopics:
- Types of intracranial hemorrhage include subdural, subarachnoid, and intraventricular bleeding.
- Symptoms may include seizures, lethargy, poor feeding, and abnormal movements.
- Diagnosis is done through imaging studies like ultrasound or MRI.
- Treatment involves monitoring, supportive care, and sometimes surgery.

As a Maternal Newborn Nurse, it is crucial to recognize signs of intracranial hemorrhage promptly. Early intervention can improve outcomes for newborns with this condition. Understanding the causes, symptoms, and treatment options is essential for providing optimal care to these vulnerable patients.

5.2.4 Neural Tube Defects:

Neural tube defects are birth defects affecting the brain, spine, or spinal cord. They occur in early pregnancy when the neural tube, which forms the baby's brain and spinal cord, doesn't close properly. The most common types are spina bifida, anencephaly, and encephalocele. Spina bifida can cause physical disabilities, while anencephaly is fatal. Encephalocele involves a sac-like protrusion of the brain through an opening in the skull. Folic acid supplementation before and during pregnancy can reduce the risk of neural tube defects. Prenatal screening and early detection are crucial for managing these conditions. Treatment may involve surgery, therapy, and ongoing medical care. Maternal newborn nurses play a vital role in educating expectant mothers about prevention and providing support to families affected by neural tube defects.

5.2.5 Substance Abused Neonate:

Substance Abused Neonate is a critical issue in newborn care. Neonates exposed to substances in utero may experience neurological and gastrointestinal complications. These infants are at risk for seizures, tremors, and feeding difficulties. They may also suffer from irritability, poor weight gain, and vomiting.

Neurologically, substance-exposed neonates may exhibit hyperactivity, hypertonia, and poor coordination. They may have difficulty with feeding, sleeping, and self-soothing. Gastrointestinal issues can include diarrhea, constipation, and reflux.

Maternal Newborn Nurses play a crucial role in caring for these vulnerable infants. They provide specialized care, monitor for withdrawal symptoms, and support breastfeeding. Early identification and intervention are key in managing the complex needs of substance-abused neonates.

5.2.6 Intestinal Obstructions and Anomalies:

Intestinal obstructions and anomalies in newborns can be serious conditions. These issues can result from a variety of factors.

One common cause is meconium ileus, where the newborn's first stool is thick and sticky. Another is malrotation, where the intestines are not in the correct position.
Symptoms may include vomiting, abdominal distension, and failure to pass stool. Diagnosis is typically made through imaging studies.
Treatment often involves surgery to correct the issue. Complications can arise if not treated promptly.

As a maternal newborn nurse, it is important to monitor newborns for signs of intestinal obstructions and anomalies. Early detection and intervention are key to ensuring the best outcomes for these infants.

5.3 Hematologic:

Hematologic complications in newborns can arise from various factors. One common issue is anemia, which can be caused by blood loss during delivery or inadequate iron stores. Another concern is polycythemia, where the baby has too many red blood cells. This can lead to complications such as jaundice or blood clots. Thrombocytopenia, a low platelet count, is also a potential problem that can result in bleeding issues. Additionally, hemolytic disease of the newborn occurs when the mother and baby have incompatible blood types, leading to the destruction of the baby's red blood cells. Maternal Newborn Nurses must be vigilant in monitoring newborns for signs of hematologic complications to provide prompt treatment and prevent further complications.

5.3.1 Anemia:

Anemia is a common condition in newborns, characterized by low red blood cell count. It can be caused by maternal iron deficiency during pregnancy. Symptoms include pale skin, fatigue, and poor feeding. Anemia can lead to developmental delays if left untreated. Treatment may involve iron supplements or blood transfusions. Regular screening for anemia is important in newborns to ensure early detection and management. Maternal Newborn Nurses play a crucial role in educating parents about the importance of iron-rich diets and proper prenatal care to prevent anemia in newborns. Monitoring the baby's growth and development is essential to identify any signs of anemia early on. Collaboration with healthcare providers is key in providing comprehensive care for newborns with anemia.

5.3.2 Vitamin K Deficiency:

Vitamin K deficiency in newborns can lead to serious hematologic complications. Newborns are at risk due to low levels of vitamin K at birth. Vitamin K is essential for blood clotting. Without enough vitamin K, newborns can experience bleeding issues. Hemorrhagic disease of the newborn is a potential complication. Administering vitamin K at birth can prevent deficiency-related complications. Maternal newborn nurses play a crucial role in educating parents about the importance of vitamin K supplementation. Monitoring newborns for signs of bleeding is essential. Early detection and treatment are key in preventing serious consequences of vitamin K deficiency.

5.3.3 Hyperbilirubinemia:

Hyperbilirubinemia is common in newborns, caused by high bilirubin levels. It can lead to jaundice. Risk factors include prematurity, breastfeeding, and blood type incompatibility. Monitoring bilirubin levels is crucial. Treatment may involve phototherapy or exchange transfusion. Complications can arise if left untreated. Education on signs and symptoms is important for parents. Maternal Newborn Nurses play a key role in assessing and managing hyperbilirubinemia. Regular monitoring and early intervention are essential. Collaboration with healthcare team members is necessary for optimal care. Understanding the causes and treatment options is vital for providing quality care to newborns with hyperbilirubinemia.

5.3.4 ABO Incompatibility:

ABO incompatibility occurs when a mother's blood type is different from her baby's. This can lead to hemolytic disease of the newborn. The mother's antibodies attack the baby's red blood cells. Symptoms include jaundice, anemia, and enlarged liver or spleen. Diagnosis is done through blood tests. Treatment may include phototherapy, blood transfusions, or intravenous immunoglobulin. Prevention methods include giving Rh immunoglobulin to Rh-negative mothers. Complications can range from mild to severe, depending on the level of incompatibility. Close monitoring and early intervention are crucial for a positive outcome. Maternal newborn nurses play a vital role in educating parents about ABO incompatibility and providing support during treatment.

5.3.5 Hemolytic Disease:

Hemolytic Disease occurs when mother and baby blood types are incompatible. Maternal antibodies attack baby's red blood cells. This can lead to anemia, jaundice, and in severe cases, brain damage or death. Rh incompatibility is a common cause. Rh-negative mother and Rh-positive baby can trigger the disease. ABO incompatibility is another cause. It happens when mother's blood type is O and baby's is A, B, or AB. Symptoms include yellowing of skin and eyes, pale skin, and fussiness. Treatment may involve phototherapy, blood transfusions, or exchange transfusions. Prevention includes giving Rh immunoglobulin to Rh-negative mothers. Early detection and management are crucial for a positive outcome. Maternal Newborn Nurses play a vital role in educating mothers about the risks and monitoring newborns for signs of Hemolytic Disease.

5.3.6 G6PD:

G6PD deficiency is a genetic condition affecting red blood cells. It can lead to hemolytic anemia. Newborns with G6PD deficiency may experience jaundice and anemia. Avoid triggers like certain foods and medications. Educate parents on signs of hemolysis. Monitor newborns closely for complications. Treat severe jaundice with phototherapy. Blood transfusions may be necessary in severe cases. Genetic counseling is important for families. Follow-up care is essential for newborns with G6PD deficiency. Maternal Newborn Nurses play a crucial role in educating families and providing care.

5.3.7 Polycythemia/Hyperviscosity:

Polycythemia/Hyperviscosity in newborns can lead to complications. It is characterized by high red blood cell count. This condition can cause increased blood thickness. Symptoms include poor feeding, lethargy, and respiratory distress. Complications may include hypoglycemia and seizures. Treatment involves monitoring blood volume and hydration status. Phototherapy may be needed for jaundice. Blood exchange transfusion is done in severe cases. Maternal factors like gestational diabetes can contribute to polycythemia. Nurses should monitor newborns closely for signs of hyperviscosity. Early detection and management are crucial for a positive outcome. Education for parents on signs and symptoms is essential. Collaboration with the healthcare team is important for optimal care.

5.3.8 Thrombocytopenia:

Thrombocytopenia is a condition where the blood has a low platelet count. Platelets help with blood clotting, so low levels can lead to excessive bleeding. In newborns, thrombocytopenia can be caused by maternal factors like gestational thrombocytopenia or immune thrombocytopenic purpura. It can also be due to neonatal factors such as sepsis, asphyxia, or prematurity.

Symptoms of thrombocytopenia in newborns may include petechiae, purpura, or bleeding from the umbilical cord. Diagnosis is done through blood tests to measure platelet levels. Treatment depends on the cause and severity, and may include platelet transfusions or medications. Nurses should monitor newborns closely for signs of bleeding and collaborate with healthcare providers to provide appropriate care.

5.4 Infectious Disease:

Infectious diseases can affect newborns, leading to complications. Newborns are more vulnerable.
Common infectious diseases include respiratory syncytial virus (RSV) and group B streptococcus (GBS).

Symptoms may include fever, poor feeding, and lethargy.
Early detection and treatment are crucial.
Prevention strategies include proper hand hygiene and vaccination.
Maternal infections during pregnancy can also pose a risk.
Newborns may require antibiotics or antiviral medications.
In severe cases, hospitalization may be necessary.
Educating parents on infection prevention is essential.
Maternal Newborn Nurses play a vital role in caring for newborns with infectious diseases.

5.4.1 Neonatal Sepsis:

Neonatal sepsis is a serious infection in newborns. It can be caused by bacteria, viruses, or fungi. Early-onset sepsis occurs within the first week of life, while late-onset sepsis occurs after the first week. Risk factors include premature birth, low birth weight, and maternal infection. Symptoms may include fever, poor feeding, and breathing problems. Diagnosis is based on blood tests and cultures. Treatment involves antibiotics and supportive care. Complications can include organ damage and even death. Prevention strategies include proper hand hygiene, sterile procedures during delivery, and early detection and treatment of maternal infections. Maternal Newborn Nurses play a crucial role in recognizing the signs of neonatal sepsis and providing prompt care to affected infants.

5.4.2 Neonatal CBC and differential:

Neonatal CBC and differential are crucial for assessing newborn health. CBC provides information on red blood cells, white blood cells, and platelets. Differential helps identify specific types of white blood cells. In infectious diseases, CBC can show signs of infection like elevated white blood cell count. Neutrophils are important in fighting infections and can be elevated in response to infection. Lymphocytes play a role in immune response and can also be affected by infections. Monitoring CBC and differential helps in early detection of newborn complications. Maternal Newborn Nurses should be familiar with interpreting these results to provide appropriate care for newborns. Understanding the significance of neonatal CBC and differential is essential in managing infectious diseases and other newborn complications.

5.4.3 Lumbar Puncture:

Lumbar puncture is a procedure to collect cerebrospinal fluid from the lower back. It helps diagnose infections like meningitis in newborns. Before the procedure, the baby is positioned on their side with knees tucked. The area is cleaned and numbed with a local anesthetic. A needle is then inserted between the vertebrae to collect the fluid. It is sent to the lab for analysis. Complications can include bleeding, infection, or headache. Nurses play a crucial role in preparing the baby and comforting them during the procedure. They monitor for any signs of infection or bleeding post-procedure. Understanding the importance of lumbar puncture in diagnosing infectious diseases in newborns is essential for maternal newborn nurses.

5.4.4 Viral Infections:

Viral infections can pose risks to newborns. Maternal transmission of viruses like HIV, herpes, and hepatitis B can lead to serious complications. These infections can be passed to the baby during pregnancy, birth, or breastfeeding. Newborns are more vulnerable to viral illnesses due to their immature immune systems. Common symptoms include fever, rash, and respiratory issues. Diagnosis may involve blood tests or cultures. Treatment focuses on managing symptoms and preventing complications. Prevention strategies include vaccination, antiviral medications, and proper hygiene practices. Maternal Newborn Nurses play a crucial role in educating mothers about the risks of viral infections and providing support and care for affected newborns. Early detection and intervention are key in ensuring the best outcomes for newborns with viral infections.

5.4.5 Bacterial Infections:

Bacterial infections in newborns can lead to serious complications. These infections can be acquired during birth or shortly after. Common bacterial infections in newborns include Group B Streptococcus, E. coli, and Listeria. Symptoms may include fever, poor feeding, and irritability. Early detection and treatment are crucial to prevent complications. Bacterial infections can be diagnosed through blood tests and cultures. Treatment usually involves antibiotics administered intravenously. Prevention strategies include proper hand hygiene and screening pregnant women for bacterial infections. Maternal vaccination can also help protect newborns from certain bacterial infections. Educating parents on the signs and symptoms of bacterial infections is essential. Maternal newborn nurses play a vital role in recognizing and managing bacterial infections in newborns.

5.4.6 Sexually Transmitted Infections:

Sexually Transmitted Infections (STIs) can pose risks to newborns. STIs can be transmitted from mother to baby during pregnancy, childbirth, or breastfeeding. Common STIs include chlamydia, gonorrhea, syphilis, HIV, and herpes. These infections can lead to serious complications for newborns, such as low birth weight, premature birth, pneumonia, eye infections, and even death. It is crucial for maternal newborn nurses to screen pregnant women for STIs, provide appropriate treatment, and educate them on prevention methods. Early detection and management of STIs can help prevent transmission to the newborn and reduce the risk of complications. Nurses play a vital role in promoting maternal and newborn health by addressing STIs effectively.

5.4.7 Anti-infectives:

Anti-infectives are used to treat infectious diseases in newborns. They help fight off bacteria, viruses, fungi, and parasites. Antibiotics are commonly prescribed for bacterial infections. Antivirals are used for viral infections. Antifungals treat fungal infections. Antiparasitics are given for parasitic infections. These medications help prevent the spread of infection and promote healing. It is important for maternal newborn nurses to understand the different types of anti-infectives and their uses. They must also be aware of potential side effects and drug interactions. Proper administration and monitoring of these medications are crucial for the well-being of newborns with infectious diseases. Maternal newborn nurses play a vital role in ensuring the safe and effective use of anti-infectives in newborns.

5.4.8 Genetic, Metabolic and Endocrine:

Genetic, Metabolic, and Endocrine issues in newborns can lead to complications. Genetic conditions can affect physical and mental development. Metabolic disorders can impact how the body processes nutrients. Endocrine problems may disrupt hormone levels. Common genetic disorders include Down syndrome and cystic fibrosis. Metabolic issues like hypoglycemia and phenylketonuria require monitoring and treatment. Endocrine disorders such as congenital hypothyroidism can affect growth and development. Maternal Newborn Nurses play a crucial role in identifying and managing these complications. Early detection and intervention are key to ensuring the best outcomes for newborns with genetic, metabolic, and endocrine issues. Regular monitoring and collaboration with healthcare providers are essential in providing comprehensive care.

5.4.9 Hypoglycemia:

Hypoglycemia is low blood sugar in newborns, often due to inadequate feeding. It can lead to neurological issues if not treated promptly. Symptoms include jitteriness, poor feeding, and lethargy. Risk factors include maternal diabetes, preterm birth, and macrosomia. Diagnosis is through blood glucose testing. Treatment involves feeding, IV glucose, or glucagon administration. Monitoring blood sugar levels is crucial. Complications can arise if hypoglycemia is not managed effectively. Education on feeding techniques and signs of hypoglycemia is essential for parents. Maternal Newborn Nurses play a vital role in recognizing and managing hypoglycemia in newborns. Early detection and intervention are key to preventing long-term consequences.

5.4.10 Inborn Errors of Metabolism:

Inborn Errors of Metabolism are genetic disorders affecting metabolism in newborns. These disorders result from enzyme deficiencies that disrupt normal metabolic processes. Common types include amino acid disorders, organic acid disorders, and fatty acid oxidation disorders. Symptoms may include poor feeding, vomiting, lethargy, and seizures. Early detection through newborn screening is crucial for prompt treatment. Treatment often involves dietary modifications, enzyme replacement therapy, and medications. Complications can arise if left untreated, leading to developmental delays, organ damage, and even death. Maternal Newborn Nurses play a vital role in educating parents about these disorders, providing support, and coordinating care with healthcare providers. Understanding the signs and symptoms of Inborn Errors of Metabolism is essential for early intervention and improved outcomes for newborns.

5.4.11 Patterns of Inheritance:

Patterns of inheritance play a crucial role in understanding genetic conditions. Inheritance can be autosomal dominant, autosomal recessive, X-linked dominant, or X-linked recessive. Autosomal dominant disorders only require one copy of the gene for the condition to be present. In contrast, autosomal recessive disorders need two copies of the gene. X-linked disorders are carried on the X chromosome and can affect males more severely. Understanding these patterns helps predict the likelihood of a newborn inheriting a genetic condition. Maternal newborn nurses must be knowledgeable about these patterns to provide appropriate care and support to families. By recognizing inheritance patterns, nurses can offer genetic counseling and help families make informed decisions about their newborn's health.

5.4.12 Infant of a Diabetic Mother:

Infants of diabetic mothers are at risk for various complications. These babies may have low blood sugar levels at birth. They are also prone to respiratory distress syndrome. Additionally, they may have an increased risk of being born prematurely. These infants may have a higher chance of developing jaundice. They are also at risk for having congenital anomalies. It is important to closely monitor these babies after birth. They may require special care and treatment in the neonatal intensive care unit. Maternal blood sugar levels during pregnancy can impact the health of the baby. Proper management of diabetes during pregnancy is crucial to reduce the risk of complications in the newborn. Regular monitoring and early intervention are key in ensuring the well-being of infants of diabetic mothers.

RNC-MNN Practice Questions

SET 1

Question 1: Mrs. Smith, a postpartum mother, is bottle-feeding her newborn. Which technique should the nurse recommend to ensure proper bottle-feeding hygiene?
A) Reusing the same bottle without washing between feedings
B) Using soap and water to wash bottles after each feeding
C) Storing unwashed bottles in the refrigerator between feedings
D) Boiling bottles once a week for sterilization

Question 2: Mrs. Smith gave birth to a newborn who is diagnosed with congenital hypothyroidism. The nurse is educating the parents about the condition. Which statement by the parents indicates a need for further teaching?
A) "We should ensure our baby takes the thyroid hormone replacement medication regularly."
B) "It is important to monitor our baby's growth and development closely."
C) "We can discontinue the medication once our baby starts showing improvement."
D) "Regular follow-up visits with the healthcare provider are necessary."

Question 3: What is a potential respiratory complication that can occur in infants of diabetic mothers?
A) Transient tachypnea of the newborn (TTN)
B) Bronchopulmonary dysplasia (BPD)
C) Meconium aspiration syndrome (MAS)
D) Persistent pulmonary hypertension of the newborn (PPHN)

Question 4: Ms. Johnson, a 28-year-old pregnant woman, is pregnant with triplets. She is at 30 weeks of gestation and complains of persistent lower back pain. Which of the following interventions is most appropriate for managing lower back pain in a pregnant woman with multiple gestation?
A) Encouraging bed rest and limited physical activity.
B) Applying heat packs to the lower back.
C) Administering nonsteroidal anti-inflammatory drugs (NSAIDs).
D) Performing regular gentle exercises and stretches.

Question 5: Scenario: Sarah, a newborn, is being assessed for circulation. The nurse notes a capillary refill time of 4 seconds. What is the most appropriate interpretation of this finding?
A) Normal circulation
B) Delayed circulation
C) Impaired circulation
D) Inadequate circulation

Question 6: Which of the following antenatal factors is associated with obesity in pregnancy?
A) Low birth weight
B) Preterm birth
C) Gestational diabetes
D) Post-term pregnancy

Question 7: Scenario: Baby Emma, a newborn, is admitted to the neonatal intensive care unit (NICU) with symptoms of feeding intolerance, abdominal distension, and bilious vomiting. Upon assessment, the nurse notes that Emma has a high-pitched cry, lethargy, and poor feeding. The healthcare provider suspects a gastrointestinal complication. What condition should be considered in this newborn?
A) Necrotizing enterocolitis (NEC)
B) Hirschsprung's disease
C) Intussusception
D) Malrotation with volvulus

Question 8: During a postpartum education session, a new mother expresses concerns about her ability to breastfeed effectively. She mentions feeling overwhelmed and anxious about not producing enough milk for her baby. Which nursing action best upholds the ethical principle of non-maleficence in this situation?
A) Dismissing the mother's concerns as common postpartum worries.
B) Providing evidence-based information and support for successful breastfeeding.
C) Ignoring the mother's worries and focusing on other postpartum topics.
D) Suggesting the mother switch to formula feeding to alleviate her anxiety.

Question 9: Mrs. Smith, a 28-year-old postpartum mother, is experiencing engorgement in her breasts. Which of the following hormones is primarily responsible for milk ejection during breastfeeding?
A) Estrogen
B) Progesterone
C) Oxytocin
D) Prolactin

Question 10: Ms. Smith, a 32-year-old pregnant woman at 38 weeks gestation, is admitted to the labor and delivery unit. During the electronic fetal monitoring (EFM), the nurse notes a baseline fetal heart rate of 160 beats per minute with minimal variability and repetitive late decelerations. What is the most appropriate interpretation of this fetal heart rate pattern?
A) Category I FHR pattern
B) Category II FHR pattern
C) Category III FHR pattern
D) Category IV FHR pattern

Question 11: Which of the following is a potential complication of circumcision in newborns?
A) Hemorrhage
B) Hypoglycemia
C) Jaundice
D) Bradycardia

Question 12: During a gestational age assessment of a newborn using the New Ballard Score, the nurse notes that the baby has lanugo covering the entire body, minimal creases on the soles of the feet, and the testes are palpable in the scrotum. What would be the most likely gestational age assessment based on these observations?
A) 28 weeks
B) 34 weeks
C) 38 weeks
D) 42 weeks

Question 13: Scenario: Sarah, a newborn, is born with poor respiratory effort and central cyanosis. The healthcare provider initiates resuscitation. Which intervention should be prioritized in this situation?
A) Administering intravenous fluids
B) Providing positive-pressure ventilation
C) Checking blood glucose levels
D) Placing a nasogastric tube

Question 14: Ms. Smith, a 32-year-old pregnant woman, presents to the antenatal clinic for a routine check-up at 32 weeks gestation. She has a history of hypertension and smoking. On ultrasound, the fetus is found to have an estimated fetal weight below the 10th percentile for gestational age. Which of the following maternal conditions is a significant risk factor for the development of intrauterine growth restriction (IUGR) in this scenario?
A) Advanced maternal age
B) Gestational diabetes
C) Smoking
D) Multiparity

Question 15: A newborn, James, is admitted to the neonatal intensive care unit with bilious vomiting, abdominal distension, and a palpable mass in the right upper quadrant. An abdominal X-ray reveals a "double-bubble" sign. Which of the following conditions is most likely causing James's symptoms?
A) Meconium ileus
B) Duodenal atresia
C) Necrotizing enterocolitis
D) Pyloric stenosis

Question 16: Which antihypertensive medication is commonly used in the postpartum period due to its safety profile for breastfeeding mothers?
A) Lisinopril
B) Atenolol
C) Methyldopa
D) Furosemide

Question 17: Which of the following factors increases the risk of wound infection in postpartum mothers?
A) Early ambulation after delivery
B) Adequate hand hygiene practices
C) Timely administration of prophylactic antibiotics
D) Prolonged rupture of membranes during labor

Question 18: Which complication in the postpartum period requires immediate medical attention?
A) Postpartum hemorrhage
B) Perineal laceration
C) Engorged breasts
D) Infant feeding difficulties

Question 19: Which of the following is a potential risk associated with a cesarean section delivery?
A) Increased risk of postpartum hemorrhage
B) Decreased risk of surgical complications
C) Lower risk of neonatal respiratory distress syndrome
D) Reduced risk of maternal infection

Question 20: How can healthcare providers support parent/infant interactions in the postpartum period?
A) Encouraging the use of pacifiers to soothe the baby
B) Promoting kangaroo care for premature infants
C) Limiting parental involvement in infant care
D) Discouraging skin-to-skin contact between the mother and baby

Question 21: Which of the following is a common sign of respiratory distress in a newborn?
A) Bradycardia
B) Nasal flaring
C) Hypoglycemia
D) Jaundice

Question 22: During breastfeeding, which action by the newborn indicates effective suck/swallow/sequence coordination?
A) Audible swallowing sounds
B) Frequent pauses and breaks
C) Shallow latch with clicking noises
D) Short, rapid sucks without swallowing

Question 23: Baby James, born at 36 weeks gestation, is diagnosed with apnea of prematurity. The healthcare provider prescribes caffeine citrate to stimulate the baby's respiratory drive. What is the rationale behind using caffeine citrate in this situation?
A) To improve feeding tolerance
B) To prevent hypothermia
C) To reduce the risk of infection
D) To stimulate the baby's respiratory drive

Question 24: Which hormone is primarily responsible for milk production in the lactating mother?
A) Estrogen
B) Progesterone
C) Prolactin
D) Oxytocin

Question 25: What is a common emotional response of siblings to the arrival of a new baby?
A) Increased feelings of independence
B) Decreased need for parental attention
C) Jealousy and regression in behavior
D) Enhanced communication skills

Question 26: During newborn assessment, the nurse observes that the newborn is cyanotic and has poor muscle tone. The nurse initiates tactile stimulation and rubs the newborn's back to stimulate breathing. After a few seconds, the newborn begins to cry and shows improved color and muscle tone. What should be the nurse's next step to assess the effectiveness of the intervention?
A) Administer oxygen via nasal cannula
B) Check the newborn's temperature
C) Assess the newborn's respiratory rate
D) Perform a blood glucose test

Question 27: Which of the following is a risk factor for the development of hyperbilirubinemia in newborns?
A) Exclusive breastfeeding
B) Term gestation

C) ABO incompatibility
D) Maternal diabetes

Question 28: Ms. Smith, a 2-day-old newborn, is diagnosed with acyanotic heart disease. Which of the following congenital heart defects is commonly associated with increased pulmonary blood flow in acyanotic heart disease?
A) Tetralogy of Fallot
B) Ventricular septal defect (VSD)
C) Coarctation of the aorta
D) Transposition of the great arteries

Question 29: Which of the following newborn complications is characterized by a blue discoloration of the skin and mucous membranes due to inadequate oxygenation?
A) Hypoglycemia
B) Hyperbilirubinemia
C) Cyanosis
D) Sepsis

Question 30: Ms. Smith brings her 2-day-old newborn to the clinic for a routine check-up. During the assessment, the nurse notices jaundice in the baby. Upon further investigation, it is revealed that the baby has glucose-6-phosphate dehydrogenase (G6PD) deficiency. Which of the following statements regarding G6PD deficiency in newborns is true?
A) G6PD deficiency is more common in female newborns.
B) Newborns with G6PD deficiency are at decreased risk of jaundice.
C) G6PD deficiency can lead to hemolytic anemia triggered by certain medications or infections.
D) G6PD deficiency has no impact on the newborn's health.

Question 31: What is a potential drug interaction to consider when administering diuretics to postpartum women?
A) Nonsteroidal anti-inflammatory drugs (NSAIDs)
B) Iron supplements
C) Prenatal vitamins
D) Antihypertensive medications

Question 32: Which of the following is a crucial step to prepare a newborn for a lumbar puncture procedure?
A) Positioning the newborn in a side-lying fetal position
B) Administering sedation to keep the newborn calm
C) Applying a warm compress to the lumbar area
D) Ensuring the newborn is well-hydrated

Question 33: Which psychosocial factor is most commonly associated with postpartum depression?
A) Advanced maternal age
B) Multiparity
C) Low socioeconomic status
D) Planned pregnancy

Question 34: At 36 weeks of gestation, Mrs. Johnson, a 25-year-old primigravida, presents to the antenatal clinic with complaints of severe itching on her palms and soles, especially at night. On further assessment, the nurse suspects intrahepatic cholestasis of pregnancy (ICP). Which antenatal factor is most closely associated with the development of ICP in pregnancy?
A) Maternal age
B) Primigravida status
C) Family history of ICP
D) Maternal body mass index (BMI)

Question 35: Which of the following is a critical congenital heart defect that results in oxygen-poor blood being pumped out to the body?
A) Transposition of the Great Arteries
B) Atrial Septal Defect
C) Hypoplastic Left Heart Syndrome
D) Pulmonary Stenosis

Question 36: Which analgesic medication is commonly used for pain relief in newborns?
A) Ibuprofen
B) Acetaminophen
C) Aspirin
D) Morphine

Question 37: Scenario: James, a 1-week-old infant, is admitted with cyanotic heart disease. He exhibits cyanosis that worsens with crying or feeding, along with clubbing of fingers and toes. An echocardiogram reveals a right-to-left shunt at the atrial level. Which of the following conditions is most likely affecting James?
A) Transposition of the Great Arteries (TGA)
B) Tricuspid Atresia
C) Total Anomalous Pulmonary Venous Connection (TAPVC)
D) Hypoplastic Left Heart Syndrome (HLHS)

Question 38: Which of the following is a common risk factor for the development of pulmonary embolus in the postpartum period?
A) Prolonged bed rest
B) Regular ambulation
C) Adequate hydration
D) Controlled breathing exercises

Question 39: Which antepartum complication is characterized by high blood pressure and proteinuria after 20 weeks of gestation?
A) Gestational diabetes
B) Placenta previa
C) Preeclampsia
D) Ectopic pregnancy

Question 40: Mrs. Smith, a 32-year-old pregnant woman at 38 weeks gestation, arrives at the labor and delivery unit with regular contractions every 5 minutes lasting 45 seconds. On examination, her cervix is dilated 4 cm. Which of the following intrapartum factors should the nurse prioritize assessing in this situation?
A) Fetal heart rate variability
B) Maternal blood pressure
C) Amniotic fluid volume
D) Maternal temperature

Question 41: Which endocrine disorder in the newborn is characterized by adrenal insufficiency

and electrolyte imbalances?
A) Neonatal Cushing's syndrome
B) Neonatal hypothyroidism
C) Neonatal hyperparathyroidism
D) Neonatal adrenal crisis

Question 42: What is a common symptom associated with Placenta Previa?
A) Severe lower back pain
B) Vaginal bleeding in the third trimester
C) Excessive fetal movement
D) High blood pressure

Question 43: During a postpartum education session, a new mother asks about ways to prevent breast engorgement. Which advice should the nurse provide to promote optimal breast health and prevent engorgement?
A) Limiting breastfeeding sessions to every 4 hours
B) Ensuring proper latch and positioning during breastfeeding
C) Supplementing breastfeeding with formula feeds
D) Wearing tight-fitting bras for support

Question 44: Which nutrient is essential for promoting postpartum wound healing and tissue repair in mothers?
A) Vitamin C
B) Iron
C) Calcium
D) Vitamin K

Question 45: Which medication is commonly used to manage postpartum hemorrhage (PPH) due to uterine atony?
A) Oxytocin
B) Magnesium sulfate
C) Misoprostol
D) Nifedipine

Question 46: Ms. Smith, a postpartum mother, expresses her desire to exclusively breastfeed her newborn. She requests not to be disturbed during the night to ensure uninterrupted breastfeeding sessions. What ethical principle is Ms. Smith exercising in this scenario?
A) Beneficence
B) Nonmaleficence
C) Autonomy
D) Justice

Question 47: Ethical principles related to autonomy in maternal newborn nursing include:
A) Coercing the mother into specific healthcare decisions
B) Providing the mother with all relevant information to make informed choices
C) Disregarding the mother's preferences in care planning
D) Restricting the mother's involvement in decision-making processes

Question 48: Which of the following is a common nursing intervention for managing vaginal lacerations postpartum?
A) Application of ice packs continuously
B) Administering oral antibiotics prophylactically
C) Encouraging sitz baths for comfort
D) Applying direct pressure on the laceration site

Question 49: Mrs. Smith, at 36 weeks gestation, is scheduled for a nonstress test (NST) to assess fetal well-being. During the NST, what would be considered a reassuring finding?
A) Fetal heart rate accelerations with fetal movement
B) Fetal heart rate decelerations with fetal movement
C) Absence of fetal heart rate variability
D) Baseline fetal heart rate of 90 bpm

Question 50: What is the initial intervention for a newborn experiencing respiratory distress immediately after birth?
A) Administering glucose
B) Providing chest compressions
C) Placing in a warm environment
D) Initiating positive-pressure ventilation

Question 51: During a postpartum education session, the nurse discusses the importance of iron-rich foods in the maternal diet. Which of the following meal options would be most beneficial for a postpartum mother to increase her iron intake?
A) Grilled cheese sandwich with a side of potato chips
B) Spinach salad with strawberries and balsamic vinaigrette
C) Plain white rice with steamed broccoli
D) Ham and cheese sandwich on white bread with mayonnaise

Question 52: Mrs. Smith, a postpartum mother, complains of mild headache and requests pain relief. As the nurse, you plan to administer acetaminophen (Tylenol). What is the primary indication for using acetaminophen in this situation?
A) To reduce fever
B) To relieve mild to moderate pain
C) To decrease inflammation
D) To provide sedation

Question 53: Mrs. Smith, a postpartum mother, presents with redness, warmth, and tenderness around her cesarean incision site. On assessment, the incision site is also oozing purulent discharge. What is the most appropriate nursing intervention in this situation?
A) Apply a warm compress to the incision site
B) Administer oral antibiotics as prescribed
C) Encourage the patient to clean the incision site with hydrogen peroxide
D) Remove the sutures from the incision site

Question 54: Scenario: Sarah, a 28-year-old pregnant woman, is concerned about the risk of neural tube defects in her baby. She asks the nurse about the importance of folic acid supplementation during pregnancy. Which of the following statements by the nurse is correct regarding folic acid and neural tube defects?
A) Folic acid supplementation is not necessary during pregnancy.
B) Folic acid supplementation should start after the first trimester.
C) Folic acid supplementation before and during early

pregnancy can help prevent neural tube defects.
D) Folic acid supplementation is only important for the mother's health, not the baby's.

Question 55: Which breastfeeding device is commonly used to assist infants with latching issues and to protect sore nipples in breastfeeding mothers?
A) Nipple shield
B) Breast pump
C) Breast shells
D) Milk storage bags

Question 56: Which of the following is a contraindication to breastfeeding in the context of breast engorgement?
A) Applying cold compresses
B) Ensuring proper latch during breastfeeding
C) Using cabbage leaves on the breasts
D) Delaying breastfeeding sessions

Question 57: Which antenatal factor is associated with an increased risk of preterm birth?
A) Maternal age over 35 years
B) Multiparity
C) Smoking during pregnancy
D) Normal BMI

Question 58: How is septic pelvic thrombophlebitis typically diagnosed in postpartum women?
A) Chest X-ray
B) Urine analysis
C) Doppler ultrasound
D) Electrocardiogram (ECG)

Question 59: What is a typical interpretation of a reactive Nonstress Test (NST) result?
A) Fetal heart rate accelerations are absent.
B) Fetal heart rate decelerations are observed.
C) At least two fetal heart rate accelerations occur within a 20-minute period.
D) Fetal heart rate remains constant throughout the test.

Question 60: Which of the following strategies is recommended to promote better sleep in postpartum women experiencing sleep disturbances?
A) Consuming caffeine before bedtime
B) Engaging in stimulating activities close to bedtime
C) Establishing a relaxing bedtime routine
D) Using electronic devices in bed

Question 61: Which of the following signs in a newborn would indicate the need for resuscitation?
A) Pink skin color
B) Strong cry
C) Respiratory rate of 40 breaths per minute
D) Poor muscle tone

Question 62: Which vaccine is contraindicated during pregnancy due to its live attenuated nature?
A) Hepatitis A vaccine
B) Tetanus toxoid vaccine
C) Yellow fever vaccine
D) Pneumococcal vaccine

Question 63: Mrs. Smith, a pregnant woman in her third trimester, is concerned about her nutrition. She asks the nurse about the importance of iron in her diet during pregnancy. Which of the following statements by the nurse is accurate regarding iron intake during pregnancy?
A) Iron is not essential during pregnancy
B) Iron requirements decrease during pregnancy
C) Iron supplements are usually not recommended during pregnancy
D) Iron is crucial for the production of hemoglobin to prevent anemia during pregnancy

Question 64: Which of the following is a risk factor for postpartum depression?
A) Previous history of depression
B) High socioeconomic status
C) Strong social support
D) Regular exercise routine

Question 65: Ms. Smith, a 32-year-old pregnant woman, is concerned about the risk of passing on a genetic disorder to her baby. She has a family history of cystic fibrosis, an autosomal recessive disorder. What is the likelihood that her baby will inherit cystic fibrosis if the father is a carrier of the gene?
A) 25%
B) 50%
C) 75%
D) 100%

Question 66: Mrs. Smith, a 32-year-old postpartum mother, presents with excessive bleeding 24 hours after a vaginal delivery. Her vital signs are stable, but she appears pale and fatigued. Laboratory results show a hemoglobin level of 8 g/dL. What is the most likely cause of Mrs. Smith's postpartum hemorrhage?
A) Uterine Atony
B) Retained Placental Fragments
C) Cervical Laceration
D) Coagulopathy

Question 67: During a routine postpartum assessment, a nurse identifies signs of mastitis in a breastfeeding mother. The healthcare provider decides to initiate antimicrobial therapy to treat the infection. Which of the following antimicrobials is typically recommended for the treatment of mastitis in breastfeeding mothers?
A) Ibuprofen
B) Amoxicillin
C) Lorazepam
D) Furosemide

Question 68: Which of the following is a common newborn complication associated with maternal diabetes during pregnancy?
A) Hypoglycemia
B) Hyperbilirubinemia
C) Respiratory distress syndrome
D) Patent ductus arteriosus

Question 69: Which of the following statements regarding cardiac disease in pregnancy is true?
A) All pregnant women with cardiac disease should avoid

physical activity.
B) Pregnant women with cardiac disease are at decreased risk of adverse outcomes.
C) Women with known cardiac disease should receive preconception counseling.
D) Cardiac disease in pregnancy has no impact on maternal or fetal outcomes.

Question 70: Which maternal postpartum complication is characterized by symptoms such as fever, abdominal pain, and abnormal vaginal discharge?
A) Postpartum depression
B) Postpartum hemorrhage
C) Endometritis
D) Mastitis

Question 71: Which fetal heart rate abnormality is characterized by a baseline heart rate above 160 beats per minute?
A) Tachycardia
B) Bradycardia
C) Altered Variability
D) Decelerations

Question 72: Mrs. Smith has just given birth to a full-term newborn who is showing signs of respiratory distress. The nurse initiates resuscitation measures, including providing positive-pressure ventilation. After a few minutes, the newborn's respiratory rate improves, and oxygen saturation levels begin to rise. What should the nurse do next to evaluate the effectiveness of the intervention?
A) Increase the rate of positive-pressure ventilation
B) Decrease the oxygen flow rate
C) Monitor the newborn's heart rate
D) Stop positive-pressure ventilation

Question 73: How can the nurse uphold the ethical principle of non-maleficence in maternal postpartum assessment?
A) Performing regular assessments of vital signs
B) Ensuring proper hygiene practices are maintained
C) Monitoring for signs of postpartum hemorrhage
D) Providing emotional support and counseling

Question 74: Ms. Smith, a 32-year-old pregnant woman at 28 weeks gestation, presents to the antenatal clinic with painless vaginal bleeding. On examination, the fundal height is higher than expected for gestational age. Which of the following is the most likely diagnosis?
A) Abruptio Placentae
B) Placenta Previa
C) Uterine Rupture
D) Cervical Insufficiency

Question 75: Which of the following is a common sign of bladder distention in postpartum women?
A) Hypotension
B) Bradycardia
C) Suprapubic pain and discomfort
D) Increased appetite

Question 76: During a newborn assessment, the nurse observes that the baby's caregiver is placing the infant on their stomach for sleep. What action should the nurse take?
A) Educate the caregiver on the importance of tummy time when the baby is awake
B) Encourage the caregiver to continue placing the baby on their stomach for sleep
C) Provide a soft pillow for the baby to sleep on their stomach
D) Demonstrate how to swaddle the baby tightly for sleep

Question 77: Mrs. Johnson, 28 years old, is undergoing fertility treatment due to unexplained infertility. She has been prescribed ovulation induction therapy. Which of the following birth risk factors is associated with ovulation induction therapy?
A) Preterm birth
B) Multiple gestation
C) Post-term pregnancy
D) Macrosomia

Question 78: During a postpartum assessment, the nurse notes that a mother is experiencing hemorrhoids. Which nursing intervention is most appropriate for managing this condition?
A) Applying ice packs to the perineal area
B) Encouraging the mother to avoid all physical activity
C) Suggesting the use of a sitz bath for comfort
D) Administering a laxative to soften stools

Question 79: Which of the following antepartum risk factors is associated with an increased risk of cardiac disease in pregnancy?
A) Gestational diabetes
B) Hypothyroidism
C) Chronic hypertension
D) Iron deficiency anemia

Question 80: Which sexually transmitted infection (STI) poses the highest risk of vertical transmission from mother to newborn during childbirth?
A) Chlamydia
B) Syphilis
C) Gonorrhea
D) Trichomoniasis

Question 81: During a postpartum education session, a nurse is discussing the preparation of formula for bottle feeding with a group of new mothers. Which of the following statements accurately describes the correct preparation of formula?
A) It is safe to prepare a large batch of formula in advance and store it in the refrigerator for up to 48 hours.
B) Formula should be prepared using hot tap water to ensure proper mixing of the powder.
C) It is important to follow the manufacturer's instructions for the correct ratio of water to formula powder.
D) Formula can be left at room temperature for up to 6 hours after preparation.

Question 82: Which intervention is essential in the postoperative care of a mother following a cesarean section to prevent deep vein thrombosis (DVT)?
A) Encouraging early ambulation
B) Administering high-dose opioids

C) Keeping the mother on strict bed rest
D) Applying heat packs to the incision site

Question 83: Ms. Smith has just given birth to a baby boy. The nurse is performing a gestational age assessment using the New Ballard Score. The baby's skin is translucent, and the nurse observes that the baby's ears are flat with a soft pinna. What is the most appropriate gestational age assessment based on these findings?
A) 32 weeks
B) 36 weeks
C) 40 weeks
D) 44 weeks

Question 84: Mrs. Smith has just given birth to a premature newborn who is showing signs of respiratory distress. The healthcare provider decides to administer a medication to help improve the baby's breathing. Which of the following drugs is commonly used in newborns for respiratory support?
A) Furosemide
B) Caffeine
C) Acetaminophen
D) Ondansetron

Question 85: Which action is essential for promoting bonding and attachment between a newborn and parents?
A) Encouraging rooming-in
B) Limiting parental visitation
C) Delaying skin-to-skin contact
D) Discouraging breastfeeding

Question 86: Which of the following is a risk factor associated with prolonged labor during the intrapartum period?
A) Maternal obesity
B) Early prenatal care
C) Multiparity
D) Normal fetal presentation

Question 87: When expressing breast milk, which method is recommended to store the milk for later use?
A) Glass containers
B) Plastic bags designed for breast milk storage
C) Regular plastic bags
D) Metal containers

Question 88: Which statement best describes the role of a nurse in supporting family dynamics during the postpartum period?
A) Encouraging the family to prioritize the newborn's needs over their own.
B) Providing education on infant care and promoting bonding between the newborn and family members.
C) Advising the family to limit visitors to reduce stress and promote rest.
D) Suggesting that the family handle all tasks independently to build self-reliance.

Question 89: Which action is recommended to prevent hypothermia in a newborn during the first few hours after birth?

A) Keeping the newborn in a cold room
B) Using a radiant warmer for an extended period
C) Drying the newborn and covering the head
D) Administering a cold bath

Question 90: What maneuver is commonly used to resolve shoulder dystocia during delivery?
A) McRoberts maneuver
B) Ritgen maneuver
C) Rubin maneuver
D) Woods' screw maneuver

Question 91: After delivery, Mrs. Johnson complains of bloating and gas. The healthcare provider recommends a medication to help with her symptoms. Which of the following GI motility drugs is commonly used to reduce bloating and gas in postpartum patients?
A) Esomeprazole
B) Loperamide
C) Simethicone
D) Ranitidine

Question 92: Which of the following signs and symptoms is characteristic of placental abruption?
A) Uterine contractions that stop with position changes
B) Bright red vaginal bleeding
C) Fetal heart rate decelerations relieved by maternal position changes
D) Decreased uterine tone between contractions

Question 93: After giving birth, Mrs. Johnson is concerned about her weight and wants to know if she can start dieting immediately to lose the extra pounds gained during pregnancy. What advice should the nurse provide regarding maternal nutritional needs in the postpartum period?
A) Start a strict diet to lose weight rapidly
B) Increase calorie intake to promote weight loss
C) Focus on nutrient-dense foods and gradual weight loss
D) Skip meals to reduce calorie intake

Question 94: Ms. Johnson, a 32-year-old postpartum patient, is diagnosed with hypertension. The healthcare provider prescribes an antihypertensive medication that is safe for breastfeeding mothers. Which antihypertensive medication is most appropriate for Ms. Johnson?
A) Lisinopril
B) Atenolol
C) Nifedipine
D) Metoprolol

Question 95: Which medication used in labor is an opioid analgesic that provides pain relief without causing significant respiratory depression in the newborn?
A) Fentanyl
B) Meperidine
C) Butorphanol
D) Nalbuphine

Question 96: Which statement regarding gestational diabetes mellitus (GDM) is true?
A) GDM is a permanent type of diabetes that persists

after pregnancy.
B) GDM can only be managed with insulin therapy.
C) GDM typically develops after the 28th week of pregnancy.
D) GDM does not pose any risks to the mother or the baby.

Question 97: Mrs. Smith, a 32-year-old woman, is admitted to the postpartum unit after delivering a healthy baby boy. She expresses concerns about her ability to breastfeed due to previous unsuccessful attempts with her older child. The nurse observes Mrs. Smith becoming emotional and anxious during breastfeeding sessions. Which action by the nurse best demonstrates the ethical principle of justice in this situation?
A) Providing Mrs. Smith with additional breastfeeding resources and support
B) Ignoring Mrs. Smith's concerns and focusing on other postpartum care tasks
C) Suggesting formula feeding as an easier alternative for Mrs. Smith
D) Limiting Mrs. Smith's access to lactation consultants due to hospital policies

Question 98: During a postpartum assessment, the nurse observes a mother experiencing nipple soreness while breastfeeding. Which equipment should the nurse recommend to alleviate nipple soreness?
A) Nipple shields
B) Breast pump
C) Nipple cream
D) Warm compress

Question 99: Ms. Smith, 32 years old, is seeking advice regarding her infertility issues. She mentions irregular menstrual cycles and a history of pelvic inflammatory disease (PID). Which of the following antenatal factors is most likely contributing to her infertility?
A) Advanced maternal age
B) History of PID
C) Obesity
D) Smoking

Question 100: Mrs. Smith, a new mother, is experiencing difficulties in bonding with her newborn baby. She expresses feelings of inadequacy and struggles to establish a connection with her infant. Which of the following factors could be a potential barrier to parent/infant interactions in this scenario?
A) Lack of social support
B) Baby's excessive crying
C) Mrs. Smith's age
D) Baby's weight

Question 101: Which breastfeeding device is designed to collect leaking breast milk from the non-nursing breast during breastfeeding or pumping?
A) Nipple shield
B) Breast pump
C) Breast shells
D) Milk storage bags

Question 102: Mrs. Smith has just given birth to a newborn baby girl. The baby is crying persistently, and Mrs. Smith is concerned about how to provide comfort. Which comfort measure is most appropriate in this situation?
A) Swaddling the baby snugly
B) Offering a pacifier
C) Placing the baby in a cold room
D) Letting the baby cry it out

Question 103: Which psychosocial/cultural factor is considered a risk factor for adverse pregnancy outcomes?
A) High socioeconomic status
B) Strong social support
C) Maternal stress
D) Positive coping mechanisms

Question 104: Which hormone is primarily responsible for milk ejection during breastfeeding?
A) Prolactin
B) Oxytocin
C) Estrogen
D) Progesterone

Question 105: During a postpartum education session, a new mother asks about the importance of burping her newborn after bottle-feeding. How should the nurse respond?
A) "Burping is not necessary after bottle-feeding."
B) "Burping helps prevent colic in newborns."
C) "Burping helps release any swallowed air during feeding."
D) "Burping should only be done if the baby seems fussy."

Question 106: Which therapeutic medication is contraindicated during breastfeeding due to its potential adverse effects on the infant?
A) Ibuprofen
B) Metoclopramide
C) Codeine
D) Acetaminophen

Question 107: Mrs. Smith, a 32-year-old postpartum patient, presents with signs of hypovolemic shock following a postpartum hemorrhage. Her blood pressure is 90/60 mmHg, heart rate is 120 bpm, and she appears pale and diaphoretic. What is the priority nursing intervention for Mrs. Smith?
A) Administering a bolus of intravenous fluids
B) Providing oxygen therapy
C) Monitoring fetal heart rate
D) Offering emotional support

Question 108: Which ethical principle guides healthcare providers to be truthful and honest with their patients, providing all necessary information for informed decision-making?
A) Autonomy
B) Beneficence
C) Nonmaleficence
D) Veracity

Question 109: After assessing a postpartum client, the nurse suspects urinary retention. Which finding is most indicative of this complication?

A) Urine output of 50 mL in the last 2 hours
B) Bladder palpable above the symphysis pubis
C) Client reports feeling the urge to void frequently
D) Complaints of lower abdominal cramping

Question 110: Which laboratory test is crucial in diagnosing hemolytic disease of the newborn (HDN)?
A) Coombs test
B) Blood glucose level
C) Serum electrolytes
D) Liver function tests

Question 111: Which viral infection poses the highest risk to newborns due to potential vertical transmission during pregnancy?
A) Influenza
B) Rubella
C) Cytomegalovirus (CMV)
D) Varicella zoster virus (VZV)

Question 112: During a postpartum assessment, the nurse observes that a new mother is experiencing nipple pain and discomfort while breastfeeding. The nurse suspects that the pain may be due to a shallow latch on. Which of the following interventions should the nurse recommend to improve the latch on and alleviate nipple pain?
A) Suggest applying a cold compress to the nipples before breastfeeding.
B) Encourage the mother to stop breastfeeding temporarily and switch to formula feeding.
C) Teach the mother to break the baby's latch by inserting a finger into the corner of the baby's mouth.
D) Instruct the mother to ensure the baby's mouth covers a large portion of the areola during latch on.

Question 113: During a newborn musculoskeletal assessment, the nurse notes asymmetry in hip abduction. Which condition should be suspected based on this finding?
A) Developmental dysplasia of the hip (DDH)
B) Osteogenesis imperfecta
C) Congenital muscular torticollis
D) Spina bifida

Question 114: During a postpartum visit, a mother asks about the benefits of breastfeeding for her newborn. Which of the following statements accurately describes a benefit of breastfeeding for newborn nutrition?
A) Formula-fed babies have fewer allergies
B) Breast milk provides antibodies for immune protection
C) Formula-fed babies gain weight faster
D) Breastfeeding increases the risk of infections

Question 115: During a lactation education session, a new mother inquires about the fat content of breast milk. Which of the following statements regarding the fat composition of breast milk is accurate?
A) Breast milk contains primarily saturated fats
B) Breast milk is low in cholesterol
C) Breast milk fat content remains constant throughout a feeding session
D) Breast milk fat aids in the absorption of fat-soluble vitamins

Question 116: Scenario: Baby Emma, a 2-day-old neonate, presents with fever and poor feeding. Her CBC shows a white blood cell count of 22,000/mm3 with a left shift. The differential count reveals 70% neutrophils, 20% lymphocytes, 5% monocytes, and 5% eosinophils. What is the most likely diagnosis based on these findings?
A) Neonatal sepsis
B) Physiological leukocytosis
C) Neonatal jaundice
D) Neonatal polycythemia

Question 117: Which of the following is a risk factor for premature rupture of membranes (PROM)?
A) Maternal age over 35 years
B) Multifetal gestation
C) Regular prenatal exercise
D) Low BMI

Question 118: During a lactation consultation, a new mother asks about the composition of colostrum. Which of the following statements accurately describes colostrum?
A) Colostrum is high in fat content and low in antibodies.
B) Colostrum is thick and yellow in color.
C) Colostrum is produced after 1 week of breastfeeding.
D) Colostrum is low in volume but rich in immune factors.

Question 119: Which of the following is a potential complication of precipitous delivery?
A) Maternal hemorrhage
B) Prolonged labor
C) Fetal macrosomia
D) Maternal hypertension

Question 120: Scenario: Sarah, a newborn, is brought to the neonatal unit for assessment. She is having difficulty breathing and appears cyanotic. The nurse notices poor chest movement and increased respiratory effort. What is the initial nursing intervention for Sarah?
A) Administering oxygen via nasal cannula
B) Performing chest compressions
C) Suctioning the airway
D) Placing an oropharyngeal airway

Question 121: Which of the following is NOT a common antepartum risk factor for developing polyhydramnios?
A) Maternal diabetes
B) Fetal anomalies
C) Oligohydramnios
D) Multiple gestation

Question 122: Ms. Johnson, a 28-year-old postpartum mother, complains of sudden onset shortness of breath and chest pain 48 hours after a cesarean section. On examination, she is tachypneic and tachycardic. A chest X-ray reveals a wedge-shaped infiltrate in the lung. What is the most likely diagnosis for Ms. Johnson's condition?
A) Pulmonary Embolism
B) Pneumonia
C) Atelectasis
D) Pleural Effusion

Question 123: Mrs. Smith, a 28-year-old postpartum mother, is experiencing engorgement in her breasts. She complains of severe pain and tightness in her breasts. Which of the following interventions should the nurse recommend to relieve engorgement?
A) Applying cold compresses
B) Massaging the breasts vigorously
C) Skipping breastfeeding sessions
D) Wearing a tight-fitting bra

Question 124: Mrs. Johnson, a 35-year-old postpartum patient, is seeking advice on long-acting reversible contraception (LARC) methods. Which LARC method provides contraception for up to 10 years and is suitable for women who desire long-term birth control?
A) Copper intrauterine device (IUD)
B) Levonorgestrel-releasing intrauterine system (IUS)
C) Contraceptive implant
D) Injectable progestin

Question 125: During a postpartum assessment, a nurse observes that a new mother, Emily, is showing signs of postpartum depression, such as persistent sadness and withdrawal from her baby. Which intervention would be most appropriate to address the barriers to parent/infant interactions in this situation?
A) Encouraging Emily to spend more time alone with her baby
B) Providing education on infant care techniques
C) Referring Emily to a mental health professional
D) Suggesting Emily to ignore her feelings and focus on the baby

Question 126: Which medication is commonly used to prevent postpartum hemorrhage by promoting uterine contractions?
A) Oxytocin
B) Magnesium sulfate
C) Methylergonovine
D) Nifedipine

Question 127: Which of the following components is NOT typically found in human breast milk?
A) Lactose
B) Casein
C) Immunoglobulins
D) Gluten

Question 128: During the assessment of a newborn delivered to a mother with meconium-stained amniotic fluid, the nurse notes that the infant has meconium aspiration syndrome. Which of the following clinical manifestations is commonly associated with this condition?
A) Hypoglycemia
B) Tachypnea
C) Bradycardia
D) Hyperthermia

Question 129: What is a key aspect of patient education regarding postpartum depression?
A) Postpartum depression is a sign of weakness in new mothers.
B) Postpartum depression is a rare condition that does not require attention.
C) Educating mothers about postpartum depression can help in early detection and intervention.
D) Postpartum depression is solely caused by hormonal changes and cannot be prevented.

Question 130: During a postpartum assessment, you find that a mother is experiencing persistent, severe headaches, visual disturbances, and epigastric pain. Which condition should be of primary concern in this situation?
A) Postpartum depression
B) Postpartum hemorrhage
C) Postpartum preeclampsia
D) Postpartum thyroiditis

Question 131: Which of the following statements regarding jitteriness in newborns is accurate?
A) Jitteriness is a normal finding in all newborns
B) Jitteriness is always a sign of a serious neurological disorder
C) Jitteriness can be a manifestation of hypoglycemia
D) Jitteriness is primarily caused by respiratory distress

Question 132: During a routine ultrasound at 18 weeks gestation, Mrs. Johnson's ultrasound report shows an increased nuchal translucency measurement of 3.5mm. What could this finding indicate?
A) Normal fetal development
B) Down syndrome
C) Neural tube defect
D) Umbilical cord abnormality

Question 133: Baby Emily, born at 38 weeks gestation, is being discharged home with her parents. The nurse is providing education on newborn care. Which statement by the parents indicates a need for further teaching?
A) "We will place Emily on her back to sleep to reduce the risk of Sudden Infant Death Syndrome (SIDS)."
B) "We will clean Emily's umbilical cord stump with alcohol at every diaper change."
C) "We will schedule Emily's first pediatrician visit within the first week of life."
D) "We will ensure Emily is securely fastened in her car seat for all travels."

Question 134: Which assessment finding should be reported immediately in the postoperative care of a mother following a cesarean section?
A) Incision site with minimal serosanguineous drainage
B) Fundus firm and midline
C) Respiratory rate of 18 breaths per minute
D) Sudden onset of shortness of breath

Question 135: Maria, a Hispanic postpartum mother, expresses distress due to the lack of Spanish-speaking staff members in the hospital. She feels isolated and misunderstood. What should the nurse prioritize to support Maria's emotional well-being?
A) Provide Maria with written instructions in English to overcome language barriers.
B) Encourage Maria to communicate in English to facilitate better understanding.
C) Offer Maria the assistance of a non-Spanish-speaking

staff member for support.
D) Arrange for a professional interpreter to communicate effectively with Maria.

Question 136: Which of the following is a contraindication to breastfeeding?
A) Maternal HIV infection
B) Maternal diabetes
C) Maternal hypertension
D) Maternal obesity

Question 137: Which of the following is a potential complication of regional anesthesia during labor?
A) Hypertension
B) Hypoglycemia
C) Urinary retention
D) Hypoxemia

Question 138: Baby Liam, born at 38 weeks gestation, is undergoing a sensory assessment. The nurse is testing his ability to track objects visually. Which of the following responses would be expected in a newborn of this gestational age?
A) Following a toy with eyes smoothly
B) Fixating on an object briefly
C) Ignoring visual stimuli
D) Inability to visually track objects

Question 139: Ms. Johnson, a 32-year-old pregnant woman, has a history of chronic hypertension. She is currently at 34 weeks of gestation. During her antenatal visit, her blood pressure is 150/95 mmHg. She complains of a headache and blurry vision. What is the most appropriate nursing intervention for Ms. Johnson?
A) Instruct her to increase her salt intake
B) Advise bed rest in a dark, quiet room
C) Administer antihypertensive medication as prescribed
D) Encourage her to perform vigorous exercise

Question 140: After a vaginal delivery, a postpartum mother is experiencing excessive bleeding. The nurse should suspect which of the following complications and take immediate action?
A) Uterine atony
B) Perineal laceration
C) Retained placental fragments
D) Cervical laceration

Question 141: Ms. Smith, a 28-year-old pregnant woman at 32 weeks gestation, presents to the antenatal clinic with complaints of regular uterine contractions, lower back pain, and pelvic pressure. On assessment, her cervix is found to be 2 cm dilated and 50% effaced. Which of the following interventions is most appropriate for managing preterm labor in this patient?
A) Administering tocolytic therapy
B) Encouraging ambulation and hydration
C) Administering oxytocin for cervical ripening
D) Scheduling an elective cesarean section

Question 142: During the postpartum assessment of Ms. Johnson, a 32-year-old G1P1 mother, the nurse observes that she is experiencing heavy vaginal bleeding with clots, saturating more than one pad per hour. What should be the nurse's immediate action based on this finding?
A) Instruct Ms. Johnson to perform perineal exercises to help control bleeding.
B) Administer pain medication to alleviate discomfort associated with bleeding.
C) Notify the healthcare provider immediately.
D) Encourage Ms. Johnson to ambulate to promote circulation.

Question 143: Which intervention is appropriate for managing severe hyperbilirubinemia in a newborn?
A) Encouraging more frequent breastfeeding
B) Initiating phototherapy
C) Administering iron supplements
D) Increasing skin-to-skin contact

Question 144: During newborn resuscitation, which intervention is essential to establish effective ventilation?
A) Administering intravenous fluids
B) Providing warmth through radiant warmer
C) Performing chest compressions
D) Clearing airway with suction and providing positive pressure ventilation

Question 145: Mrs. Smith, a 28-year-old pregnant woman with obesity, is scheduled for a cesarean section due to fetal macrosomia. Which of the following statements regarding obesity and birth risk factors is correct?
A) Obesity does not increase the risk of cesarean section.
B) Women with obesity are at lower risk of developing gestational hypertension.
C) Fetal macrosomia is not associated with maternal obesity.
D) Women with obesity have a higher risk of postpartum hemorrhage.

Question 146: Which of the following is a common variation in the genitourinary system of a newborn that may require further evaluation?
A) Presence of milia on the genitalia
B) Labial adhesions in female newborns
C) Umbilical hernia
D) Mongolian spots on the buttocks

Question 147: Mrs. Smith, a 28-year-old postpartum mother, complains of excessive vaginal bleeding after giving birth. On assessment, her vital signs are stable, and she reports passing clots. What is the most appropriate nursing intervention in this situation?
A) Encourage ambulation to help decrease bleeding
B) Administer oxytocin to help control bleeding
C) Apply ice packs to the perineum to reduce bleeding
D) Perform fundal massage to promote uterine contractions

Question 148: Mrs. Smith, a postpartum mother, asks the nurse about the importance of breastfeeding for her newborn. Which of the following statements by the nurse is most appropriate for patient education?
A) "Breastfeeding provides essential nutrients and antibodies that help protect your baby from infections."

B) "Formula feeding is a better option as it is more convenient and ensures the baby gets enough to eat."
C) "Breastfeeding is only beneficial for a short period after birth, and then you should switch to formula."
D) "It is not necessary to breastfeed; formula feeding is equally beneficial for your baby."

Question 149: Which screening method is commonly used to detect inborn errors of metabolism in newborns?
A) Electrocardiogram (ECG)
B) Chest X-ray
C) Newborn screening blood test
D) Urinalysis

Question 150: Which of the following maternal complications is associated with preexisting diabetes in pregnancy?
A) Preterm labor
B) Preeclampsia
C) Placental abruption
D) Gestational hypertension

ANSWERS WITH DETAILED EXPLANATION (SET 1)

Question 1: Correct Answer: B) Using soap and water to wash bottles after each feeding
Rationale: Proper bottle-feeding hygiene is essential to prevent infections in newborns. Reusing unwashed bottles can introduce harmful bacteria to the baby. Storing unwashed bottles in the refrigerator can promote bacterial growth. Boiling bottles once a week is not sufficient to maintain cleanliness. Washing bottles with soap and water after each feeding is the most effective way to ensure proper hygiene and reduce the risk of infections.

Question 2: Correct Answer: C) "We can discontinue the medication once our baby starts showing improvement."
Rationale: Congenital hypothyroidism requires lifelong thyroid hormone replacement therapy to prevent complications such as developmental delays and intellectual disabilities. Discontinuing the medication can lead to serious consequences. Options A, B, and D are correct statements that emphasize the importance of medication adherence, monitoring growth and development, and regular follow-up care.

Question 3: Correct Answer: A) Transient tachypnea of the newborn (TTN)
Rationale: Infants of diabetic mothers are at increased risk of developing transient tachypnea of the newborn (TTN) due to delayed clearance of lung fluid. While bronchopulmonary dysplasia (BPD), meconium aspiration syndrome (MAS), and persistent pulmonary hypertension of the newborn (PPHN) are respiratory complications seen in neonates, they are not specifically associated with infants of diabetic mothers, making them incorrect choices.

Question 4: Correct Answer: D) Performing regular gentle exercises and stretches.
Rationale: Lower back pain is common in multiple gestation pregnancies due to the increased strain on the back from the growing uterus. Encouraging bed rest and limited physical activity (Option A) may exacerbate the pain and lead to muscle weakness. Heat packs (Option B) can provide temporary relief but do not address the underlying cause. NSAIDs (Option C) are contraindicated in pregnancy due to potential risks to the fetus. Performing regular gentle exercises and stretches (Option D) can help strengthen the muscles supporting the back, alleviate pain, and improve overall comfort.

Question 5: Correct Answer: B) Delayed circulation
Rationale: A capillary refill time of 4 seconds in a newborn indicates delayed circulation, which may be a sign of decreased cardiac output or peripheral vasoconstriction. This finding warrants further assessment and intervention to improve perfusion. Options A, C, and D are incorrect as they do not accurately reflect the significance of a prolonged capillary refill time in a newborn.

Question 6: Correct Answer: C) Gestational diabetes
Rationale: Obesity in pregnancy is a risk factor for developing gestational diabetes. This condition can lead to complications for both the mother and the baby, such as macrosomia and birth injuries. Low birth weight and preterm birth are more commonly associated with factors like smoking or poor maternal nutrition. Post-term pregnancy, while potentially a concern, is not directly linked to obesity in the same way that gestational diabetes is. Therefore, the correct answer is C) Gestational diabetes.

Question 7: Correct Answer: A) Necrotizing enterocolitis (NEC)
Rationale: The correct answer is A) Necrotizing enterocolitis (NEC). NEC is a serious gastrointestinal emergency in newborns characterized by feeding intolerance, abdominal distension, bilious vomiting, lethargy, and a high-pitched cry. It is crucial to consider NEC in newborns presenting with these symptoms. Hirschsprung's disease, Intussusception, and Malrotation with volvulus are also gastrointestinal conditions but typically present with different clinical manifestations, making them less likely in this scenario.

Question 8: Correct Answer: B) Providing evidence-based information and support for successful breastfeeding.
Rationale: Providing evidence-based information and support for successful breastfeeding aligns with the ethical principle of non-maleficence by ensuring the mother receives appropriate guidance and support to prevent harm to herself and her baby. Option A dismisses her concerns, potentially causing distress. Option C ignores her worries, which could lead to further anxiety. Option D may not address the underlying issue and could potentially harm the mother-baby bonding and breastfeeding relationship.

Question 9: Correct Answer: C) Oxytocin
Rationale: Oxytocin is the hormone responsible for milk ejection or let-down reflex during breastfeeding. It causes the muscles around the milk-producing cells to contract, pushing milk into the ducts. Estrogen and progesterone play a role in preparing the breasts for lactation during pregnancy, while prolactin is responsible for milk production.

Question 10: Correct Answer: C) Category III FHR pattern
Rationale: A Category III FHR pattern indicates abnormal fetal acid-base status and is associated with an increased risk of fetal hypoxia and metabolic acidosis. In this scenario, the presence of minimal variability and repetitive late decelerations suggests fetal distress, requiring immediate intervention to improve fetal oxygenation and prevent adverse outcomes. Options A and B are incorrect as they do not reflect the severity of the FHR pattern observed. Option D is not a recognized category in fetal heart rate monitoring classification.

Question 11: Correct Answer: A) Hemorrhage
Rationale: Hemorrhage is a potential complication of circumcision in newborns due to the vascular nature of the tissue involved. It is essential to monitor for bleeding post-circumcision to prevent excessive blood loss. Hypoglycemia, jaundice, and bradycardia are not directly associated with circumcision and are more commonly related to other newborn care aspects.

Question 12: Correct Answer: B) 34 weeks
Rationale: The presence of lanugo, minimal creases on the soles of the feet, and palpable testes in the scrotum are consistent with a gestational age of around 34

weeks. Option A (28 weeks) is incorrect as the described features are more indicative of a later gestational age. Option C (38 weeks) is incorrect as the findings suggest a preterm infant. Option D (42 weeks) is incorrect as it exceeds a full-term gestational age.

Question 13: Correct Answer: B) Providing positive-pressure ventilation
Rationale: In newborns with poor respiratory effort and central cyanosis, the priority intervention is to provide positive-pressure ventilation to support adequate oxygenation. Administering intravenous fluids, checking blood glucose levels, and placing a nasogastric tube are important interventions in neonatal care but are not the priority in this scenario. Positive-pressure ventilation helps establish effective ventilation and oxygenation, crucial for newborn resuscitation.

Question 14: Correct Answer: C) Smoking
Rationale: Smoking is a well-established risk factor for IUGR due to its vasoconstrictive effects on the placental circulation, leading to reduced oxygen and nutrient delivery to the fetus. Advanced maternal age, gestational diabetes, and multiparity are also risk factors for IUGR, but in this scenario, smoking is the most significant risk factor based on the patient's history.

Question 15: Correct Answer: B) Duodenal atresia
Rationale: Duodenal atresia is a congenital condition where there is a complete or partial obstruction of the duodenum. The "double-bubble" sign on X-ray is characteristic of this condition, with dilated stomach and duodenum. Symptoms include bilious vomiting and abdominal distension. Meconium ileus is associated with cystic fibrosis and presents with meconium obstruction in the distal ileum. Necrotizing enterocolitis is a gastrointestinal emergency in premature infants, characterized by abdominal distension, bloody stools, and systemic signs of sepsis. Pyloric stenosis is a condition where the muscle of the pylorus is thickened, leading to projectile non-bilious vomiting, typically in the first few weeks of life.

Question 16: Correct Answer: C) Methyldopa
Rationale: Methyldopa is often the preferred antihypertensive medication in the postpartum period for breastfeeding mothers due to its safety profile. Lisinopril (A) is contraindicated during breastfeeding due to its potential adverse effects on the infant. Atenolol (B) is also not recommended as it can lead to neonatal bradycardia and hypoglycemia. Furosemide (D) is a diuretic and not typically used as a first-line agent for postpartum hypertension.

Question 17: Correct Answer: D) Prolonged rupture of membranes during labor
Rationale: Prolonged rupture of membranes during labor increases the risk of ascending bacterial infection, leading to postpartum wound infections. Early ambulation, adequate hand hygiene, and timely administration of prophylactic antibiotics are actually preventive measures that help reduce the risk of wound infections. Therefore, option D is the correct answer as it directly correlates with an increased risk of wound infection.

Question 18: Correct Answer: A) Postpartum hemorrhage
Rationale: Postpartum hemorrhage is a life-threatening complication that requires immediate medical attention to prevent severe blood loss. It is essential for nurses to monitor for signs of hemorrhage such as excessive bleeding, changes in vital signs, and signs of shock. Perineal laceration, engorged breasts, and infant feeding difficulties are important postpartum issues but do not require immediate medical attention like postpartum hemorrhage.

Question 19: Correct Answer: A) Increased risk of postpartum hemorrhage
Rationale: Cesarean section deliveries are associated with an increased risk of postpartum hemorrhage due to factors such as reduced uterine tone and delayed contraction of the uterus post-delivery. This can lead to excessive bleeding and necessitate interventions to control hemorrhage. While cesarean sections may be necessary in certain situations, it is essential to be aware of the potential risks involved, including postpartum hemorrhage.

Question 20: Correct Answer: B) Promoting kangaroo care for premature infants
Rationale: Promoting kangaroo care, which involves skin-to-skin contact between the parent and premature infant, is a beneficial practice to enhance parent/infant interactions. Kangaroo care has been shown to improve bonding, regulate the baby's temperature and heart rate, and support breastfeeding. Options A, C, and D are not conducive to fostering positive parent/infant interactions as they involve practices that may hinder bonding, disrupt natural soothing mechanisms, and limit parental involvement in infant care, which are essential for establishing a strong parent-child relationship.

Question 21: Correct Answer: B) Nasal flaring
Rationale: Nasal flaring is a common sign of respiratory distress in newborns, indicating increased work of breathing. Bradycardia refers to a slow heart rate and is not specific to respiratory distress. Hypoglycemia is low blood sugar levels and is not directly related to respiratory distress. Jaundice is the yellowing of the skin and eyes due to high bilirubin levels, unrelated to respiratory distress.

Question 22: Correct Answer: A) Audible swallowing sounds
Rationale: Audible swallowing sounds during breastfeeding indicate effective suck/swallow/sequence coordination. This demonstrates that the newborn is effectively transferring milk from the breast. Frequent pauses and breaks (Option B) may suggest inefficient feeding. A shallow latch with clicking noises (Option C) indicates improper latch and potential air intake. Short, rapid sucks without swallowing (Option D) may signify a shallow latch or ineffective milk transfer. Therefore, the correct answer is A as it reflects proper breastfeeding technique and milk transfer.

Question 23: Correct Answer: D) To stimulate the baby's respiratory drive
Rationale: Caffeine citrate is commonly used in premature infants with apnea of prematurity to stimulate the respiratory drive and reduce the frequency of apneic episodes. It is not indicated for improving feeding tolerance, preventing hypothermia, or reducing the risk of infection. Caffeine citrate acts as a respiratory stimulant by affecting the central nervous system, enhancing diaphragmatic contractility, and increasing minute ventilation.

Question 24: Correct Answer: C) Prolactin
Rationale: Prolactin is the hormone responsible for milk production in the lactating mother. Estrogen and progesterone play a role in preparing the breast for

lactation during pregnancy but do not directly produce milk. Oxytocin is responsible for milk ejection or let-down, not milk production. Therefore, the correct answer is Prolactin as it is the primary hormone involved in milk synthesis.

Question 25: Correct Answer: C) Jealousy and regression in behavior
Rationale: Siblings often experience jealousy and regression in behavior when a new baby arrives due to feelings of displacement and the need to compete for parental attention. This response is a normal part of adjusting to a new family dynamic. Increased independence and enhanced communication skills are less common immediate responses, as the focus is often on adapting to the changes and emotions associated with the new sibling.

Question 26: Correct Answer: C) Assess the newborn's respiratory rate
Rationale: Assessing the newborn's respiratory rate is essential to determine the effectiveness of the tactile stimulation in initiating breathing. Improved respiratory effort and oxygenation are key indicators of successful intervention. Options A, B, and D are important aspects of newborn assessment but are not directly related to evaluating the effectiveness of the breathing stimulation.

Question 27: Correct Answer: C) ABO incompatibility
Rationale: ABO incompatibility between the mother and baby can lead to the breakdown of red blood cells in the newborn, causing an increase in bilirubin levels and subsequent hyperbilirubinemia. Exclusive breastfeeding, term gestation, and maternal diabetes are not direct risk factors for hyperbilirubinemia. Term gestation is actually a protective factor as preterm infants are at higher risk for jaundice due to immature liver function.

Question 28: Correct Answer: B) Ventricular septal defect (VSD)
Rationale: In acyanotic heart disease, a ventricular septal defect (VSD) is commonly associated with increased pulmonary blood flow due to the left-to-right shunt. This results in increased workload on the right side of the heart and pulmonary congestion. Tetralogy of Fallot, coarctation of the aorta, and transposition of the great arteries are not typically associated with increased pulmonary blood flow in acyanotic heart disease.

Question 29: Correct Answer: C) Cyanosis
Rationale: Cyanosis is a clinical sign of inadequate oxygenation in newborns, leading to a bluish discoloration of the skin and mucous membranes. It can be caused by various conditions such as respiratory distress syndrome, congenital heart defects, or transient tachypnea of the newborn. Hypoglycemia, hyperbilirubinemia, and sepsis are important newborn complications but do not present with cyanosis as a primary symptom. Early recognition and management of cyanosis are crucial to prevent further complications and ensure optimal newborn outcomes.

Question 30: Correct Answer: C) G6PD deficiency can lead to hemolytic anemia triggered by certain medications or infections.
Rationale: G6PD deficiency is an X-linked genetic disorder that primarily affects males. Newborns with G6PD deficiency are at an increased risk of jaundice due to hemolysis triggered by oxidative stressors such as certain medications or infections. This condition can lead to hemolytic anemia, characterized by the destruction of red blood cells. Therefore, option C is the correct answer as it accurately reflects the implications of G6PD deficiency in newborns.

Question 31: Correct Answer: A) Nonsteroidal anti-inflammatory drugs (NSAIDs)
Rationale: Nonsteroidal anti-inflammatory drugs (NSAIDs) can reduce the effectiveness of diuretics when used concomitantly. It is important to monitor for this interaction as NSAIDs can interfere with the diuretic's ability to promote diuresis. Iron supplements, prenatal vitamins, and antihypertensive medications do not typically interact significantly with diuretics. Monitoring for potential drug interactions is crucial to ensure the optimal therapeutic effect of diuretics in postpartum women.

Question 32: Correct Answer: A) Positioning the newborn in a side-lying fetal position
Rationale: Positioning the newborn in a side-lying fetal position is essential for a successful lumbar puncture procedure as it helps to open up the spaces between the vertebrae, making it easier to access the lumbar region. Administering sedation is generally not recommended for lumbar punctures in newborns due to the risks involved. Applying a warm compress may cause vasodilation and increase the risk of bleeding. Ensuring hydration is important but not directly related to the lumbar puncture procedure.

Question 33: Correct Answer: C) Low socioeconomic status
Rationale: Postpartum depression is more prevalent among women with low socioeconomic status due to factors such as financial stress, lack of social support, and limited access to healthcare resources. Advanced maternal age (option A) and multiparity (option B) are not directly linked to postpartum depression. While a planned pregnancy (option D) may contribute to a more stable emotional state postpartum, it is not the most commonly associated factor with postpartum depression.

Question 34: Correct Answer: C) Family history of ICP
Rationale: Family history of ICP is a significant risk factor for developing the condition during pregnancy. While maternal age, primigravida status, and maternal BMI are important antenatal factors, they are not as closely associated with the development of ICP as a positive family history.

Question 35: Correct Answer: A) Transposition of the Great Arteries
Rationale: Transposition of the Great Arteries is a critical congenital heart defect where the aorta and pulmonary artery are switched, leading to oxygen-poor blood being pumped out to the body. This condition requires immediate medical intervention after birth. Options B, C, and D are also congenital heart defects but do not specifically result in oxygen-poor blood being pumped out to the body, making them incorrect choices for this question.

Question 36: Correct Answer: B) Acetaminophen
Rationale: Acetaminophen is the preferred analgesic for pain relief in newborns due to its safety profile and effectiveness. Ibuprofen and aspirin are generally avoided in newborns due to potential adverse effects on the gastrointestinal system and bleeding risks. Morphine is a potent opioid analgesic that may be used in specific cases under close monitoring, but it is not typically the first-line choice for routine pain management in newborns.

Question 37: Correct Answer: B) Tricuspid Atresia
Rationale: Tricuspid atresia is a cyanotic congenital

heart defect where the tricuspid valve is absent, leading to a right-to-left shunt at the atrial level. This condition presents with cyanosis that worsens with crying or feeding, clubbing of fingers and toes, and requires immediate medical intervention. While other conditions like TGA, TAPVC, and HLHS also present with cyanosis, the presence of a right-to-left shunt at the atrial level points towards tricuspid atresia in James' case.

Question 38: Correct Answer: A) Prolonged bed rest
Rationale: Prolonged bed rest is a significant risk factor for the development of pulmonary embolus in the postpartum period due to stasis of blood flow in the lower extremities, leading to the formation of blood clots. Regular ambulation, adequate hydration, and controlled breathing exercises are actually preventive measures against pulmonary embolus as they help in maintaining blood circulation and preventing clot formation.

Question 39: Correct Answer: C) Preeclampsia
Rationale: Preeclampsia is a serious antepartum complication characterized by high blood pressure and proteinuria after 20 weeks of gestation. It can lead to severe complications for both the mother and the baby if left untreated. Gestational diabetes is a condition where blood sugar levels rise during pregnancy but is not related to high blood pressure and proteinuria. Placenta previa involves the abnormal placement of the placenta in the uterus and does not present with the symptoms described. Ectopic pregnancy is a potentially life-threatening condition where the fertilized egg implants outside the uterus, unrelated to the symptoms of preeclampsia.

Question 40: Correct Answer: A) Fetal heart rate variability
Rationale: Assessing fetal heart rate variability is crucial in this scenario as it provides valuable information about fetal well-being and response to labor. Monitoring for any signs of fetal distress is essential during labor. Maternal blood pressure, amniotic fluid volume, and maternal temperature are also important parameters to monitor, but fetal heart rate variability takes precedence in assessing fetal status during labor.

Question 41: Correct Answer: D) Neonatal adrenal crisis
Rationale: Neonatal adrenal crisis is a life-threatening condition caused by adrenal insufficiency, leading to electrolyte imbalances such as hyponatremia and hyperkalemia. Neonatal Cushing's syndrome (Option A) is excessive cortisol production. Neonatal hypothyroidism (Option B) is the underproduction of thyroid hormone. Neonatal hyperparathyroidism (Option C) is excessive parathyroid hormone production, affecting calcium levels. Therefore, the correct answer is Neonatal adrenal crisis, characterized by adrenal insufficiency and electrolyte imbalances.

Question 42: Correct Answer: B) Vaginal bleeding in the third trimester
Rationale: Vaginal bleeding in the third trimester, especially after 28 weeks of gestation, is a common symptom of Placenta Previa. This bleeding occurs due to the abnormal placement of the placenta near or over the cervix. Options A, C, and D are not typically associated with Placenta Previa. Severe lower back pain could be indicative of other conditions such as preterm labor, while excessive fetal movement and high blood pressure are not specific symptoms of Placenta Previa.

Question 43: Correct Answer: B) Ensuring proper latch and positioning during breastfeeding
Rationale: Proper latch and positioning during breastfeeding are essential to ensure effective milk removal and prevent engorgement. Limiting breastfeeding sessions or supplementing with formula can lead to decreased milk supply and exacerbate engorgement. Tight-fitting bras can constrict milk flow and increase the risk of engorgement. By emphasizing proper latch and positioning, the nurse can help the mother establish a successful breastfeeding routine and prevent complications like breast engorgement.

Question 44: Correct Answer: A) Vitamin C
Rationale: Vitamin C plays a crucial role in collagen synthesis, which is essential for wound healing and tissue repair postpartum. Adequate intake of Vitamin C helps in strengthening the immune system and promoting overall healing. Iron is important for replenishing maternal stores after childbirth, but it is not directly involved in wound healing. Calcium is essential for bone health but does not directly impact wound healing. Vitamin K is important for blood clotting but is not primarily involved in tissue repair.

Question 45: Correct Answer: A) Oxytocin
Rationale: Oxytocin is the first-line medication for managing postpartum hemorrhage (PPH) caused by uterine atony, which is the most common cause of PPH. Oxytocin helps stimulate uterine contractions, which can aid in controlling bleeding. While magnesium sulfate, misoprostol, and nifedipine may have other obstetric uses, they are not the primary medications used for managing PPH due to uterine atony. It is essential to promptly administer oxytocin and other interventions to address uterine atony and prevent further complications associated with PPH.

Question 46: Correct Answer: C) Autonomy
Rationale: In this scenario, Ms. Smith is exercising autonomy by making decisions about her own body and care based on her personal values and beliefs. Autonomy refers to the right of individuals to make their own choices and decisions regarding their health care. Beneficence focuses on doing good for the patient, nonmaleficence on avoiding harm, and justice on fairness in healthcare delivery. While all these principles are important in nursing care, autonomy specifically emphasizes respecting the patient's right to self-determination.

Question 47: Correct Answer: B) Providing the mother with all relevant information to make informed choices
Rationale: Ethical principles in maternal newborn nursing emphasize the importance of autonomy, which involves providing mothers with comprehensive information to enable them to make informed decisions about their care and the care of their newborn. Option A is incorrect as coercion is unethical and violates the principle of autonomy. Option C is incorrect as disregarding the mother's preferences goes against the concept of autonomy. Option D is incorrect as limiting the mother's involvement in decision-making processes undermines her autonomy and right to self-determination.

Question 48: Correct Answer: C) Encouraging sitz baths for comfort
Rationale: Sitz baths are commonly recommended for women with vaginal lacerations postpartum to promote healing, reduce swelling, and provide comfort. Continuous application of ice packs may cause vasoconstriction and impair healing. Prophylactic oral antibiotics are not routinely indicated for vaginal

lacerations unless signs of infection are present. Applying direct pressure on the laceration site may increase the risk of infection and hinder healing.

Question 49: Correct Answer: A) Fetal heart rate accelerations with fetal movement
Rationale: A reassuring finding during a nonstress test (NST) includes fetal heart rate accelerations with fetal movement, indicating a responsive and healthy fetal nervous system. Fetal heart rate decelerations with fetal movement (Option B) are concerning and may indicate fetal distress. Absence of fetal heart rate variability (Option C) is also a non-reassuring finding as variability is a sign of fetal well-being. A baseline fetal heart rate of 90 bpm (Option D) is abnormally low and would be concerning.

Question 50: Correct Answer: D) Initiating positive-pressure ventilation
Rationale: The initial intervention for a newborn experiencing respiratory distress is to initiate positive-pressure ventilation to support breathing. Administering glucose is not the first-line intervention for respiratory distress. Chest compressions are indicated for cardiac arrest, not respiratory distress. Placing the newborn in a warm environment is important but not the initial intervention for respiratory distress.

Question 51: Correct Answer: B) Spinach salad with strawberries and balsamic vinaigrette
Rationale: Spinach is a rich source of iron, which is essential for postpartum mothers to replenish iron stores after childbirth. Strawberries provide vitamin C, which enhances iron absorption. Potato chips, white rice, and white bread are low in iron and do not support postpartum recovery. Including iron-rich foods like spinach in meals can help prevent postpartum anemia and support overall maternal health.

Question 52: Correct Answer: B) To relieve mild to moderate pain
Rationale: Acetaminophen (Tylenol) is commonly used to relieve mild to moderate pain, such as headaches, in postpartum patients. It is not typically used for reducing fever, decreasing inflammation, or providing sedation. It is important to assess the patient's pain level and provide appropriate pain relief medication.

Question 53: Correct Answer: B) Administer oral antibiotics as prescribed
Rationale: In the scenario described, the signs and symptoms indicate a wound infection. The most appropriate nursing intervention would be to administer oral antibiotics as prescribed by the healthcare provider to treat the infection. Applying a warm compress may worsen the infection, cleaning with hydrogen peroxide can be too harsh on the wound, and removing sutures should only be done by a healthcare provider.

Question 54: Correct Answer: C) Folic acid supplementation before and during early pregnancy can help prevent neural tube defects.
Rationale: Folic acid supplementation before conception and during early pregnancy is crucial in preventing neural tube defects in the baby. It is recommended that women of childbearing age take a daily folic acid supplement of 400-800 mcg to reduce the risk of these birth defects. Options A, B, and D are incorrect as they provide inaccurate information regarding the importance and timing of folic acid supplementation.

Question 55: Correct Answer: A) Nipple shield
Rationale: A nipple shield is a thin, flexible silicone cover that is placed over the nipple during breastfeeding. It can help infants latch onto the breast more easily and can protect sore or cracked nipples. Breast pumps are used to express breast milk, breast shells are used to protect nipples from friction, and milk storage bags are used to store expressed breast milk. Therefore, the correct option is A) Nipple shield as it directly relates to assisting with latching and protecting sore nipples during breastfeeding.

Question 56: Correct Answer: D) Delaying breastfeeding sessions
Rationale: Delaying breastfeeding sessions can exacerbate breast engorgement by causing further swelling and discomfort. It is important to initiate breastfeeding early and frequently to prevent engorgement. Applying cold compresses, ensuring proper latch, and using cabbage leaves are all recommended strategies to alleviate breast engorgement. By delaying breastfeeding sessions, the milk accumulates in the breasts, leading to increased engorgement.

Question 57: Correct Answer: C) Smoking during pregnancy
Rationale: Smoking during pregnancy is a well-established antenatal factor that significantly increases the risk of preterm birth. Nicotine and other harmful chemicals in cigarettes can lead to placental insufficiency, reduced oxygen supply to the fetus, and premature labor. Maternal age over 35 years (option A) is a risk factor for other pregnancy complications but not specifically preterm birth. Multiparity (option B) and having a normal BMI (option D) are not directly linked to an increased risk of preterm birth.

Question 58: Correct Answer: C) Doppler ultrasound
Rationale: Doppler ultrasound is the preferred diagnostic tool for septic pelvic thrombophlebitis as it can visualize thrombi in the pelvic veins. Chest X-ray (option A) is not useful for this diagnosis. Urine analysis (option B) and ECG (option D) are not relevant to identifying this condition, making them incorrect choices.

Question 59: Correct Answer: C) At least two fetal heart rate accelerations occur within a 20-minute period.
Rationale: A reactive NST result is characterized by the presence of at least two fetal heart rate accelerations within a 20-minute period, indicating a healthy fetal central nervous system and oxygenation. Options A, B, and D are incorrect as they do not reflect the expected findings of a reactive NST, highlighting the importance of understanding the interpretation criteria for this test in maternal newborn nursing practice.

Question 60: Correct Answer: C) Establishing a relaxing bedtime routine
Rationale: Establishing a relaxing bedtime routine, such as taking a warm bath, reading a book, or practicing relaxation techniques, can help promote better sleep in postpartum women experiencing sleep disturbances. Options A, B, and D are incorrect as consuming caffeine before bedtime, engaging in stimulating activities close to bedtime, and using electronic devices in bed can all exacerbate sleep issues by interfering with the ability to fall asleep. Therefore, recommending a calming bedtime routine is essential in improving sleep quality for postpartum women.

Question 61: Correct Answer: D) Poor muscle tone
Rationale: Poor muscle tone in a newborn is a concerning sign that may indicate the need for resuscitation. It suggests potential central nervous

system depression or hypoxia, requiring immediate intervention to support the newborn's respiratory and circulatory functions. Pink skin color, a strong cry, and a respiratory rate of 40 breaths per minute are generally positive indicators of newborn health and may not necessarily warrant resuscitative measures. Therefore, identifying poor muscle tone is crucial in determining the need for prompt resuscitation in a newborn.

Question 62: Correct Answer: C) Yellow fever vaccine
Rationale: The correct option is C) Yellow fever vaccine. This vaccine is contraindicated during pregnancy due to its live attenuated nature, which poses a theoretical risk to the developing fetus. The other options, A) Hepatitis A vaccine, B) Tetanus toxoid vaccine, and D) Pneumococcal vaccine, are considered safe for administration during pregnancy. It is important to avoid live vaccines during pregnancy to prevent any potential harm to the fetus.

Question 63: Correct Answer: D) Iron is crucial for the production of hemoglobin to prevent anemia during pregnancy
Rationale: Iron is essential during pregnancy as it is needed for the production of hemoglobin to prevent anemia, which is common in pregnant women due to increased blood volume. Anemia can lead to adverse outcomes for both the mother and the baby. Therefore, adequate iron intake through diet and supplements if necessary is crucial during pregnancy. Options A, B, and C are incorrect as they provide inaccurate information about the importance of iron during pregnancy.

Question 64: Correct Answer: A) Previous history of depression
Rationale: Postpartum depression is more likely to occur in women with a history of depression. This is due to the hormonal changes, lack of sleep, and stress associated with childbirth, which can exacerbate pre-existing mental health conditions. High socioeconomic status (option B) and strong social support (option C) are actually protective factors against postpartum depression. While regular exercise (option D) can help improve mood, it is not a significant risk factor for postpartum depression compared to a history of depression.

Question 65: Correct Answer: A) 25%
Rationale: In the scenario described, since cystic fibrosis is an autosomal recessive disorder, both parents must be carriers of the gene for there to be a 25% chance that the baby will inherit the disorder. If the father is a carrier, the Punnett square analysis shows a 25% chance of the baby inheriting cystic fibrosis. Options B, C, and D are incorrect as they do not align with the principles of autosomal recessive inheritance.

Question 66: Correct Answer: A) Uterine Atony
Rationale: Postpartum hemorrhage is commonly caused by uterine atony, which is the failure of the uterus to contract adequately after delivery. This results in the inability of the blood vessels at the placental site to constrict, leading to excessive bleeding. Retained placental fragments, cervical lacerations, and coagulopathy can also cause postpartum hemorrhage, but in this scenario, the presentation of stable vital signs and the timing of the bleeding point towards uterine atony as the primary cause.

Question 67: Correct Answer: B) Amoxicillin
Rationale: Amoxicillin is commonly prescribed for mastitis in breastfeeding mothers due to its safety profile for both the mother and the infant. Ibuprofen is a nonsteroidal anti-inflammatory drug, Lorazepam is a benzodiazepine used for anxiety, and Furosemide is a diuretic, none of which are indicated for mastitis treatment.

Question 68: Correct Answer: A) Hypoglycemia
Rationale: Newborns born to mothers with diabetes are at risk of hypoglycemia due to excessive insulin production in response to maternal hyperglycemia during pregnancy. Hypoglycemia can occur within the first few hours after birth and requires close monitoring and prompt intervention to prevent complications such as seizures and long-term neurological damage. Hyperbilirubinemia, respiratory distress syndrome, and patent ductus arteriosus are also common newborn complications but are not directly linked to maternal diabetes.

Question 69: Correct Answer: C) Women with known cardiac disease should receive preconception counseling.
Rationale: Preconception counseling is crucial for women with known cardiac disease to assess risks, optimize health, and plan for a safe pregnancy. Avoiding physical activity is not always necessary and can be determined on a case-by-case basis. Pregnant women with cardiac disease are at increased risk of adverse outcomes, and cardiac disease can have significant impacts on both maternal and fetal health outcomes.

Question 70: Correct Answer: C) Endometritis
Rationale: Endometritis is an infection of the uterine lining that commonly occurs after childbirth. Symptoms include fever, abdominal pain, abnormal vaginal discharge, and uterine tenderness. Postpartum depression is a mood disorder, postpartum hemorrhage is excessive bleeding, and mastitis is inflammation of the breast tissue. Endometritis requires prompt diagnosis and treatment to prevent serious complications.

Question 71: Correct Answer: A) Tachycardia
Rationale: Tachycardia is defined as a baseline fetal heart rate above 160 beats per minute. It can be caused by maternal fever, fetal hypoxia, or maternal dehydration. Tachycardia is a concerning finding that requires prompt evaluation and management to prevent adverse outcomes. Bradycardia, on the other hand, is characterized by a baseline heart rate below 110 beats per minute and is associated with fetal distress. Altered variability refers to irregular fluctuations in the fetal heart rate pattern, while decelerations are temporary decreases in heart rate during contractions.

Question 72: Correct Answer: C) Monitor the newborn's heart rate
Rationale: Monitoring the newborn's heart rate is crucial in evaluating the effectiveness of resuscitation interventions. An increase in heart rate indicates improved perfusion and response to ventilation. Options A and B are not directly related to assessing the effectiveness of the intervention. Stopping positive-pressure ventilation without proper evaluation could compromise the newborn's condition.

Question 73: Correct Answer: C) Monitoring for signs of postpartum hemorrhage
Rationale: Monitoring for signs of postpartum hemorrhage is crucial in upholding the ethical principle of non-maleficence as it involves early detection and intervention to prevent harm to the mother. Postpartum hemorrhage is a life-threatening complication that requires prompt recognition and management to prevent

adverse outcomes. While performing regular assessments, ensuring hygiene, and providing emotional support are essential aspects of care, monitoring for postpartum hemorrhage directly addresses the prevention of harm and aligns with the principle of non-maleficence.

Question 74: Correct Answer: B) Placenta Previa
Rationale: Placenta Previa is characterized by painless vaginal bleeding in the third trimester, often associated with a fundal height that is higher than expected for gestational age. This condition occurs when the placenta partially or completely covers the cervix, leading to bleeding as the cervix begins to efface and dilate in preparation for labor. Abruptio Placentae presents with painful bleeding, uterine rupture is associated with severe abdominal pain and fetal distress, while cervical insufficiency typically presents as painless cervical dilation in the second trimester.

Question 75: Correct Answer: C) Suprapubic pain and discomfort
Rationale: Bladder distention in postpartum women commonly presents with suprapubic pain and discomfort due to the pressure exerted by the distended bladder against surrounding structures. Hypotension and bradycardia are not typical signs of bladder distention. Increased appetite is not a specific indicator of bladder distention and is not directly related to this condition. Therefore, option C is the correct answer as it aligns with the expected clinical manifestation of bladder distention.

Question 76: Correct Answer: A) Educate the caregiver on the importance of tummy time when the baby is awake
Rationale: Placing the baby on their stomach for sleep increases the risk of SIDS. Educating the caregiver on the importance of tummy time when the baby is awake helps promote healthy development and prevents positional plagiocephaly. Providing a soft pillow for stomach sleeping is unsafe and increases the risk of suffocation. Swaddling tightly for sleep is not recommended as it can also increase the risk of SIDS.

Question 77: Correct Answer: B) Multiple gestation
Rationale: Ovulation induction therapy can increase the chances of multiple gestation (twins, triplets, etc.), which is a known risk factor associated with fertility treatments. While preterm birth, post-term pregnancy, and macrosomia are potential birth risk factors, multiple gestation is specifically linked to ovulation induction therapy in the context of infertility treatment.

Question 78: Correct Answer: C) Suggesting the use of a sitz bath for comfort
Rationale: Hemorrhoids are a common postpartum issue due to increased intra-abdominal pressure during pregnancy and childbirth. Sitz baths can help reduce swelling and discomfort associated with hemorrhoids. Applying ice packs can also provide relief, but it is not the primary intervention. Encouraging physical activity is important for overall recovery, and administering a laxative may not directly address the hemorrhoids.

Question 79: Correct Answer: C) Chronic hypertension
Rationale: Chronic hypertension is a significant antepartum risk factor for cardiac disease during pregnancy. It can lead to complications such as preeclampsia and exacerbate existing cardiac conditions. Gestational diabetes, hypothyroidism, and iron deficiency anemia, although important in pregnancy, are not directly linked to an increased risk of cardiac disease.

Question 80: Correct Answer: B) Syphilis
Rationale: Syphilis is the STI that poses the highest risk of vertical transmission from mother to newborn during childbirth. Untreated syphilis in pregnancy can lead to adverse outcomes such as stillbirth, neonatal death, and congenital syphilis. Chlamydia, gonorrhea, and trichomoniasis can also be transmitted from mother to newborn but are not associated with as high a risk of vertical transmission as syphilis. It is crucial to screen and treat pregnant women for syphilis to prevent these serious complications.

Question 81: Correct Answer: C) It is important to follow the manufacturer's instructions for the correct ratio of water to formula powder.
Rationale: It is crucial to follow the manufacturer's instructions for the correct ratio of water to formula powder to ensure the infant receives the appropriate nutrition. Preparing a large batch of formula in advance is not recommended due to the risk of bacterial contamination. Formula should be prepared using water that has been boiled and then cooled to the appropriate temperature, not hot tap water. Additionally, prepared formula should not be left at room temperature for more than 2 hours to prevent bacterial growth.

Question 82: Correct Answer: A) Encouraging early ambulation
Rationale: Encouraging early ambulation is crucial in postoperative care to prevent DVT as it helps in promoting circulation and preventing blood stasis. High-dose opioids can lead to respiratory depression and delay mobilization, increasing the risk of DVT. Keeping the mother on strict bed rest can also contribute to stasis and DVT formation. Applying heat packs to the incision site is not recommended postoperatively as it can increase inflammation and discomfort, hindering early mobilization.

Question 83: Correct Answer: A) 32 weeks
Rationale: The translucent skin and flat ears with a soft pinna are characteristic findings in a newborn with a gestational age of around 32 weeks. Option B (36 weeks) is incorrect as the described features are more indicative of an earlier gestational age. Option C (40 weeks) is incorrect as the findings suggest a preterm infant. Option D (44 weeks) is incorrect as it exceeds a full-term gestational age.

Question 84: Correct Answer: B) Caffeine
Rationale: Caffeine is a commonly used medication in newborns for respiratory support, especially in premature infants with apnea of prematurity. It helps stimulate the baby's respiratory drive and can reduce the episodes of apnea. Furosemide is a diuretic, acetaminophen is a pain reliever, and ondansetron is an antiemetic, none of which are used for respiratory support in newborns.

Question 85: Correct Answer: A) Encouraging rooming-in
Rationale: Encouraging rooming-in, where the newborn stays in the same room as the parents, promotes bonding and attachment by allowing for frequent interaction, feeding, and care. Limiting parental visitation can hinder bonding opportunities. Skin-to-skin contact immediately after birth enhances bonding and breastfeeding initiation. Breastfeeding is encouraged as it fosters bonding through close physical contact and nurturing interaction between the newborn and parents.

Question 86: Correct Answer: A) Maternal obesity
Rationale: Maternal obesity is a known risk factor for

prolonged labor during the intrapartum period due to factors such as increased adipose tissue affecting uterine contractions and the progress of labor. Early prenatal care (Option B) is actually beneficial in identifying and managing risk factors early, reducing complications. Multiparity (Option C) may lead to shorter labors due to the body's previous experience. Normal fetal presentation (Option D) refers to the baby positioned head-down, which is the optimal position for labor progress, not a risk factor for prolonged labor.

Question 87: Correct Answer: B) Plastic bags designed for breast milk storage
Rationale: Storing expressed breast milk in plastic bags specifically designed for this purpose is the recommended method. These bags are sterile, BPA-free, and designed to preserve the nutrients in breast milk. Using glass containers (option A) can increase the risk of breakage and contamination. Regular plastic bags (option C) are not suitable for storing breast milk as they may not be sterile and can leach harmful chemicals. Metal containers (option D) are also not recommended as they can react with the breast milk and alter its composition.

Question 88: Correct Answer: B) Providing education on infant care and promoting bonding between the newborn and family members.
Rationale: During the postpartum period, it is crucial for the nurse to support family dynamics by providing education on infant care and facilitating bonding between the newborn and family members. This helps in enhancing the family's confidence in caring for the newborn and promotes a strong emotional connection. Options A, C, and D are incorrect as they do not focus on the essential role of the nurse in promoting family bonding and education, which are vital aspects of postpartum care.

Question 89: Correct Answer: C) Drying the newborn and covering the head
Rationale: Drying the newborn and covering the head with a cap are essential steps to prevent hypothermia by reducing evaporative heat loss. Placing the newborn in a cold room or administering a cold bath can further decrease the baby's body temperature, leading to hypothermia. Using a radiant warmer for an extended period may cause overheating and should be used judiciously to maintain the newborn's temperature within the normal range.

Question 90: Correct Answer: A) McRoberts maneuver
Rationale: The McRoberts maneuver is a well-known technique used to alleviate shoulder dystocia during delivery. This maneuver involves hyperflexing the mother's legs tightly against her abdomen to help rotate the pelvis and release the impacted shoulder. The Ritgen maneuver, Rubin maneuver, and Woods' screw maneuver are not specifically indicated for managing shoulder dystocia and are not considered standard interventions for this obstetric emergency.

Question 91: Correct Answer: C) Simethicone
Rationale: Simethicone is an anti-gas medication that helps break up gas bubbles in the gut, providing relief from bloating and gas. Esomeprazole and Ranitidine are used for acid-related conditions, while Loperamide is an antidiarrheal agent, making them inappropriate choices for bloating and gas relief in this case.

Question 92: Correct Answer: B) Bright red vaginal bleeding

Rationale: Placental abruption often presents with sudden-onset, painful uterine contractions that may not stop with position changes, accompanied by dark red or occasionally bright red vaginal bleeding. Fetal heart rate decelerations are typically persistent and not relieved by maternal position changes. Decreased uterine tone between contractions is not a typical sign of placental abruption, as the uterus may remain firm due to continuous bleeding and lack of relaxation.

Question 93: Correct Answer: C) Focus on nutrient-dense foods and gradual weight loss
Rationale: Postpartum mothers should focus on consuming nutrient-dense foods to support healing and milk production. Gradual weight loss is recommended to ensure an adequate nutrient supply for both the mother and the baby. Starting a strict diet or skipping meals can lead to nutrient deficiencies and may affect milk production. Increasing calorie intake is not advised for weight loss; instead, a balanced diet with appropriate portion sizes is key for postpartum nutrition.

Question 94: Correct Answer: C) Nifedipine
Rationale: Nifedipine is a calcium channel blocker commonly used as a first-line antihypertensive medication in breastfeeding mothers due to its minimal excretion in breast milk. Lisinopril (Option A) and Atenolol (Option B) are contraindicated during breastfeeding due to potential adverse effects on the infant. Metoprolol (Option D) is also not recommended as it can pass into breast milk in significant amounts, potentially affecting the infant.

Question 95: Correct Answer: C) Butorphanol
Rationale: Butorphanol is a commonly used opioid analgesic in labor that provides pain relief to the mother without causing significant respiratory depression in the newborn. Fentanyl (Option A) is a potent opioid that can cause respiratory depression in the newborn. Meperidine (Option B) crosses the placenta and can accumulate in the newborn, causing respiratory depression. Nalbuphine (Option D) is an opioid agonist-antagonist that can also lead to respiratory depression in the newborn. Therefore, Butorphanol is the safest option among the choices provided.

Question 96: Correct Answer: C) GDM typically develops after the 28th week of pregnancy.
Rationale: Gestational diabetes mellitus (GDM) is a type of diabetes that develops during pregnancy, usually after the 28th week. It is characterized by high blood sugar levels and can pose risks to both the mother and the baby if not properly managed. Options A, B, and D are incorrect as GDM is not a permanent type of diabetes, can be managed through diet, exercise, and sometimes medication (not just insulin), and does pose risks such as macrosomia (large birth weight) for the baby and increased risk of developing type 2 diabetes for the mother postpartum.

Question 97: Correct Answer: A) Providing Mrs. Smith with additional breastfeeding resources and support
Rationale: The correct answer demonstrates the ethical principle of justice by ensuring that Mrs. Smith receives equitable access to resources and support to overcome her breastfeeding challenges. Options B, C, and D do not align with the principle of justice as they either ignore Mrs. Smith's concerns, suggest an alternative without addressing her needs, or restrict her access to necessary support.

Question 98: Correct Answer: C) Nipple cream

Rationale: Nipple soreness is a common issue during breastfeeding. Nipple shields may interfere with proper latch and milk transfer. A breast pump is not necessary for alleviating nipple soreness. Warm compress can help with milk flow but may not directly address soreness. Nipple cream is specifically designed to soothe and protect sore nipples, making it the most appropriate choice for this situation.

Question 99: Correct Answer: B) History of PID
Rationale: Pelvic inflammatory disease (PID) can lead to scarring and damage to the fallopian tubes, increasing the risk of infertility. While advanced maternal age, obesity, and smoking are also risk factors for infertility, in this scenario, the history of PID is the most likely contributing factor based on the patient's history.

Question 100: Correct Answer: A) Lack of social support
Rationale: Lack of social support can significantly impact a mother's ability to bond with her baby. In this scenario, Mrs. Smith's feelings of inadequacy and difficulty in establishing a connection with her infant may be exacerbated by the absence of a strong support system. While the baby's excessive crying or weight can be challenging, they are not direct barriers to parent/infant interactions. Mrs. Smith's age alone is not a determining factor in bonding with her baby.

Question 101: Correct Answer: C) Breast shells
Rationale: Breast shells are worn inside the bra to collect leaking breast milk from the non-nursing breast. They are not used for latching assistance or milk expression like nipple shields or breast pumps. Nipple shields are used for latching issues, breast pumps are used for expressing milk, and milk storage bags are used to store expressed breast milk. Therefore, the correct option is C) Breast shells as they serve the specific purpose of collecting leaking breast milk during breastfeeding.

Question 102: Correct Answer: A) Swaddling the baby snugly
Rationale: Swaddling the baby snugly helps recreate the womb environment, providing a sense of security and comfort to the newborn. This practice can help soothe the baby and promote better sleep. Offering a pacifier can also provide comfort by satisfying the baby's natural sucking reflex. Placing the baby in a cold room is not recommended as newborns need to be kept warm. Letting the baby cry it out is not a recommended comfort measure for newborns as it can lead to increased stress and feelings of abandonment.

Question 103: Correct Answer: C) Maternal stress
Rationale: Maternal stress is a significant risk factor for adverse pregnancy outcomes. High levels of stress during pregnancy have been associated with preterm birth, low birth weight, and developmental delays in infants. While high socioeconomic status and strong social support are generally considered protective factors, positive coping mechanisms can help mitigate the effects of stress but do not eliminate it as a risk factor. Therefore, maternal stress stands out as the correct option among the choices provided.

Question 104: Correct Answer: B) Oxytocin
Rationale: Oxytocin is the hormone responsible for milk ejection or let-down reflex during breastfeeding. It causes the muscles around the milk-producing cells to contract, pushing milk into the ducts. Prolactin, on the other hand, is responsible for milk production. Estrogen and progesterone play roles in preparing the breast for lactation during pregnancy but are not directly involved in milk ejection.

Question 105: Correct Answer: C) "Burping helps release any swallowed air during feeding."
Rationale: Burping is essential after bottle-feeding to release any trapped air that the baby may have swallowed during feeding, reducing the risk of discomfort and colic. Option A is incorrect as burping is recommended for bottle-fed babies. Option B is partially true but does not encompass the main reason for burping. Option D is incorrect as burping should be done routinely, not just based on fussiness.

Question 106: Correct Answer: C) Codeine
Rationale: Codeine is contraindicated during breastfeeding due to its potential to cause respiratory depression and sedation in infants, especially those who are ultra-rapid metabolizers of codeine to morphine. Ibuprofen and acetaminophen are considered safe for use during breastfeeding as they have minimal excretion into breast milk and are unlikely to harm the infant. Metoclopramide is also generally safe for use during breastfeeding as it enhances lactation without significant adverse effects on the infant.

Question 107: Correct Answer: A) Administering a bolus of intravenous fluids
Rationale: In hypovolemic shock, the priority intervention is to restore intravascular volume by administering intravenous fluids to improve tissue perfusion. Oxygen therapy may be necessary but is not the priority in this situation. Monitoring fetal heart rate is not relevant in the management of hypovolemic shock in a postpartum patient. While emotional support is important, addressing the physiological needs takes precedence in this critical situation.

Question 108: Correct Answer: D) Veracity
Rationale: Veracity is the ethical principle that emphasizes the importance of truthfulness and honesty in healthcare interactions. It involves providing accurate information to patients to enable them to make informed decisions about their care. Autonomy relates to respecting patients' rights to make their own decisions, beneficence focuses on doing good for the patient, and nonmaleficence pertains to avoiding harm. By choosing veracity as the correct answer, healthcare providers uphold transparency and foster trust in the patient-provider relationship.

Question 109: Correct Answer: B) Bladder palpable above the symphysis pubis
Rationale: A palpable bladder above the symphysis pubis indicates significant urine retention. Option A suggests decreased urine output, which may be a sign of inadequate fluid intake. Option C indicates a normal sensation postpartum. Lower abdominal cramping (Option D) is a common postpartum discomfort and not specific to urinary retention.

Question 110: Correct Answer: A) Coombs test
Rationale: The Coombs test, also known as direct antiglobulin test (DAT), is essential in diagnosing hemolytic disease of the newborn (HDN) by detecting the presence of maternal antibodies on the surface of fetal red blood cells. This test helps confirm the immune-mediated destruction of red blood cells in the newborn. Options B, C, and D are not specific to HDN diagnosis. While monitoring blood glucose levels, serum electrolytes, and liver function tests are important in neonatal care, they do not directly aid in diagnosing

HDN, making them incorrect choices in this context.

Question 111: Correct Answer: C) Cytomegalovirus (CMV)
Rationale: Cytomegalovirus (CMV) is the most common viral cause of congenital infection, posing a significant risk to newborns due to potential vertical transmission during pregnancy. CMV can lead to serious complications such as hearing loss, developmental delays, and microcephaly in newborns. Influenza, Rubella, and Varicella zoster virus (VZV) are also important viral infections, but CMV stands out as the highest risk due to its prevalence and potential impact on newborn health.

Question 112: Correct Answer: D) Instruct the mother to ensure the baby's mouth covers a large portion of the areola during latch on.
Rationale: Option A may provide temporary relief but does not address the root cause of the issue. Option B is not the best solution as breastfeeding is beneficial for both the mother and the baby. Option C is incorrect as breaking the latch improperly can cause further discomfort. Option D is the correct intervention as ensuring a deep latch on can help prevent nipple pain and improve breastfeeding effectiveness.

Question 113: Correct Answer: A) Developmental dysplasia of the hip (DDH)
Rationale: Asymmetry in hip abduction is a common clinical finding in newborns with developmental dysplasia of the hip (DDH). DDH is a condition where the hip joint does not develop properly, leading to instability and potential dislocation. Osteogenesis imperfecta is a genetic disorder causing brittle bones, congenital muscular torticollis is a condition characterized by neck muscle tightness, and spina bifida is a neural tube defect. However, these conditions do not typically present with asymmetry in hip abduction as seen in DDH.

Question 114: Correct Answer: B) Breast milk provides antibodies for immune protection
Rationale: Breast milk contains antibodies that help protect newborns from infections and provide essential nutrients for growth and development. Formula-fed babies are not necessarily less prone to allergies, and breastfeeding is associated with optimal weight gain. Contrary to the statement, breastfeeding actually reduces the risk of infections due to the immune-boosting properties of breast milk.

Question 115: Correct Answer: D) Breast milk fat aids in the absorption of fat-soluble vitamins
Rationale: Breast milk contains a higher proportion of unsaturated fats rather than saturated fats, promoting healthy growth and development in infants. It is also rich in cholesterol, essential for brain development. The fat content of breast milk varies during a feeding session, with hindmilk having a higher fat content than foremilk. The fat in breast milk plays a crucial role in helping the baby absorb fat-soluble vitamins like A, D, E, and K.

Question 116: Correct Answer: A) Neonatal sepsis
Rationale: The elevated white blood cell count with a left shift, along with increased neutrophils, is indicative of an inflammatory response seen in neonatal sepsis. Physiological leukocytosis, seen in the first few days of life, typically resolves without intervention and is characterized by a left shift as well. Neonatal jaundice is characterized by elevated bilirubin levels, not by changes in the CBC. Neonatal polycythemia is marked by an elevated hematocrit level, not an elevated white blood cell count.

Question 117: Correct Answer: B) Multifetal gestation
Rationale: Multifetal gestation, such as twins or triplets, is a known risk factor for PROM due to increased pressure on the amniotic sac. Maternal age over 35 years is a risk factor for other complications but not specifically for PROM. Regular prenatal exercise and low BMI are actually associated with a decreased risk of PROM.

Question 118: Correct Answer: D) Colostrum is low in volume but rich in immune factors.
Rationale: Colostrum is the first milk produced by the breasts after childbirth. It is low in volume but rich in immune factors such as antibodies, white blood cells, and growth factors, providing essential protection and nutrition to the newborn. Colostrum is often described as thin and yellowish in color, unlike mature milk which is higher in fat content. It is produced in the initial days after birth, not after 1 week of breastfeeding.

Question 119: Correct Answer: A) Maternal hemorrhage
Rationale: Precipitous delivery, defined as labor lasting less than 3 hours from the onset of contractions to delivery, can lead to maternal hemorrhage due to rapid expulsion of the baby, causing inadequate uterine contractions to control bleeding. Maternal hemorrhage is a significant concern in precipitous deliveries and requires prompt management to prevent complications such as hypovolemic shock. Prolonged labor (option B) is not a complication of precipitous delivery, as it refers to labor lasting more than 20 hours for first-time mothers and more than 14 hours for multiparous women. Fetal macrosomia (option C) is excessive fetal growth, not directly related to precipitous delivery. Maternal hypertension (option D) is a separate condition that can occur during pregnancy but is not specific to precipitous delivery.

Question 120: Correct Answer: C) Suctioning the airway
Rationale: In this scenario, Sarah is presenting with signs of airway obstruction, which can be due to secretions or mucus. The initial nursing intervention should be to suction the airway to clear any obstructions and improve air exchange. Administering oxygen, performing chest compressions, or placing an oropharyngeal airway would not address the underlying issue of airway obstruction in this case.

Question 121: Correct Answer: C) Oligohydramnios
Rationale: Oligohydramnios refers to a decreased amniotic fluid volume, which is opposite to polyhydramnios. Polyhydramnios, on the other hand, is often associated with maternal diabetes, fetal anomalies, and multiple gestation. It is crucial to differentiate between these two conditions as they have different implications for maternal and fetal health. While oligohydramnios can lead to fetal growth restriction and compression-related deformities, polyhydramnios can increase the risk of preterm labor, placental abruption, and postpartum hemorrhage.

Question 122: Correct Answer: A) Pulmonary Embolism
Rationale: The clinical presentation of sudden onset shortness of breath, chest pain, tachypnea, tachycardia, and a wedge-shaped infiltrate on chest X-ray is highly suggestive of a pulmonary embolism. While pneumonia, atelectasis, and pleural effusion can also present with similar symptoms, the combination of findings in this scenario points towards a pulmonary embolism, which is a serious postpartum complication associated with

increased risk in the peripartum period.

Question 123: Correct Answer: A) Applying cold compresses
Rationale: Engorgement is a common issue in lactating mothers due to an overabundance of milk. Applying cold compresses can help reduce swelling and provide relief. Massaging the breasts vigorously can lead to further milk production and exacerbate the engorgement. Skipping breastfeeding sessions can worsen the condition, leading to more discomfort. Wearing a tight-fitting bra can constrict the breasts and increase discomfort.

Question 124: Correct Answer: A) Copper intrauterine device (IUD)
Rationale: The copper IUD is a highly effective LARC method that can provide contraception for up to 10 years. The levonorgestrel-releasing IUS is effective for up to 5 years. While the contraceptive implant and injectable progestin are also LARC methods, they do not provide contraception for as long as the copper IUD. It is important to consider the patient's preferences and medical history when recommending a LARC method.

Question 125: Correct Answer: C) Referring Emily to a mental health professional
Rationale: Postpartum depression can significantly hinder parent/infant interactions. Referring Emily to a mental health professional for evaluation and support is crucial in addressing this barrier. Encouraging Emily to spend more time alone with her baby may not be effective if she is struggling with depression. Providing education on infant care techniques is important but may not directly address the underlying mental health issue. Suggesting Emily to ignore her feelings can worsen the situation and is not a recommended approach in managing postpartum depression.

Question 126: Correct Answer: A) Oxytocin
Rationale: Oxytocin is the medication of choice for preventing postpartum hemorrhage due to its ability to stimulate uterine contractions, helping the uterus to contract and reduce bleeding. Magnesium sulfate is used for preventing seizures in preeclampsia and eclampsia, not for postpartum hemorrhage. Methylergonovine is used to treat postpartum hemorrhage but not as commonly as oxytocin. Nifedipine is a calcium channel blocker used for hypertension in pregnancy, not for preventing postpartum hemorrhage.

Question 127: Correct Answer: D) Gluten
Rationale: Human breast milk does not contain gluten, as it is a protein found in grains like wheat, barley, and rye. Breast milk is rich in lactose, a carbohydrate, casein, a protein, and immunoglobulins, which are antibodies that help protect the infant from infections. Gluten is not a component of breast milk and is not recommended for infants until they are developmentally ready to digest it, usually around 6 months of age.

Question 128: Correct Answer: B) Tachypnea
Rationale: Meconium aspiration syndrome is characterized by respiratory distress due to meconium aspiration into the lungs. Tachypnea, or rapid breathing, is a common clinical manifestation of this condition as the meconium can obstruct the airways and lead to breathing difficulties. Hypoglycemia, bradycardia, and hyperthermia are not typically associated with meconium aspiration syndrome and are less specific to this condition.

Question 129: Correct Answer: C) Educating mothers about postpartum depression can help in early detection and intervention.
Rationale: Patient education on postpartum depression is vital as it enables mothers to recognize the signs and symptoms, seek help early, and receive appropriate support and treatment. Option A is incorrect as postpartum depression is a common mental health condition and not a sign of weakness. Option B is incorrect as postpartum depression affects a significant number of women and requires attention. Option D is incorrect as postpartum depression is multifactorial, and education can play a role in prevention and management by promoting awareness and seeking help.

Question 130: Correct Answer: C) Postpartum preeclampsia
Rationale: The symptoms described are indicative of postpartum preeclampsia, a serious condition characterized by high blood pressure, protein in the urine, and often involving headaches, visual changes, and epigastric pain. Postpartum depression is characterized by persistent feelings of sadness and worthlessness, postpartum hemorrhage involves excessive bleeding, and postpartum thyroiditis affects the thyroid gland. Postpartum preeclampsia is the most critical concern in this scenario due to the potential risks associated with uncontrolled hypertension post-delivery.

Question 131: Correct Answer: C) Jitteriness can be a manifestation of hypoglycemia
Rationale: Jitteriness in newborns can be a clinical manifestation of hypoglycemia, which is a common metabolic issue in the neonatal period. It is crucial for healthcare providers to recognize jitteriness as a potential sign of low blood sugar levels in newborns. While jitteriness can be a benign finding in some newborns, it should never be dismissed without further evaluation, especially in the context of potential hypoglycemia. Options A, B, and D are incorrect as jitteriness is not always normal, not always indicative of a serious neurological disorder, and not primarily caused by respiratory distress in newborns.

Question 132: Correct Answer: B) Down syndrome
Rationale: An increased nuchal translucency measurement (>3mm) is associated with an increased risk of chromosomal abnormalities, particularly Down syndrome. Options A, C, and D are incorrect as they do not correlate with the specific implication of an increased nuchal translucency measurement for Down syndrome risk assessment.

Question 133: Correct Answer: B) "We will clean Emily's umbilical cord stump with alcohol at every diaper change."
Rationale: Cleaning the umbilical cord stump with alcohol at every diaper change is an outdated practice that can delay the natural healing process. Parents should be taught to keep the cord stump clean and dry, allowing it to fall off on its own. Options A, C, and D are correct statements that promote newborn safety and well-being.

Question 134: Correct Answer: D) Sudden onset of shortness of breath
Rationale: Sudden onset of shortness of breath postoperatively could indicate pulmonary embolism, a life-threatening complication. While minimal serosanguineous drainage from the incision site, a firm and midline fundus, and a respiratory rate of 18 breaths per minute are expected findings, sudden shortness of breath requires immediate attention to rule out pulmonary embolism and ensure the mother's safety.

Question 135: Correct Answer: D) Arrange for a professional interpreter to communicate effectively with Maria.
Rationale: Effective communication is crucial for addressing emotional needs. Providing a professional interpreter ensures accurate understanding, enhances trust, and promotes emotional support. This approach respects Maria's cultural background, fosters a therapeutic relationship, and aligns with ethical principles of patient-centered care, emphasizing the importance of language access for quality healthcare delivery.

Question 136: Correct Answer: A) Maternal HIV infection
Rationale: Maternal HIV infection is a contraindication to breastfeeding due to the risk of transmission of the virus to the infant through breast milk. It is essential to prevent the vertical transmission of HIV from mother to child. Maternal diabetes, hypertension, and obesity are not contraindications to breastfeeding. In fact, breastfeeding is beneficial for mothers with these conditions as it can help improve maternal health outcomes and provide numerous benefits to the infant.

Question 137: Correct Answer: C) Urinary retention
Rationale: Urinary retention is a common complication of regional anesthesia during labor, such as epidurals, due to the effects of the anesthesia on bladder function. Hypertension (Option A) is not typically associated with regional anesthesia during labor. Hypoglycemia (Option B) is more related to maternal metabolic changes during labor. Hypoxemia (Option D) is not a common complication of regional anesthesia but can occur in certain situations like respiratory depression from opioids.

Question 138: Correct Answer: B) Fixating on an object briefly
Rationale: At 38 weeks gestation, newborns are typically able to briefly fixate on objects but may not smoothly track them yet. The ability to smoothly track objects develops over the first few months of life. Ignoring visual stimuli or inability to track objects may indicate visual impairment or developmental delay.

Question 139: Correct Answer: C) Administer antihypertensive medication as prescribed
Rationale: In the scenario described, Ms. Johnson is exhibiting signs of worsening chronic hypertension, which can lead to complications such as preeclampsia. The most appropriate nursing intervention in this situation is to administer antihypertensive medication as prescribed to help lower her blood pressure and prevent further complications. Increasing salt intake, advising bed rest, or encouraging vigorous exercise are not recommended and could potentially worsen her condition.

Question 140: Correct Answer: A) Uterine atony
Rationale: Excessive bleeding post-vaginal delivery can be indicative of uterine atony, a condition where the uterus fails to contract effectively. This can lead to postpartum hemorrhage, a life-threatening complication. While perineal and cervical lacerations can also cause bleeding, uterine atony is the most common cause of postpartum hemorrhage and requires immediate intervention to prevent further complications. Retained placental fragments can also lead to bleeding but are usually associated with a delayed onset compared to uterine atony.

Question 141: Correct Answer: A) Administering tocolytic therapy
Rationale: Tocolytic therapy is the first-line treatment for preterm labor to inhibit uterine contractions and delay delivery. Encouraging ambulation and hydration may be helpful but not the primary intervention. Administering oxytocin for cervical ripening and scheduling an elective cesarean section are not appropriate in the management of preterm labor.

Question 142: Correct Answer: C) Notify the healthcare provider immediately.
Rationale: Heavy vaginal bleeding with clots exceeding one pad per hour in the postpartum period is indicative of postpartum hemorrhage, a potentially life-threatening complication. The nurse should promptly notify the healthcare provider to initiate appropriate interventions and prevent further complications. Options A, B, and D are incorrect as they do not address the urgency of the situation and the need for immediate medical attention in the case of postpartum hemorrhage.

Question 143: Correct Answer: B) Initiating phototherapy
Rationale: Phototherapy is the mainstay treatment for severe hyperbilirubinemia in newborns. It helps convert bilirubin into a form that can be excreted by the body. Encouraging more frequent breastfeeding, administering iron supplements, and increasing skin-to-skin contact are not primary interventions for managing severe hyperbilirubinemia. Iron supplements can actually exacerbate jaundice in some cases.

Question 144: Correct Answer: D) Clearing airway with suction and providing positive pressure ventilation
Rationale: During newborn resuscitation, the priority is to establish effective ventilation to ensure oxygenation. Administering intravenous fluids (Option A) is not a primary intervention during resuscitation. Providing warmth through a radiant warmer (Option B) is important but not the initial step in establishing ventilation. Performing chest compressions (Option C) is indicated if the newborn's heart rate remains below 60 bpm despite adequate ventilation. Clearing the airway with suction and providing positive pressure ventilation (Option D) is crucial to ensure air exchange and oxygen delivery, making it the correct answer.

Question 145: Correct Answer: D) Women with obesity have a higher risk of postpartum hemorrhage.
Rationale: Maternal obesity is a significant risk factor for postpartum hemorrhage due to factors such as increased blood volume, difficulty in assessing blood loss accurately, and impaired uterine contractility. Women with obesity are also at higher risk for cesarean section, gestational hypertension, gestational diabetes, macrosomia, and other complications. It is essential to provide comprehensive care and closely monitor these patients during pregnancy and childbirth to optimize outcomes and reduce risks.

Question 146: Correct Answer: B) Labial adhesions in female newborns
Rationale: Labial adhesions in female newborns are a common variation in the genitourinary system that may require further evaluation. This condition occurs when the labia minora stick together, often due to exposure to maternal hormones. It is important to assess the extent of adhesion and monitor for any complications such as urinary retention or recurrent urinary tract infections. The other options, presence of milia on the genitalia, umbilical hernia, and Mongolian spots on the buttocks, are unrelated to genitourinary variations in newborns.

Question 147: Correct Answer: D) Perform fundal massage to promote uterine contractions
Rationale: Fundal massage is a crucial nursing intervention to promote uterine contractions and control postpartum bleeding. Ambulation, oxytocin, and ice packs are not the first-line interventions for excessive postpartum bleeding. Ambulation may be encouraged later, oxytocin can be administered if fundal massage is ineffective, and ice packs are used for perineal discomfort, not to reduce bleeding.

Question 148: Correct Answer: A) "Breastfeeding provides essential nutrients and antibodies that help protect your baby from infections."
Rationale: Breastfeeding is highly recommended for newborns as it provides essential nutrients and antibodies that help protect them from infections. Option B is incorrect as breastfeeding is the optimal choice for infant nutrition. Option C is incorrect as breastfeeding is recommended for at least the first six months of life. Option D is incorrect as breastfeeding offers unique health benefits for both the baby and the mother.

Question 149: Correct Answer: C) Newborn screening blood test
Rationale: Newborn screening blood tests are routinely performed on newborns to detect various inborn errors of metabolism. These tests help identify conditions such as phenylketonuria, congenital hypothyroidism, and galactosemia early, allowing for prompt intervention and management. Electrocardiograms and chest X-rays are not typically used for screening metabolic disorders in newborns. While urinalysis can provide valuable information, it is not the primary method for detecting most inborn errors of metabolism in the neonatal period.

Question 150: Correct Answer: B) Preeclampsia
Rationale: Preexisting diabetes in pregnancy, such as type 1 or type 2 diabetes, increases the risk of developing preeclampsia. Preeclampsia is a serious condition characterized by high blood pressure and signs of damage to other organ systems, typically occurring after 20 weeks of pregnancy. Women with preexisting diabetes are at a higher risk of developing preeclampsia compared to those without diabetes due to the underlying vascular and metabolic changes associated with diabetes. Monitoring and managing blood pressure and other parameters are crucial in pregnant women with preexisting diabetes to prevent and manage complications like preeclampsia effectively.

RNC-MNN Practice Questions (SET 2)

Question 1: Ms. Smith brings her 2-day-old newborn to the clinic for a routine check-up. During the assessment, the nurse notices a bluish discoloration of the skin on the baby's hands and feet. What is the most likely cause of this finding?
A) Physiological jaundice
B) Acrocyanosis
C) Erythema toxicum
D) Mongolian spots

Question 2: Mrs. Smith, a postpartum mother, asks the nurse about receiving the influenza vaccine. Which statement by Mrs. Smith indicates a need for further education regarding the influenza vaccine during the postpartum period?
A) "I should wait until next year to get the influenza vaccine."
B) "I can receive the influenza vaccine while breastfeeding."
C) "It is important for me to protect myself and my baby from the flu."
D) "I should consult my healthcare provider before getting the influenza vaccine."

Question 3: Which of the following is a common sign of inadequate circulation in a newborn?
A) Capillary refill time less than 2 seconds
B) Warm extremities
C) Strong peripheral pulses
D) Pallor

Question 4: Baby James, a newborn, is diagnosed with early-onset neonatal sepsis and requires antibiotic therapy. Which anti-infective medication is commonly used as the first-line treatment for neonatal sepsis?
A) Vancomycin
B) Ampicillin
C) Ciprofloxacin
D) Clindamycin

Question 5: Which of the following is a risk factor for developing thrombophlebitis in the postpartum period?
A) Multiparity
B) Young maternal age
C) Regular ambulation
D) Low body mass index

Question 6: Which action is essential for newborn skin care to prevent heat loss and maintain skin integrity?
A) Applying lotion immediately after birth
B) Keeping the newborn uncovered
C) Delaying the first bath for 24 hours
D) Using a soft, warm blanket for swaddling

Question 7: Mrs. Smith, a 32-year-old primigravida at 39 weeks gestation, is admitted to the labor and delivery unit in active labor. After a prolonged second stage of labor, the fetal head is at +2 station, and the maternal pushing efforts are ineffective. The obstetrician decides to proceed with an operative vaginal delivery. Which method of operative delivery would be most appropriate in this situation?
A) Vacuum extraction
B) Forceps delivery
C) Cesarean section
D) Zavanelli maneuver

Question 8: Which component is not included in the Biophysical Profile (BPP) for fetal assessment?
A) Nonstress test
B) Amniotic fluid volume
C) Fetal heart rate monitoring
D) Maternal blood pressure monitoring

Question 9: Which intervention is a priority in the management of a newborn with pneumothorax?
A) Administering antibiotics
B) Providing oxygen therapy
C) Performing needle decompression
D) Initiating enteral feeding

Question 10: Which of the following is a risk factor for developing endometritis in the postpartum period?
A) Cesarean section delivery
B) Exclusive breastfeeding
C) Maternal age below 25 years
D) Pre-pregnancy BMI of 30

Question 11: Mrs. Smith, a 32-year-old pregnant woman, presents to the antenatal clinic for her routine check-up at 28 weeks of gestation. She has a history of chronic hypertension. During assessment, her blood pressure is 150/95 mmHg. Which of the following antepartum risk factors is most likely associated with Mrs. Smith's condition?
A) Gestational diabetes
B) Preterm labor
C) Placenta previa
D) Preeclampsia

Question 12: Which laboratory finding should be monitored closely in a newborn to assess for polycythemia?
A) Platelet count
B) Blood glucose level
C) Hematocrit level
D) Serum bilirubin level

Question 13: Which fetal factor may necessitate a cesarean delivery instead of a vaginal birth?
A) Fetal heart rate variability
B) Fetal macrosomia
C) Vertex presentation
D) Fetal scalp pH within normal range

Question 14: Baby James is born with phenylketonuria (PKU), a metabolic disorder. The nurse is discussing dietary management with the

parents. What should be the primary focus of the baby's diet?
A) High protein intake
B) Low carbohydrate intake
C) Low phenylalanine intake
D) High fat intake

Question 15: Which of the following is a characteristic feature of hypovolemic shock in postpartum women?
A) Bradycardia
B) Hypertension
C) Cool, clammy skin
D) Increased urine output

Question 16: What is the purpose of administering Rh Immune Globulin (RhoGAM) to an Rh-negative pregnant woman at 28 weeks gestation?
A) To prevent Rh incompatibility in the current pregnancy.
B) To treat Rh-positive antibodies already present in the mother's blood.
C) To prevent sensitization to Rh-positive blood cells in future pregnancies.
D) To stimulate the production of Rh antibodies in the mother.

Question 17: Which maternal age group is associated with an increased risk of chromosomal abnormalities in newborns?
A) 20-25 years
B) 30-35 years
C) 40-45 years
D) 50-55 years

Question 18: During a postpartum assessment, a nurse observes a new mother experiencing engorgement and nipple pain. The mother mentions that she has been using a breast pump to relieve the engorgement. What education should the nurse provide to address the nipple pain associated with engorgement?
A) Advise the mother to pump more frequently to empty the breasts completely
B) Recommend applying ice packs to the breasts before breastfeeding
C) Encourage the use of nipple shields to reduce pain during breastfeeding
D) Suggest warm compresses and gentle massage before breastfeeding

Question 19: Sarah, a 30-year-old mother, is worried about her milk supply as she feels her breasts are not engorged and her baby seems hungry after feeds. She mentions that she has been under a lot of stress lately. What intervention would be most beneficial in this situation?
A) Suggest using a breast pump after each feeding session
B) Recommend starting solid foods for the baby
C) Advise Sarah to drink herbal teas for milk production
D) Encourage relaxation techniques and stress management

Question 20: How can nurses demonstrate beneficence in maternal postpartum care?
A) Encouraging skin-to-skin contact between the mother and newborn.
B) Restricting visitation hours for family members.
C) Delaying essential vaccinations for the newborn.
D) Dismissing maternal concerns without discussion.

Question 21: Ms. Smith, a 38-year-old G2P1 at 39 weeks gestation, presents to the labor and delivery unit in active labor. She has a history of gestational diabetes and is a known smoker. During labor, thick meconium-stained amniotic fluid is noted. Fetal heart rate monitoring shows variable decelerations. The nurse should prioritize which intervention in the management of this situation?
A) Administer oxygen via face mask
B) Prepare for immediate delivery
C) Perform an amnioinfusion
D) Position the patient on her left side

Question 22: Which of the following antepartum risk factors is associated with an increased risk of preterm birth?
A) Maternal age over 35 years
B) Multiparity
C) Smoking during pregnancy
D) Normal BMI

Question 23: What is the recommended interval between a cesarean delivery and a trial of labor for a VBAC?
A) Less than 6 months
B) 12-18 months
C) 24-36 months
D) More than 48 months

Question 24: Which of the following statements best describes the importance of patient education in the postpartum period?
A) Patient education is not necessary in the postpartum period.
B) Patient education helps in promoting self-care and recovery.
C) Patient education should only be provided to first-time mothers.
D) Patient education is solely the responsibility of the healthcare provider.

Question 25: Scenario: Sarah, a full-term newborn, is exhibiting signs of respiratory distress shortly after birth. She is tachypneic with a respiratory rate of 70 breaths per minute, grunting, and mild retractions. Upon assessment, her oxygen saturation is 92%. The healthcare provider suspects Transient Tachypnea of the Newborn (TTN). What is the most appropriate initial nursing intervention for Sarah?
A) Initiate oxygen therapy
B) Perform chest physiotherapy
C) Administer intravenous antibiotics
D) Encourage breastfeeding

Question 26: Mrs. Smith, a postpartum mother, complains of urinary incontinence when she coughs or sneezes. Which of the following interventions would be most appropriate for her condition?
A) Encouraging her to limit fluid intake
B) Instructing her to perform Kegel exercises regularly

C) Administering diuretics to reduce urine production
D) Suggesting she avoids emptying her bladder frequently

Question 27: Mrs. Smith, a postpartum mother, asks the nurse about the importance of nutrition during breastfeeding. Which of the following statements by the nurse is accurate regarding maternal nutrition during lactation?
A) "Consuming caffeine in moderation can help increase milk production."
B) "It is essential to limit fluid intake to avoid engorgement."
C) "Including sources of Omega-3 fatty acids in your diet can benefit your baby's brain development."
D) "Skipping meals can help with weight loss while breastfeeding."

Question 28: During the postpartum period, which gastrointestinal change is commonly observed in women?
A) Increased gastric motility
B) Decreased gastric motility
C) Increased gastric acid secretion
D) Decreased gastric acid secretion

Question 29: Mrs. Johnson, a 35-year-old postpartum mother, is experiencing sleep disturbances characterized by frequent awakenings during the night to breastfeed her newborn. Which of the following strategies is most appropriate for improving Mrs. Johnson's sleep quality?
A) Co-sleeping with the baby to facilitate nighttime feedings
B) Limiting fluid intake before bedtime
C) Using over-the-counter sleep aids to promote sleep
D) Implementing a consistent bedtime routine for both herself and the baby

Question 30: Scenario: Baby James, born at 38 weeks gestation, is diagnosed with polycythemia. The nurse is educating the parents about the potential complications of polycythemia in newborns. Which statement by the parents indicates a need for further teaching?
A) "We should monitor James for signs of respiratory distress."
B) "We will ensure James stays well-hydrated."
C) "Polycythemia can increase the risk of blood clot formation."
D) "We will limit James' feedings to prevent complications."

Question 31: Which of the following is a potential risk associated with diagnostic ultrasound during pregnancy?
A) Increased risk of miscarriage
B) Fetal growth restriction
C) Development of fetal anomalies
D) Thermal effects on fetal tissues

Question 32: Which of the following statements regarding meconium aspiration syndrome (MAS) is true?
A) MAS occurs when the newborn inhales amniotic fluid contaminated with meconium during delivery.
B) MAS is more common in preterm infants than in term infants.
C) MAS is typically a benign condition with no potential for respiratory distress.
D) MAS is diagnosed based on the presence of clear amniotic fluid during delivery.

Question 33: Which insulin is typically administered 30 minutes before a meal?
A) Regular insulin
B) NPH insulin
C) Lispro insulin
D) Glargine insulin

Question 34: Which maternal postpartum assessment finding should raise concern for a potential cardiopulmonary complication?
A) Mild diaphoresis
B) Respiratory rate of 18 breaths per minute
C) Oxygen saturation of 98%
D) Sudden onset of shortness of breath

Question 35: During labor, a 28-year-old multiparous woman with a history of opioid use disorder requests pain relief. The healthcare provider decides to administer a non-opioid analgesic. Which of the following non-opioid analgesics is commonly used in labor due to its effectiveness in reducing pain without affecting the fetus?
A) Ibuprofen
B) Acetaminophen
C) Ketorolac
D) Aspirin

Question 36: Which of the following genetic disorders is characterized by an extra copy of chromosome 21?
A) Turner syndrome
B) Klinefelter syndrome
C) Down syndrome
D) Fragile X syndrome

Question 37: Mrs. Smith, a 28-year-old primiparous woman, gave birth to a healthy baby girl via spontaneous vaginal delivery. She appears tearful and expresses feelings of inadequacy in caring for her newborn. Which action by the nurse is most appropriate in supporting Mrs. Smith during her maternal role transition?
A) Encouraging Mrs. Smith to compare her experiences with those of other mothers
B) Providing Mrs. Smith with information on postpartum depression support groups
C) Advising Mrs. Smith to spend more time alone with her baby to build confidence
D) Suggesting Mrs. Smith to resume her pre-pregnancy activities immediately

Question 38: Afterpains are caused by:
A) Increased estrogen levels
B) Decreased uterine contractions
C) Relaxation of uterine muscles
D) Contractions of the uterus

Question 39: Mrs. Smith, a 32-year-old pregnant woman, is expecting twins. She is at 32 weeks of

gestation and presents to the antenatal clinic for a routine check-up. During the assessment, the nurse notes that Mrs. Smith has gained 40 pounds since the beginning of her pregnancy. Which of the following statements regarding weight gain in multiple gestation pregnancies is accurate?
A) Weight gain in multiple gestation pregnancies should be around 25-35 pounds.
B) Weight gain in multiple gestation pregnancies should be around 40-50 pounds.
C) Weight gain in multiple gestation pregnancies is not a significant factor to monitor.
D) Weight gain in multiple gestation pregnancies should be around 15-20 pounds.

Question 40: A new mother expresses concerns about her ability to breastfeed successfully. Which of the following actions by the nurse would best support the mother's maternal role transition in this situation?
A) Dismissing the mother's concerns and emphasizing the importance of breastfeeding.
B) Providing reassurance, guidance, and practical tips on breastfeeding techniques.
C) Criticizing the mother for her doubts and lack of confidence in breastfeeding.
D) Suggesting the mother switch to formula feeding to avoid stress and anxiety.

Question 41: Mrs. Smith, a postpartum mother, is considering introducing supplementary feedings to her newborn. Which statement by Mrs. Smith indicates a need for further education regarding the use of supplementary feedings?
A) "I plan to introduce a bottle of formula at every feeding to ensure my baby is getting enough nutrition."
B) "I will continue to breastfeed my baby on demand and offer a small amount of expressed breast milk after each feeding."
C) "I understand that introducing supplementary feedings too early can interfere with establishing a good breastfeeding relationship."
D) "I will consult with a lactation consultant before introducing any supplementary feedings to ensure proper guidance."

Question 42: During a postpartum assessment, the nurse notes that a patient who received oxytocin (Pitocin) is experiencing uterine atony and increased vaginal bleeding. The healthcare provider suspects uterine atony and prescribes methylergonovine (Methergine). What nursing intervention is essential when administering methylergonovine?
A) Administer methylergonovine intravenously.
B) Monitor for signs of hypertension during methylergonovine administration.
C) Encourage the patient to ambulate immediately after methylergonovine administration.
D) Administer methylergonovine to patients with a history of migraines.

Question 43: Ms. Johnson, a 32-year-old pregnant woman at 34 weeks gestation, presents to the labor and delivery unit with regular contractions every 5 minutes. She has a history of preterm labor in a previous pregnancy. The healthcare provider decides to administer a tocolytic medication to inhibit uterine contractions and delay preterm birth. Which of the following medications is commonly used as a tocolytic agent in this scenario?
A) Oxytocin
B) Magnesium sulfate
C) Misoprostol
D) Dinoprostone

Question 44: Mrs. Smith, a 28-year-old pregnant woman, is diagnosed with a urinary tract infection (UTI) during her third trimester. Which anti-infective medication is considered safe for use in pregnancy to treat UTIs?
A) Tetracycline
B) Trimethoprim
C) Nitrofurantoin
D) Fluconazole

Question 45: Emily, a 32-year-old woman, presents with symptoms of postpartum psychosis, including hallucinations, delusions, and disorganized behavior, one week after giving birth. What is the priority nursing intervention for Emily?
A) Administer antipsychotic medication as prescribed.
B) Encourage her to practice relaxation techniques.
C) Provide education on infant care and breastfeeding.
D) Refer her to outpatient counseling services.

Question 46: Ms. Smith, a 32-year-old pregnant woman at 34 weeks gestation, presents with excessive amniotic fluid accumulation. Which of the following maternal conditions is commonly associated with polyhydramnios?
A) Gestational diabetes
B) Chronic hypertension
C) Hypothyroidism
D) Iron-deficiency anemia

Question 47: Which anti-infective medication is commonly used to treat newborns with suspected or confirmed sepsis?
A) Acyclovir
B) Vancomycin
C) Ceftriaxone
D) Gentamicin

Question 48: What is the recommended route of administration for vitamin K in newborns to prevent hemorrhagic disease?
A) Intramuscular injection
B) Oral administration
C) Intravenous infusion
D) Subcutaneous injection

Question 49: During a routine newborn assessment, the nurse observes signs of pain and distress in a newborn prior to a minor procedure. The nurse decides to administer oral sucrose to help manage the newborn's pain. How soon before the procedure should the nurse administer the oral sucrose?
A) Immediately after the procedure
B) 30 minutes before the procedure
C) 15 minutes before the procedure
D) Just before the procedure

Question 50: Which of the following is a common complication seen in infants of diabetic mothers?
A) Hypoglycemia
B) Hypernatremia
C) Hypocalcemia
D) Hypokalemia

Question 51: Which endocrine disorder in the newborn is characterized by excessive production of thyroid hormone?
A) Congenital hypothyroidism
B) Neonatal diabetes mellitus
C) Neonatal Graves' disease
D) Neonatal hypoparathyroidism

Question 52: Ms. Johnson, a 32-year-old pregnant woman at 36 weeks gestation, presents with a decreased amniotic fluid index on ultrasound examination. She reports no leakage of fluid. Fetal monitoring shows no signs of distress. What is the most appropriate nursing intervention for Ms. Johnson?
A) Encourage increased fluid intake
B) Administer tocolytic therapy
C) Prepare for immediate delivery
D) Monitor fetal well-being closely

Question 53: Which equipment is essential for maternal postpartum assessment?
A) Baby monitor
B) Breast pump
C) Blood pressure cuff
D) Diaper changing station

Question 54: Which maternal factor can significantly impact the success of 'Latch On' during breastfeeding?
A) Engorged breasts
B) Using a nipple shield from the beginning
C) Feeding the baby on a strict schedule
D) Avoiding skin-to-skin contact with the baby

Question 55: During a newborn assessment, which finding would require immediate intervention?
A) Acrocyanosis
B) Heart rate of 180 beats per minute
C) Respiratory rate of 40 breaths per minute
D) Caput succedaneum

Question 56: During a postpartum assessment, Nurse Kelly observes that a new mother's breasts are engorged and tender. The mother is experiencing difficulty latching her baby due to the breast fullness. What advice should Nurse Kelly provide to help alleviate the mother's discomfort?
A) Use a breast pump to completely empty the breasts
B) Apply warm compresses before breastfeeding
C) Limit the baby's feeding time to prevent overstimulation
D) Massage the breasts vigorously to break up the engorgement

Question 57: Ms. Smith, a 2-day-old newborn, is admitted to the neonatal intensive care unit (NICU) with a diagnosis of apnea. The nurse is assessing the infant and notes that the baby is experiencing periodic breathing with pauses lasting less than 20 seconds. Which action should the nurse prioritize?
A) Administering oxygen therapy
B) Placing the infant in a prone position
C) Providing tactile stimulation to the baby
D) Initiating cardiopulmonary resuscitation (CPR)

Question 58: During labor, Mrs. Rodriguez, a multiparous woman, requests pain relief due to intense contractions. The healthcare provider decides to administer a medication that provides analgesia without affecting the progress of labor. Which medication is commonly used in labor for pain relief without impacting uterine contractions?
A) Fentanyl
B) Misoprostol
C) Butorphanol
D) Dinoprostone

Question 59: Mrs. Smith, a postpartum mother, is experiencing sore nipples while breastfeeding. Which intervention is most appropriate for her to promote healing and comfort?
A) Applying soap to nipples before each feeding
B) Using a lanolin-based nipple cream after each feeding
C) Wearing tight-fitting bras to reduce friction
D) Skipping feedings to allow nipples to rest

Question 60: During a postpartum education session, a new mother expresses concern about the type of formula to use for bottle-feeding her newborn. Which information should the nurse prioritize in guiding the mother's decision?
A) Choosing a formula with added sugars for taste.
B) Selecting a formula based on the baby's weight.
C) Opting for a formula with iron for newborns.
D) Using a formula with cow's milk for quicker growth.

Question 61: Which of the following is a crucial component of a comprehensive postpartum health assessment?
A) Assessing the newborn's vital signs
B) Evaluating the mother's emotional well-being
C) Measuring the newborn's weight
D) Checking the mother's blood type

Question 62: Which medication is typically administered to newborns to prevent ophthalmia neonatorum?
A) Erythromycin ointment
B) Acyclovir
C) Gentamicin
D) Nystatin

Question 63: Which screening tool is commonly used to assess for Congenital Heart Defects (CHD) in newborns?
A) Denver Developmental Screening Test
B) Apgar Score
C) Pulse Oximetry
D) Ballard Score

Question 64: Which statement is true regarding post-term pregnancy?
A) Post-term pregnancies are defined as those lasting beyond 42 weeks of gestation.

B) Post-term pregnancies are associated with a decreased risk of fetal complications.
C) Induction of labor is not recommended in post-term pregnancies.
D) Post-term pregnancies have a lower incidence of meconium-stained amniotic fluid.

Question 65: Which of the following is a characteristic feature of Cyanotic Heart Disease in newborns?
A) Increased pulmonary blood flow
B) Decreased oxygen saturation in the blood
C) Normal heart size on chest X-ray
D) Bradycardia

Question 66: During a postpartum assessment, Nurse Jones observes a mother struggling with engorged breasts and her baby showing signs of poor latch such as clicking noises while feeding. What could be a possible management strategy for this situation?
A) Encouraging the mother to pump milk before feedings
B) Suggesting the mother to switch to formula feeding
C) Advising the mother to stop breastfeeding temporarily
D) Recommending the use of nipple shields

Question 67: Which fetal heart rate pattern is indicative of fetal distress during labor?
A) Category I
B) Category II
C) Category III
D) Category IV

Question 68: A 28-year-old postpartum patient is diagnosed with septic shock secondary to endometritis. She presents with a temperature of 39.5℃, heart rate of 130 bpm, and hypotension. Which intervention is essential in the management of septic shock in this patient?
A) Administering a vasopressor medication
B) Initiating broad-spectrum antibiotics
C) Encouraging ambulation
D) Providing warm blankets for comfort

Question 69: Mrs. Smith, a 32-year-old pregnant woman at 36 weeks gestation, presents with symptoms of DIC (Disseminated Intravascular Coagulation). Which of the following findings is consistent with DIC in pregnancy?
A) Decreased platelet count
B) Elevated blood pressure
C) Increased fetal movements
D) Decreased uterine contractions

Question 70: Ms. Smith, a 28-year-old postpartum mother, complains of difficulty falling asleep and staying asleep since giving birth to her baby two weeks ago. She reports feeling anxious and overwhelmed. Which of the following interventions is most appropriate for managing her sleep disturbances?
A) Prescribing a sedative medication
B) Encouraging relaxation techniques before bedtime
C) Suggesting Ms. Smith to consume caffeine in the evening
D) Advising Ms. Smith to watch TV in bed to help her fall asleep

Question 71: Mrs. Smith gave birth to a full-term baby boy, John, who is now 3 days old. During the assessment, the nurse notes that John's skin appears slightly yellow. His total serum bilirubin level is 12 mg/dL. Which of the following interventions is most appropriate for managing John's hyperbilirubinemia?
A) Encouraging frequent breastfeeding sessions
B) Initiating phototherapy
C) Administering intravenous antibiotics
D) Supplementing with iron drops

Question 72: Which of the following is a common neurological complication in newborns?
A) Meconium Aspiration Syndrome
B) Necrotizing Enterocolitis
C) Hypoxic-Ischemic Encephalopathy
D) Patent Ductus Arteriosus

Question 73: After delivery, Ms. Johnson is prescribed oxytocin to prevent postpartum hemorrhage. Which of the following statements about oxytocin administration is correct?
A) Oxytocin should be administered rapidly as a bolus injection to ensure immediate effect.
B) Oxytocin can be safely given intramuscularly for faster absorption.
C) Oxytocin may cause hypotension as a side effect, so blood pressure should be monitored closely.
D) Oxytocin can be administered orally for convenience in postpartum patients.

Question 74: Baby James, born at 36 weeks gestation, is exhibiting signs of respiratory distress shortly after birth. The nurse observes nasal flaring, grunting, and chest retractions in the infant. Which of the following conditions is most likely causing these respiratory symptoms in Baby James?
A) Transient Tachypnea of the Newborn
B) Meconium Aspiration Syndrome
C) Respiratory Distress Syndrome
D) Pneumothorax

Question 75: Scenario: Baby James is scheduled for a circumcision procedure. The nurse is preparing the parents for the procedure and provides preoperative instructions. What information should the nurse include in the preoperative teaching?
A) Feeding the baby immediately before the procedure.
B) Administering aspirin to the baby for pain relief.
C) Bringing a pacifier to soothe the baby after the procedure.
D) Checking the circumcision site for bleeding every hour.

Question 76: Which maternal factor is a contraindication for a vaginal delivery?
A) Previous cesarean section
B) Maternal age over 35 years
C) Gestational diabetes
D) Maternal height less than 5 feet

Question 77: Ms. Smith, a 28-year-old postpartum

patient, asks the nurse about contraceptive options. She is breastfeeding her newborn. Which contraceptive method would be most suitable for Ms. Smith at this time?
A) Combined oral contraceptives
B) Progestin-only pills
C) Condoms
D) Intrauterine device (IUD)

Question 78: Baby James is a preterm newborn who requires special attention to his skin care needs. Which of the following practices is most appropriate for caring for the skin of a preterm newborn?
A) Avoiding the use of emollients or moisturizers on the skin.
B) Keeping the preterm newborn's skin exposed to air as much as possible.
C) Using a mild, fragrance-free soap for bathing the preterm newborn.
D) Applying alcohol-based products to disinfect the skin.

Question 79: At 36 weeks of gestation, Mrs. Johnson, a 28-year-old pregnant woman, reports experiencing persistent lower back pain and occasional contractions. She mentions feeling increasingly fatigued and notices swelling in her hands and face. Which of the following birth risk factors should the nurse consider in Mrs. Johnson's case?
A) Gestational diabetes
B) Preterm labor
C) Preeclampsia
D) Placenta previa

Question 80: Scenario: Emily, a 32-year-old postpartum mother, is diagnosed with postpartum psychosis and requires pharmacological intervention. Which psychotropic drug is often prescribed as a first-line treatment for postpartum psychosis?
A) Fluoxetine
B) Quetiapine
C) Alprazolam
D) Bupropion

Question 81: During a routine postpartum assessment, the nurse notices that a newborn baby girl is exhibiting signs of respiratory distress, including grunting and nasal flaring. Which of the following actions should the nurse prioritize in this situation?
A) Administering oral glucose gel
B) Placing the baby in a prone position
C) Providing oxygen therapy
D) Offering a pacifier for comfort

Question 82: Which of the following statements best describes perinatal grief?
A) Perinatal grief is only experienced by mothers.
B) Perinatal grief is a normal response to a significant loss during pregnancy or after birth.
C) Perinatal grief is always resolved within a few weeks after the loss.
D) Perinatal grief is solely influenced by biological factors.

Question 83: Mrs. Smith, a 28-year-old pregnant woman, is in labor after a previous cesarean section. She is considering a VBAC but is concerned about the risk of uterine rupture. Which of the following is a risk factor that may increase the likelihood of uterine rupture during a VBAC?
A) Maternal age over 35 years
B) Induction of labor with prostaglandins
C) Fetal macrosomia
D) Spontaneous onset of labor

Question 84: Which of the following is a risk factor for placental abruption?
A) Maternal hypertension
B) Prolonged rupture of membranes
C) Fetal macrosomia
D) Maternal age under 20 years

Question 85: Mrs. Smith has just given birth to a healthy baby boy. As part of the newborn care, the nurse explains the importance of administering Vitamin K to prevent a potential bleeding disorder. Which of the following statements regarding Vitamin K administration in newborns is accurate?
A) Vitamin K is given orally to newborns to prevent hemorrhagic disease of the newborn.
B) Intramuscular administration of Vitamin K is the preferred route for newborns.
C) Topical application of Vitamin K is the most effective method for absorption in newborns.
D) Vitamin K is not necessary for newborns as they receive enough from breast milk.

Question 86: Which endocrine gland is responsible for producing oxytocin and vasopressin, important hormones during labor and lactation?
A) Thyroid gland
B) Adrenal gland
C) Pituitary gland
D) Pancreas

Question 87: During a postpartum education session, a new mother expresses her wish to delay the administration of routine vaccinations to her newborn due to concerns about potential side effects. Which ethical principle is most relevant in this situation?
A) Fidelity
B) Veracity
C) Autonomy
D) Paternalism

Question 88: Which type of shock is most commonly associated with amniotic fluid embolism in the postpartum period?
A) Cardiogenic shock
B) Distributive shock
C) Obstructive shock
D) Hypovolemic shock

Question 89: What is a common risk factor for the development of a hematoma in the postpartum period?
A) Prolonged bed rest
B) Regular application of cold packs
C) Adequate intake of vitamin C
D) Instrument-assisted delivery

Question 90: Which of the following is a common variation in newborn integumentary assessment that is considered normal and typically resolves within a few weeks after birth?
A) Milia
B) Petechiae
C) Jaundice
D) Mongolian spots

Question 91: Mrs. Smith, a postpartum mother, complains of severe breast pain and swelling. On assessment, her breasts are warm, tender, and firm. She mentions that her baby is having difficulty latching. What is the most appropriate nursing intervention for Mrs. Smith's condition?
A) Encourage frequent breastfeeding sessions
B) Apply ice packs to the breasts
C) Advise Mrs. Smith to avoid breastfeeding until the engorgement resolves
D) Suggest using a breast pump to empty the breasts

Question 92: What is the primary purpose of performing a lumbar puncture in a newborn?
A) To administer intrathecal medications
B) To measure intracranial pressure
C) To obtain cerebrospinal fluid for analysis
D) To assess for spinal cord abnormalities

Question 93: Mrs. Smith, a postpartum mother, is bottle-feeding her newborn. She asks the nurse about the appropriate feeding schedule for her baby. What is the nurse's best response?
A) "Feed your baby every 4 hours during the day and every 6 hours at night."
B) "Offer your baby formula every 2 hours to ensure adequate nutrition."
C) "Let your baby decide when they are hungry and feed on demand."
D) "Feed your baby every 3 hours around the clock."

Question 94: Ms. Johnson, a 32-year-old postpartum mother, is diagnosed with a urinary tract infection (UTI) following a cesarean section. Which nursing intervention is essential to prevent UTI recurrence in Ms. Johnson?
A) Encourage frequent voiding
B) Administer prophylactic antibiotics
C) Promote cranberry juice consumption
D) Educate on proper hand hygiene

Question 95: Which of the following is a potential complication of amniocentesis?
A) Maternal hemorrhage
B) Fetal macrosomia
C) Placental abruption
D) Polyhydramnios

Question 96: During a postpartum assessment, a nurse observes that a 25-year-old mother is experiencing afterpains. The mother asks why she is feeling these cramps. How should the nurse best explain the cause of afterpains to the mother?
A) "Afterpains occur due to excessive fluid intake during labor."
B) "Afterpains are caused by the stretching of the uterus during pregnancy."
C) "Afterpains happen as a result of hormonal changes after childbirth."
D) "Afterpains are due to the baby's movements inside the uterus."

Question 97: Which action is most appropriate for the nurse to take when facilitating maternal/newborn bonding and preventing separation immediately after birth?
A) Encouraging skin-to-skin contact between the mother and newborn
B) Placing the newborn in a separate bassinet for observation
C) Allowing only brief contact between the mother and newborn
D) Initiating formula feeding to establish a routine

Question 98: Which antenatal factor is a protective factor against the development of gestational diabetes mellitus (GDM)?
A) Family history of diabetes
B) Obesity
C) Regular physical activity
D) Previous history of GDM

Question 99: Which postpartum infection is characterized by red, tender, warm, and swollen breasts, often accompanied by flu-like symptoms such as fever and chills?
A) Endometritis
B) Mastitis
C) Wound infection
D) Urinary tract infection

Question 100: Mrs. Smith, a 32-year-old postpartum mother, complains of rectal pain and discomfort during defecation. On assessment, you notice swollen, tender masses around her anus. What is the most appropriate nursing intervention for Mrs. Smith's condition?
A) Encourage a high-fiber diet and adequate fluid intake
B) Apply ice packs to the affected area
C) Administer a stool softener medication
D) Suggest warm sitz baths for relief

Question 101: During the assessment of a postpartum mother who had an epidural, the nurse notes the presence of a postural headache that improves when the patient lies flat. What intervention should the nurse prioritize?
A) Encourage increased caffeine intake
B) Administer a muscle relaxant
C) Initiate intravenous fluid hydration
D) Perform a blood patch procedure

Question 102: Mrs. Smith, a postpartum mother, complains of sore and cracked nipples while breastfeeding her newborn. Upon assessment, the nurse notes that the nipples appear red, cracked, and painful. What is the most appropriate nursing intervention for Mrs. Smith's condition?
A) Encourage the use of a nipple shield during breastfeeding
B) Apply lanolin cream to the nipples after each feeding
C) Suggest using soap to clean the nipples before

breastfeeding
D) Advise Mrs. Smith to continue breastfeeding despite the pain

Question 103: Which ethical issue is crucial to address when providing postpartum education to a culturally diverse population?
A) Respect for autonomy
B) Confidentiality
C) Justice
D) Beneficence

Question 104: Which antepartum risk factor is commonly associated with multiple gestation pregnancies?
A) Maternal age over 35 years
B) History of infertility treatments
C) Low pre-pregnancy body mass index (BMI)
D) History of previous uncomplicated singleton pregnancy

Question 105: Which of the following statements best describes a hematoma in the context of maternal postpartum complications?
A) A collection of blood outside blood vessels
B) A benign skin condition
C) Excessive hair loss postpartum
D) A type of bacterial infection

Question 106: Which ethical principle involves the healthcare provider's obligation to do no harm and prevent harm to the patient?
A) Autonomy
B) Beneficence
C) Nonmaleficence
D) Justice

Question 107: Which of the following is a correct technique for bottle feeding a newborn?
A) Holding the bottle parallel to the floor
B) Using a fast-flow nipple to speed up feeding
C) Allowing the baby to feed while lying flat on their back
D) Holding the baby in an upright position during feeding

Question 108: Scenario: Mrs. Smith, a postpartum mother, requests not to have her newborn baby receive any vaccinations due to personal beliefs. She expresses concerns about the potential risks associated with vaccinations. What ethical principle should the nurse prioritize in this situation?
A) Autonomy
B) Beneficence
C) Nonmaleficence
D) Justice

Question 109: Mrs. Smith, a 32-year-old postpartum mother, presents with unilateral leg pain, swelling, and redness. She is diagnosed with superficial thrombophlebitis. What is the most appropriate nursing intervention for Mrs. Smith?
A) Apply warm compresses to the affected leg
B) Administer anticoagulant therapy
C) Encourage ambulation and leg elevation
D) Perform a venous Doppler ultrasound

Question 110: Mrs. Smith, a 28-year-old postpartum mother, complains of feeling lightheaded and dizzy when standing up. Which of the following physiological changes contributes to this symptom in the postpartum period?
A) Increased blood pressure
B) Decreased cardiac output
C) Elevated estrogen levels
D) Reduced blood volume

Question 111: Mrs. Smith, a G2P1 mother, gave birth to a newborn baby boy. The baby is diagnosed with ABO incompatibility due to the mother being blood type O positive and the baby being blood type A positive. Which of the following signs and symptoms is most likely to be observed in the newborn with ABO incompatibility?
A) Jaundice within 24 hours of birth
B) Hypoglycemia
C) Respiratory distress
D) Bradycardia

Question 112: Mrs. Smith, a 38-year-old pregnant woman, is concerned about the potential risks associated with her age during pregnancy. Which of the following statements regarding advanced maternal age is true?
A) Advanced maternal age is defined as 35 years or older.
B) Advanced maternal age is defined as 40 years or older.
C) Advanced maternal age is defined as 30 years or older.
D) Advanced maternal age is defined as 45 years or older.

Question 113: During a postpartum assessment, the nurse notes that a mother's episiotomy site is red, swollen, and has purulent drainage. What is the priority nursing action in this situation?
A) Apply ice packs to the episiotomy site
B) Instruct the mother to perform sitz baths
C) Notify the healthcare provider immediately
D) Administer over-the-counter pain medication

Question 114: Mrs. Johnson, a 34-year-old G2P2 postpartum patient, presents with a first-degree vaginal laceration following a spontaneous vaginal delivery. Which of the following statements regarding first-degree vaginal lacerations is accurate?
A) They involve the perineal muscles and extend into the anal sphincter.
B) Repair of first-degree lacerations requires suturing in the operating room.
C) First-degree lacerations are the most severe type of vaginal lacerations.
D) These lacerations involve only the vaginal mucosa and do not extend into the underlying tissues.

Question 115: What is a potential risk associated with the early introduction of complementary feedings in newborns?
A) Improved weight gain
B) Reduced risk of allergies
C) Increased risk of gastrointestinal infections
D) Enhanced breastfeeding success

Question 116: Mrs. Smith has just given birth to a healthy newborn baby boy. During the assessment, the nurse notes that the baby has not passed meconium within the first 24 hours after birth. What action should the nurse take?
A) Encourage the mother to breastfeed more frequently
B) Administer a glycerin suppository to stimulate bowel movement
C) Monitor the baby closely and document findings
D) Perform a rectal stimulation to help the baby pass meconium

Question 117: Scenario: Baby James, a term newborn, is brought to the pediatric clinic by his parents for a routine check-up. During the assessment, the nurse observes that James has poor muscle tone, weak suck, and diminished reflexes. The healthcare provider suspects a neurological complication. Which condition should be considered in this newborn?
A) Spina bifida
B) Hypoxic-ischemic encephalopathy
C) Intraventricular hemorrhage
D) Kernicterus

Question 118: A newborn infant is admitted to the neonatal intensive care unit (NICU) with respiratory distress shortly after birth. The infant is receiving oxygen therapy via nasal cannula. Despite oxygen supplementation, the infant's respiratory distress worsens, and chest X-ray shows a collapsed lung with mediastinal shift. What is the most appropriate initial nursing intervention for this infant?
A) Increase the oxygen flow rate
B) Notify the healthcare provider immediately
C) Perform chest physiotherapy
D) Position the infant on the affected side

Question 119: After giving birth, a new mother reports experiencing pain and burning sensation while urinating. Which of the following assessments should the nurse prioritize?
A) Checking for signs of urinary retention
B) Assessing for signs of urinary tract infection (UTI)
C) Monitoring for symptoms of kidney stones
D) Evaluating for pelvic organ prolapse

Question 120: Which statement regarding Hepatitis B Immunoglobulin (HBIG) administration in newborns is accurate?
A) HBIG is given to newborns within 12 hours of birth if the mother is HBsAg positive.
B) HBIG is routinely administered to all newborns regardless of maternal HBsAg status.
C) HBIG is contraindicated in newborns with low birth weight.
D) HBIG is administered orally to newborns for better absorption.

Question 121: Which maternal factor is NOT associated with an increased risk of shoulder dystocia during labor?
A) Maternal diabetes
B) Maternal obesity
C) Maternal age <20 years
D) Maternal pelvic anatomy

Question 122: Scenario: Emily, a 28-year-old woman with pre-existing diabetes, delivered a baby girl at 39 weeks of gestation. The infant is at risk for respiratory distress syndrome due to maternal diabetes. Which of the following statements regarding respiratory distress syndrome in infants of diabetic mothers is accurate?
A) Infants of diabetic mothers are at decreased risk for respiratory distress syndrome.
B) The risk of respiratory distress syndrome in infants of diabetic mothers is not influenced by maternal glycemic control.
C) Surfactant production is typically increased in infants of diabetic mothers, reducing the risk of respiratory distress syndrome.
D) Infants of diabetic mothers may require surfactant replacement therapy to manage respiratory distress syndrome.

Question 123: What intervention is essential in managing polycythemia/hyperviscosity in newborns?
A) Encouraging increased fluid intake
B) Administering iron supplements
C) Initiating phototherapy
D) Performing partial exchange transfusion

Question 124: During a postpartum education session, a new mother asks about the safety of using acetaminophen while breastfeeding. How should the nurse respond?
A) "Acetaminophen is safe to use while breastfeeding."
B) "You should avoid using acetaminophen while breastfeeding."
C) "Breastfeeding is safe only if you pump and discard the milk for 24 hours after using acetaminophen."
D) "You should stop breastfeeding completely while using acetaminophen."

Question 125: When should the cord stump typically fall off in a newborn?
A) Within 24 hours after birth
B) Within 1 week after birth
C) Within 2 weeks after birth
D) Within 4 weeks after birth

Question 126: Which of the following is a common musculoskeletal variation in newborns that typically resolves on its own without intervention?
A) Polydactyly
B) Syndactyly
C) Talipes equinovarus
D) Physiologic flexion contractures

Question 127: Mrs. Smith, a postpartum mother, is breastfeeding her newborn. She asks the nurse about her nutritional needs during lactation. Which of the following nutrients is essential for Mrs. Smith to consume in increased amounts while breastfeeding?
A) Iron
B) Vitamin C
C) Calcium
D) Protein

Question 128: Mrs. Smith, a 28-year-old pregnant woman, presents to the clinic with symptoms of fever, rash, and joint pain. She reports recent travel to an area with a Zika virus outbreak. What is the most appropriate nursing intervention for Mrs. Smith?
A) Administering antibiotics
B) Providing supportive care and monitoring fetal ultrasound
C) Initiating antiviral therapy
D) Recommending bed rest

Question 129: During a postpartum assessment, the nurse observes cracked nipples on a breastfeeding mother, Mrs. Johnson. Which action should the nurse recommend to promote healing and prevent infection?
A) Applying alcohol-based solutions to nipples before feeding
B) Air-drying nipples after each feeding
C) Using scented lotions on nipples for fragrance
D) Applying breast milk to nipples after feeding

Question 130: During a prenatal visit, Mrs. Johnson inquires about the benefits of cell-free DNA testing. Which of the following statements accurately describes cell-free DNA testing in pregnancy?
A) It can detect all types of birth defects
B) It is recommended for all pregnant women regardless of risk factors
C) It analyzes fetal DNA circulating in the mother's blood
D) It is a diagnostic test that provides definitive results

Question 131: Baby James is born to a 28-year-old G1P0 mother at 41 weeks gestation. He is delivered via emergency cesarean section due to fetal distress secondary to meconium-stained amniotic fluid. Upon assessment, Baby James presents with respiratory distress, cyanosis, and coarse breath sounds. The nurse should suspect which complication in this newborn?
A) Transient tachypnea of the newborn
B) Pneumothorax
C) Meconium aspiration syndrome
D) Respiratory distress syndrome

Question 132: Which of the following is a common problem in the postpartum period that requires nursing intervention?
A) Breast engorgement
B) Delayed cord clamping
C) Newborn jaundice
D) Maternal hypertension

Question 133: Which assessment finding in a newborn requires immediate intervention?
A) Presence of milia on the nose
B) Absence of red reflex in the eyes
C) Slight ear asymmetry
D) Nasal flaring during breathing

Question 134: What is a key nursing intervention for a woman experiencing precipitous delivery?
A) Encouraging slow breathing techniques
B) Administering oxytocin to speed up labor
C) Supporting the perineum to prevent tearing
D) Preparing for rapid delivery in a safe environment

Question 135: Ms. Johnson, a 28-year-old pregnant woman at 32 weeks gestation, presents to the antenatal clinic with complaints of fatigue, weakness, and shortness of breath. Her blood work reveals a hemoglobin level of 9 g/dL. Which type of anemia is most likely affecting Ms. Johnson?
A) Iron-deficiency anemia
B) Folate deficiency anemia
C) Vitamin B12 deficiency anemia
D) Hemolytic anemia

Question 136: Which of the following is a risk factor for cord prolapse during labor?
A) Multiple gestation
B) Post-term pregnancy
C) Maternal obesity
D) Premature rupture of membranes

Question 137: Ms. Johnson, a postpartum mother, is experiencing severe postpartum depression. She is hesitant to seek help due to fear of being judged. As a nurse, what is the most appropriate action to take in this situation?
A) Encourage Ms. Johnson to keep her feelings to herself
B) Provide Ms. Johnson with resources for mental health support
C) Disregard Ms. Johnson's concerns as they are common postpartum
D) Advise Ms. Johnson to ignore her emotions and focus on the baby

Question 138: Which of the following medications should be avoided in postpartum women with GI motility issues due to its potential to worsen constipation?
A) Bisacodyl
B) Psyllium
C) Docusate sodium
D) Loperamide

Question 139: Which of the following best describes a Nonstress Test (NST) in fetal assessment during pregnancy?
A) It assesses fetal heart rate in response to fetal movement.
B) It measures amniotic fluid volume around the fetus.
C) It evaluates uterine contractions during labor.
D) It monitors maternal blood pressure changes during pregnancy.

Question 140: Which maternal antibody is responsible for causing hemolysis in newborns with ABO incompatibility?
A) Anti-Rh(D)
B) Anti-A
C) Anti-B
D) Anti-D

Question 141: Baby James is born with a congenital heart defect and requires medication to help manage his condition. Which of the following drugs is commonly used in newborns with congenital heart

defects to improve cardiac function?
A) Albuterol
B) Digoxin
C) Ibuprofen
D) Loratadine

Question 142: Ms. Smith, a 28-year-old woman, gave birth to a baby girl two days ago. The newborn is diagnosed with hemolytic disease of the newborn due to ABO incompatibility. The nurse assesses the baby and notes pallor, jaundice, and hepatosplenomegaly. The baby's hemoglobin level is 10 g/dL. What type of anemia is the newborn most likely experiencing?
A) Iron-deficiency anemia
B) Aplastic anemia
C) Hemolytic anemia
D) Sickle cell anemia

Question 143: During a newborn assessment, which finding would require immediate intervention?
A) Acrocyanosis
B) Heart rate of 180 bpm
C) Respiratory rate of 40 breaths per minute
D) Caput succedaneum

Question 144: Scenario: Baby Emma is born at 38 weeks gestation via spontaneous vaginal delivery. She is placed skin-to-skin with her mother immediately after birth. What is the most appropriate action by the nurse to promote thermoregulation in this newborn?
A) Delay drying the baby to enhance skin-to-skin contact
B) Place a hat on the baby's head
C) Wrap the baby in a warm blanket
D) Transfer the baby to a radiant warmer

Question 145: During a lactation consultation, a new mother expresses concerns about the color of her stored breast milk. She mentions that the milk she pumped earlier looks different from the milk she pumped later in the day. What information should the nurse provide to address the mother's concerns?
A) Assure the mother that changes in breast milk color are normal and can vary throughout the day.
B) Advise the mother to discard the milk that looks different as it may be spoiled.
C) Suggest the mother consume more water to improve the color consistency of her breast milk.
D) Recommend the mother switch to formula feeding to avoid variations in breast milk color.

Question 146: Ms. Johnson, a 28-year-old postpartum woman, complains of sudden chest pain and difficulty breathing after a cesarean section. She is 2 days postpartum. On examination, she has tachycardia, tachypnea, and low-grade fever. What diagnostic test is most appropriate to confirm suspected pulmonary embolus in Ms. Johnson?
A) D-dimer assay
B) Pulmonary angiography
C) Chest CT angiography
D) Ventilation-perfusion scan

Question 147: Which nutrient is crucial for the prevention of neural tube defects in the fetus during pregnancy?
A) Vitamin C
B) Iron
C) Folic Acid
D) Vitamin D

Question 148: During a routine antenatal visit, Mrs. Johnson, a 25-year-old pregnant woman at 36 weeks gestation, complains of feeling lightheaded and dizzy. Her blood pressure is 100/60 mmHg, and her hemoglobin level is 10 g/dL. Which of the following lab values is most likely to be decreased in this scenario?
A) Serum Calcium
B) Serum Potassium
C) Hematocrit
D) Platelet Count

Question 149: During a newborn integumentary assessment, the nurse notices a bluish discoloration of the hands and feet. This finding is most likely indicative of:
A) Acrocyanosis
B) Erythema toxicum
C) Harlequin color change
D) Cutis marmorata

Question 150: Ms. Smith brings her newborn to the clinic for a routine check-up. During the musculoskeletal assessment, the nurse notes asymmetry in the gluteal skinfolds. Which condition should the nurse suspect in the newborn?
A) Developmental Dysplasia of the Hip (DDH)
B) Clubfoot (Talipes Equinovarus)
C) Osteogenesis Imperfecta
D) Congenital Torticollis

ANSWERS WITH DETAILED EXPLANATION (SET 2)

Question 1: Correct Answer: B) Acrocyanosis
Rationale: Acrocyanosis is a common finding in newborns characterized by a bluish discoloration of the hands and feet due to peripheral vasoconstriction. It is considered a normal finding in the immediate newborn period and typically resolves within a few days without any intervention. Physiological jaundice (Option A) presents as yellowing of the skin and sclera due to elevated bilirubin levels. Erythema toxicum (Option C) is a benign rash that appears as pink or red blotches with small pustules. Mongolian spots (Option D) are blue-gray pigmented areas often seen in darker-skinned infants.

Question 2: Correct Answer: A) "I should wait until next year to get the influenza vaccine."
Rationale: Mrs. Smith should not wait until next year to get the influenza vaccine, as it is recommended for postpartum mothers to receive the vaccine during flu season to protect themselves and their newborns. Option B is correct as postpartum mothers can safely receive the influenza vaccine while breastfeeding. Option C highlights the importance of flu protection for both mother and baby. Option D emphasizes the importance of consulting a healthcare provider before vaccination.

Question 3: Correct Answer: D) Pallor
Rationale: Pallor is a common sign of inadequate circulation in a newborn, indicating poor oxygenation and blood flow. Pallor can be observed in the skin, mucous membranes, and nail beds. In contrast, options A, B, and C are signs of good circulation. Capillary refill time less than 2 seconds, warm extremities, and strong peripheral pulses are indicative of adequate perfusion and oxygenation in newborns.

Question 4: Correct Answer: B) Ampicillin
Rationale: Ampicillin is commonly used as the first-line treatment for neonatal sepsis due to its effectiveness against the most common pathogens causing neonatal sepsis, such as Group B Streptococcus. Vancomycin (Option A) is reserved for penicillin-allergic patients or in cases of resistant organisms. Ciprofloxacin (Option C) is not recommended in neonates due to potential adverse effects on cartilage development. Clindamycin (Option D) is not typically used as a first-line agent for neonatal sepsis.

Question 5: Correct Answer: A) Multiparity
Rationale: Multiparity, or having multiple pregnancies, is a known risk factor for developing thrombophlebitis in the postpartum period due to the increased strain on the venous system. Young maternal age (Option B) is not a significant risk factor for thrombophlebitis. Regular ambulation (Option C) is actually a preventive measure against thrombophlebitis as it promotes circulation. A low body mass index (Option D) is not directly linked to an increased risk of thrombophlebitis.

Question 6: Correct Answer: D) Using a soft, warm blanket for swaddling
Rationale: Newborns are at risk for heat loss due to their high surface area to body weight ratio. Using a soft, warm blanket for swaddling helps to prevent heat loss by providing insulation. Applying lotion immediately after birth (Option A) can interfere with the natural vernix on the skin, which serves as a protective barrier. Keeping the newborn uncovered (Option B) exposes them to heat loss. Delaying the first bath for 24 hours (Option C) is beneficial to allow for the absorption of vernix, which helps in skin protection.

Question 7: Correct Answer: A) Vacuum extraction
Rationale: Vacuum extraction is a suitable method in this scenario due to the fetal head being at +2 station and the ineffective maternal pushing efforts. Forceps delivery may be challenging at this station, and a Cesarean section is usually reserved for cases where vacuum or forceps delivery are contraindicated. The Zavanelli maneuver involves pushing the fetal head back into the uterus, which is not indicated in this case.

Question 8: Correct Answer: D) Maternal blood pressure monitoring
Rationale: The Biophysical Profile (BPP) assesses five components: fetal breathing movements, fetal movements, fetal tone, amniotic fluid volume, and fetal heart rate monitoring. Maternal blood pressure monitoring is not a part of the BPP. This assessment focuses solely on evaluating the fetal well-being and does not involve monitoring the mother's blood pressure.

Question 9: Correct Answer: C) Performing needle decompression
Rationale: Performing needle decompression is a priority intervention in the management of a newborn with pneumothorax. This procedure involves inserting a needle into the pleural space to release trapped air and relieve pressure on the lungs and heart. Administering antibiotics may be necessary if there is an infection present, oxygen therapy can support respiratory function, and enteral feeding is important for nutrition but not a priority in the acute management of pneumothorax.

Question 10: Correct Answer: A) Cesarean section delivery
Rationale: Endometritis is more commonly associated with cesarean section deliveries due to the increased risk of infection during the surgical procedure. The incision made during a cesarean section provides a potential entry point for bacteria, leading to an increased risk of endometritis. Exclusive breastfeeding, maternal age, and pre-pregnancy BMI are not direct risk factors for developing endometritis.

Question 11: Correct Answer: D) Preeclampsia
Rationale: Chronic hypertension is a significant antepartum risk factor for developing preeclampsia. Preeclampsia is characterized by new-onset hypertension after 20 weeks of gestation along with proteinuria or end-organ dysfunction. While gestational diabetes, preterm labor, and placenta previa are also important antepartum complications, they are not directly linked to chronic hypertension as preeclampsia is.

Question 12: Correct Answer: C) Hematocrit level
Rationale: Hematocrit level should be monitored closely in newborns to assess for polycythemia, a condition characterized by an elevated red blood cell count. Monitoring platelet count, blood glucose level, or serum bilirubin level is not specific for assessing polycythemia in newborns. Polycythemia can lead to complications such as hyperviscosity and thrombosis, making hematocrit monitoring essential.

Question 13: Correct Answer: B) Fetal macrosomia
Rationale: Fetal macrosomia, which refers to a larger-than-average baby, can increase the risk of shoulder dystocia and birth complications, often necessitating a

cesarean delivery. Fetal heart rate variability (option A) is a reassuring sign of fetal well-being. Vertex presentation (option C) is the ideal fetal position for a vaginal birth. Fetal scalp pH within the normal range (option D) indicates fetal well-being and is not a factor that would require a cesarean delivery.

Question 14: Correct Answer: C) Low phenylalanine intake
Rationale: Phenylketonuria (PKU) is managed by restricting phenylalanine intake through a special low-protein diet. High protein intake (Option A) is contraindicated as it can lead to the accumulation of phenylalanine. Low carbohydrate intake (Option B) and high fat intake (Option D) are not the primary focus of the diet in PKU management. By limiting phenylalanine intake, the baby can prevent intellectual disabilities and other complications associated with PKU.

Question 15: Correct Answer: C) Cool, clammy skin
Rationale: Hypovolemic shock in postpartum women is characterized by cool, clammy skin due to vasoconstriction and decreased perfusion. Bradycardia is not typically seen in hypovolemic shock as the body compensates by increasing heart rate. Hypertension is also not a common finding in hypovolemic shock, as blood pressure tends to decrease. Additionally, in hypovolemic shock, urine output decreases as the body tries to conserve fluid, so increased urine output is an incorrect option.

Question 16: Correct Answer: C) To prevent sensitization to Rh-positive blood cells in future pregnancies.
Rationale: Administering Rh Immune Globulin (RhoGAM) to an Rh-negative pregnant woman at 28 weeks gestation is done to prevent sensitization to Rh-positive blood cells in future pregnancies. By receiving RhoGAM at this stage, the mother's immune system is suppressed from producing antibodies against Rh-positive blood cells, reducing the risk of complications in subsequent pregnancies. Options A, B, and D are incorrect as RhoGAM does not prevent Rh incompatibility in the current pregnancy, treat existing Rh-positive antibodies, or stimulate the production of Rh antibodies in the mother.

Question 17: Correct Answer: C) 40-45 years
Rationale: Maternal age is a crucial factor in determining the risk of chromosomal abnormalities in newborns. Women aged 40-45 years have a higher risk due to the increased likelihood of errors in chromosomal division during egg formation. This age group faces a higher incidence of conditions such as Down syndrome in newborns. Options A, B, and D are incorrect as they represent younger age groups where the risk of chromosomal abnormalities is comparatively lower due to more robust reproductive health and lower chances of genetic errors during cell division.

Question 18: Correct Answer: D) Suggest warm compresses and gentle massage before breastfeeding
Rationale: Warm compresses help to promote milk flow and reduce discomfort associated with engorgement. Gentle massage can help to soften the breasts and facilitate milk removal. Pumping more frequently may exacerbate engorgement, while ice packs can decrease milk supply and worsen the issue. Nipple shields are not recommended for engorgement and may lead to further complications.

Question 19: Correct Answer: D) Encourage relaxation techniques and stress management
Rationale: Stress can negatively impact milk supply. Encouraging relaxation techniques and stress management can help improve milk production. Using a breast pump after each feeding session may signal the body to produce more milk than needed, leading to oversupply. Starting solid foods for the baby is not recommended before 6 months of age. Herbal teas may have limited evidence in increasing milk supply and should be used with caution.

Question 20: Correct Answer: A) Encouraging skin-to-skin contact between the mother and newborn.
Rationale: Encouraging skin-to-skin contact between the mother and newborn promotes bonding, breastfeeding, and emotional well-being, aligning with the ethical principle of beneficence. Options B, C, and D do not uphold beneficence as they involve restricting family involvement, delaying necessary vaccinations, and dismissing maternal concerns, which can negatively impact the mother and newborn's health and relationship-building.

Question 21: Correct Answer: B) Prepare for immediate delivery
Rationale: In the scenario of meconium-stained amniotic fluid with variable decelerations, immediate delivery is crucial to prevent further complications such as meconium aspiration syndrome. Administering oxygen, performing an amnioinfusion, and positioning the patient on her left side are important interventions but do not take precedence over the need for prompt delivery in this critical situation.

Question 22: Correct Answer: C) Smoking during pregnancy
Rationale: Smoking during pregnancy is a well-established risk factor for preterm birth. Nicotine and other harmful chemicals in cigarettes can lead to placental insufficiency, which may result in preterm labor. Maternal age over 35 years, multiparity, and normal BMI are not directly linked to preterm birth. While advanced maternal age can pose other risks, such as chromosomal abnormalities, it is not a primary risk factor for preterm birth. Multiparity and normal BMI are generally considered favorable factors in pregnancy outcomes.

Question 23: Correct Answer: B) 12-18 months
Rationale: The recommended interval between a cesarean delivery and a trial of labor for a VBAC is 12-18 months. This timeframe allows for optimal healing of the uterine incision, reducing the risk of uterine rupture during a subsequent vaginal birth. Options A, C, and D do not align with the recommended interval for VBAC and may increase the risk of complications such as uterine rupture or other adverse outcomes.

Question 24: Correct Answer: B) Patient education helps in promoting self-care and recovery.
Rationale: Patient education plays a crucial role in the postpartum period as it empowers mothers to take care of themselves and their newborns effectively. By providing education on topics such as breastfeeding, postpartum care, emotional well-being, and newborn care, healthcare providers enable mothers to make informed decisions, recognize warning signs, and promote a faster recovery. Option A is incorrect as patient education is essential for optimal postpartum outcomes. Option C is incorrect as all mothers, regardless of parity, benefit from education. Option D is incorrect as patient education is a collaborative effort

between healthcare providers and mothers.

Question 25: Correct Answer: A) Initiate oxygen therapy
Rationale: In the scenario described, the most appropriate initial nursing intervention for a newborn suspected of having TTN is to initiate oxygen therapy to ensure adequate oxygenation. Oxygen therapy helps alleviate respiratory distress and improves oxygen saturation levels. Chest physiotherapy, antibiotics, and breastfeeding are not the primary interventions for TTN. Antibiotics are not indicated as TTN is a self-limiting condition related to delayed clearance of lung fluid.

Question 26: Correct Answer: B) Instructing her to perform Kegel exercises regularly
Rationale: Kegel exercises help strengthen the pelvic floor muscles, which can improve urinary incontinence. Limiting fluid intake or avoiding emptying the bladder frequently can exacerbate the issue. Diuretics may further increase urine production, worsening the symptoms.

Question 27: Correct Answer: C) "Including sources of Omega-3 fatty acids in your diet can benefit your baby's brain development."
Rationale: Omega-3 fatty acids, found in fish like salmon and flaxseeds, are crucial for infant brain development during breastfeeding. Caffeine should be limited as it can be passed to the baby through breast milk. Adequate fluid intake is important to prevent dehydration and maintain milk supply. Skipping meals can lead to nutrient deficiencies and decreased milk production.

Question 28: Correct Answer: B) Decreased gastric motility
Rationale: During the postpartum period, women commonly experience a decrease in gastric motility. This can lead to issues such as constipation and bloating. Option A is incorrect as gastric motility typically decreases. Option C is incorrect as there is usually no significant increase in gastric acid secretion postpartum. Option D is incorrect as gastric acid secretion is not typically decreased during this time.

Question 29: Correct Answer: D) Implementing a consistent bedtime routine for both herself and the baby
Rationale: Implementing a consistent bedtime routine for both Mrs. Johnson and the baby can help establish healthy sleep patterns and improve sleep quality for both. Co-sleeping may increase the risk of Sudden Infant Death Syndrome (SIDS) and disrupt maternal sleep. Limiting fluid intake before bedtime can help reduce nighttime awakenings for bathroom trips. Using sleep aids should be avoided, especially while breastfeeding, due to potential risks to the baby and dependency issues for the mother.

Question 30: Correct Answer: D) "We will limit James' feedings to prevent complications."
Rationale: Limiting feedings is not recommended in newborns with polycythemia as it can lead to hypoglycemia. Adequate feeding is essential to prevent complications. Monitoring for signs of respiratory distress (Option A), ensuring hydration (Option B), and understanding the increased risk of blood clot formation (Option C) are all appropriate actions in managing polycythemia in newborns.

Question 31: Correct Answer: D) Thermal effects on fetal tissues
Rationale: Diagnostic ultrasound is considered safe for fetal assessment during pregnancy. However, one potential risk is the thermal effects on fetal tissues due to prolonged exposure to high-intensity ultrasound waves. This can lead to a rise in temperature in the fetal tissues, potentially causing harm. Options A, B, and C are incorrect as there is no conclusive evidence linking diagnostic ultrasound to increased risk of miscarriage, fetal growth restriction, or development of fetal anomalies.

Question 32: Correct Answer: A) MAS occurs when the newborn inhales amniotic fluid contaminated with meconium during delivery.
Rationale: Meconium aspiration syndrome (MAS) occurs when the newborn inhales meconium-stained amniotic fluid during delivery, leading to respiratory complications. This can result in airway obstruction, inflammation, and chemical pneumonitis. Preterm infants are at higher risk for MAS due to immature lung development. MAS is a serious condition that can cause significant respiratory distress, requiring prompt intervention. The presence of meconium in the amniotic fluid is a key diagnostic indicator for MAS, not clear amniotic fluid.

Question 33: Correct Answer: A) Regular insulin
Rationale: Regular insulin is a short-acting insulin that is typically administered 30 minutes before a meal to help control postprandial blood glucose levels. NPH insulin is usually taken before breakfast to cover the morning rise in blood glucose. Lispro insulin is a rapid-acting insulin given just before or immediately after meals. Glargine insulin is a long-acting insulin usually administered once daily at the same time each day. Therefore, Regular insulin is the correct option for administration before a meal.

Question 34: Correct Answer: D) Sudden onset of shortness of breath
Rationale: A sudden onset of shortness of breath in the postpartum period should raise concern for a potential cardiopulmonary complication such as pulmonary embolism or cardiac issues. Options A, B, and C are normal findings in the postpartum period and do not necessarily indicate a cardiopulmonary complication. It is crucial to promptly assess and intervene in cases of sudden onset of shortness of breath to prevent adverse outcomes.

Question 35: Correct Answer: B) Acetaminophen
Rationale: Acetaminophen is a non-opioid analgesic commonly used in labor as it effectively reduces pain without significant adverse effects on the fetus. Ibuprofen, Ketorolac, and Aspirin are nonsteroidal anti-inflammatory drugs (NSAIDs) that are generally avoided during labor due to their potential adverse effects on the fetus, such as premature closure of the ductus arteriosus and increased bleeding risk.

Question 36: Correct Answer: C) Down syndrome
Rationale: Down syndrome, also known as trisomy 21, is caused by the presence of an extra copy of chromosome 21. Turner syndrome is characterized by a missing or partially missing X chromosome, Klinefelter syndrome involves an extra X chromosome in males, and Fragile X syndrome is caused by a mutation in the FMR1 gene, not an extra chromosome.

Question 37: Correct Answer: B) Providing Mrs. Smith with information on postpartum depression support groups
Rationale: It is crucial to recognize signs of postpartum depression and provide appropriate support. Option A may lead to further feelings of inadequacy by fostering comparison. Option C may increase Mrs. Smith's anxiety,

and option D does not address her emotional needs.
Question 38: Correct Answer: D) Contractions of the uterus
Rationale: Afterpains, also known as involutional pains, are caused by the contractions of the uterus as it returns to its pre-pregnancy size. These contractions help control bleeding by compressing blood vessels at the site where the placenta was attached. Increased estrogen levels do not directly cause afterpains. Decreased uterine contractions and relaxation of uterine muscles are incorrect as they are not associated with the physiological process of afterpains.
Question 39: Correct Answer: B) Weight gain in multiple gestation pregnancies should be around 40-50 pounds.
Rationale: In multiple gestation pregnancies, the recommended weight gain is higher compared to singleton pregnancies. This is due to the increased demands on the mother's body to support the growth and development of multiple fetuses. Monitoring weight gain is crucial to assess the overall health and well-being of both the mother and the fetuses. Option A is incorrect as it suggests a lower weight gain range suitable for singleton pregnancies. Option C is incorrect as weight gain is an important factor to monitor in all pregnancies. Option D is incorrect as it suggests a weight gain range that is too low for multiple gestation pregnancies.
Question 40: Correct Answer: B) Providing reassurance, guidance, and practical tips on breastfeeding techniques.
Rationale: When a new mother expresses concerns about breastfeeding, it is essential for the nurse to provide reassurance, guidance, and practical tips on breastfeeding techniques. This approach helps build the mother's confidence, enhances her breastfeeding skills, and fosters a positive maternal role transition. By offering support and education, the nurse empowers the mother to overcome challenges and succeed in breastfeeding, promoting bonding and maternal well-being. Options A, C, and D are incorrect as they do not address the mother's concerns effectively and may hinder her maternal role transition by neglecting her need for support and guidance.
Question 41: Correct Answer: A) "I plan to introduce a bottle of formula at every feeding to ensure my baby is getting enough nutrition."
Rationale: Mrs. Smith's plan to introduce formula at every feeding may lead to a decrease in her milk supply and interfere with successful breastfeeding. Option B is the correct approach as it supports breastfeeding while providing additional nutrition if needed. Options C and D demonstrate understanding of the importance of breastfeeding and seeking professional guidance.
Question 42: Correct Answer: B) Monitor for signs of hypertension during methylergonovine administration.
Rationale: Methylergonovine is typically administered orally or intramuscularly, not intravenously. It is crucial to monitor the patient for signs of hypertension, as methylergonovine can cause vasoconstriction leading to increased blood pressure. Encouraging immediate ambulation after methylergonovine administration is not recommended due to the risk of dizziness or lightheadedness. Methylergonovine is contraindicated in patients with a history of migraines due to its vasoconstrictive effects, which can trigger migraine headaches.
Question 43: Correct Answer: B) Magnesium sulfate
Rationale: Magnesium sulfate is a commonly used tocolytic agent to inhibit uterine contractions and delay preterm birth. It works by relaxing smooth muscle, including the uterus. Oxytocin, Misoprostol, and Dinoprostone are not used as tocolytics; instead, they are used for labor induction or cervical ripening.
Question 44: Correct Answer: C) Nitrofurantoin
Rationale: Nitrofurantoin is considered safe for use in pregnancy to treat UTIs as it has a low risk of teratogenic effects on the fetus. Tetracycline (Option A) is contraindicated in pregnancy due to its potential to cause discoloration of fetal teeth. Trimethoprim (Option B) is associated with an increased risk of neural tube defects. Fluconazole (Option D) is not recommended in pregnancy due to its association with birth defects.
Question 45: Correct Answer: A) Administer antipsychotic medication as prescribed.
Rationale: The priority in managing postpartum psychosis is ensuring the safety and stabilization of the mother. Administering antipsychotic medication as prescribed is crucial to manage the acute symptoms and prevent harm to the mother or infant. Options B, C, and D are incorrect as relaxation techniques, education on infant care, and outpatient counseling are important but secondary interventions compared to the immediate need for pharmacological treatment in postpartum psychosis.
Question 46: Correct Answer: A) Gestational diabetes
Rationale: Polyhydramnios is often linked to gestational diabetes due to increased fetal urine production from the fetus's exposure to high glucose levels in the amniotic fluid. Chronic hypertension, hypothyroidism, and iron-deficiency anemia are not typically associated with polyhydramnios.
Question 47: Correct Answer: D) Gentamicin
Rationale: Gentamicin is a commonly used aminoglycoside antibiotic in newborns to treat sepsis due to its broad-spectrum coverage against common pathogens. Acyclovir is an antiviral medication used for herpes infections, not bacterial sepsis. Vancomycin is a glycopeptide antibiotic used for resistant Gram-positive infections, not typically first-line for sepsis. Ceftriaxone is a third-generation cephalosporin more commonly used in older children and adults, not typically first-line in newborns due to potential side effects.
Question 48: Correct Answer: A) Intramuscular injection
Rationale: The recommended route for administering vitamin K to newborns to prevent hemorrhagic disease is through an intramuscular injection. This route ensures optimal absorption and effectiveness of the vitamin. Options B, C, and D are incorrect as oral administration, intravenous infusion, and subcutaneous injection are not the preferred routes for vitamin K administration in newborns due to varying absorption rates and effectiveness.
Question 49: Correct Answer: D) Just before the procedure
Rationale: Oral sucrose should be administered to newborns just before the procedure to maximize its effectiveness in reducing pain and distress. Administering it too early may result in decreased efficacy by the time the procedure begins. Administering it immediately after the procedure may not provide adequate pain relief during the procedure itself. Therefore, giving oral sucrose just before the procedure ensures optimal pain management for the newborn.
Question 50: Correct Answer: A) Hypoglycemia

Rationale: Infants born to diabetic mothers are at risk of hypoglycemia due to the abrupt cessation of the maternal glucose supply at birth. This condition requires close monitoring and prompt intervention to prevent long-term neurological sequelae. Hypernatremia, hypocalcemia, and hypokalemia are not typically associated with infants of diabetic mothers, making them incorrect choices.

Question 51: Correct Answer: C) Neonatal Graves' disease

Rationale: Neonatal Graves' disease is caused by transplacental transfer of maternal thyroid-stimulating immunoglobulins, leading to hyperthyroidism in the newborn. Congenital hypothyroidism (Option A) is the underproduction of thyroid hormone. Neonatal diabetes mellitus (Option B) is a rare condition characterized by hyperglycemia in the newborn. Neonatal hypoparathyroidism (Option D) is the underproduction of parathyroid hormone, leading to hypocalcemia. Therefore, the correct answer is Neonatal Graves' disease due to excessive thyroid hormone production.

Question 52: Correct Answer: D) Monitor fetal well-being closely

Rationale: In cases of oligohydramnios where there is no evidence of fetal distress, the primary nursing intervention is to closely monitor fetal well-being through methods such as non-stress tests, biophysical profiles, and ultrasound assessments. This allows for timely detection of any changes in fetal status and guides further management. Encouraging increased fluid intake, administering tocolytic therapy, or immediate delivery are not indicated without clear indications of fetal compromise.

Question 53: Correct Answer: C) Blood pressure cuff

Rationale: A blood pressure cuff is crucial for maternal postpartum assessment to monitor for signs of preeclampsia or other postpartum complications. A baby monitor (option A) is used for monitoring the newborn and not for maternal assessment. A breast pump (option B) is used for lactation purposes. A diaper changing station (option D) is essential for newborn care but not for maternal postpartum assessment.

Question 54: Correct Answer: A) Engorged breasts

Rationale: Engorged breasts can make it challenging for the baby to latch on properly due to the increased firmness of the breast tissue. This can lead to difficulties in achieving a deep latch and effective milk transfer. Options B, C, and D are incorrect as using a nipple shield from the beginning can hinder direct nipple stimulation, feeding on a strict schedule may not align with the baby's hunger cues, and avoiding skin-to-skin contact can impact bonding and breastfeeding success.

Question 55: Correct Answer: B) Heart rate of 180 beats per minute

Rationale: A heart rate of 180 beats per minute in a newborn is considered tachycardia and requires immediate intervention as it may indicate underlying cardiac issues or distress. Acrocyanosis is a common finding in newborns and does not require immediate intervention. A respiratory rate of 40 breaths per minute is within the normal range for a newborn. Caput succedaneum is swelling of the soft tissues of the scalp and typically resolves on its own without intervention.

Question 56: Correct Answer: B) Apply warm compresses before breastfeeding

Rationale: Warm compresses can help improve blood flow to the breasts, making it easier for the mother to breastfeed and relieve engorgement. Using a breast pump to completely empty the breasts can lead to oversupply issues. Limiting feeding time can hinder milk removal and exacerbate engorgement. Vigorous breast massage can cause discomfort and may not effectively resolve engorgement.

Question 57: Correct Answer: C) Providing tactile stimulation to the baby

Rationale: In newborns experiencing apnea with brief pauses, providing tactile stimulation is the initial intervention to stimulate breathing. Administering oxygen therapy may be necessary for prolonged apnea. Placing the infant in a prone position is not recommended due to the risk of sudden infant death syndrome (SIDS). Initiating CPR is indicated for severe apnea with bradycardia or cyanosis.

Question 58: Correct Answer: C) Butorphanol

Rationale: Butorphanol is a synthetic opioid agonist-antagonist that provides analgesia without significantly affecting uterine contractions, making it a suitable choice for pain relief during labor. Fentanyl is a potent opioid analgesic that can affect the fetus and labor progress. Misoprostol and Dinoprostone are prostaglandins used for cervical ripening and induction of labor, not for pain relief during labor.

Question 59: Correct Answer: B) Using a lanolin-based nipple cream after each feeding

Rationale: Applying a lanolin-based nipple cream after each feeding helps soothe and protect sore nipples. Soap can dry out the skin, exacerbating the issue. Tight-fitting bras can increase friction and worsen discomfort. Skipping feedings can lead to engorgement and affect milk supply.

Question 60: Correct Answer: C) Opting for a formula with iron for newborns.

Rationale: It is essential to prioritize guiding the mother to choose a formula with iron for newborns as iron is crucial for the baby's growth and development. Formula with added sugars (Option A) is not recommended as it can lead to early childhood obesity and dental issues. Selecting a formula based on the baby's weight (Option B) is not a standard practice, and it is more important to focus on the baby's nutritional needs. Using a formula with cow's milk (Option D) is not suitable for newborns as their digestive systems are not ready to process cow's milk proteins.

Question 61: Correct Answer: B) Evaluating the mother's emotional well-being

Rationale: A comprehensive postpartum health assessment includes evaluating the mother's emotional well-being to screen for postpartum depression or anxiety, which are common concerns during this period. Assessing the newborn's vital signs and weight are important but are part of the newborn assessment, not the maternal assessment. Checking the mother's blood type is relevant for prenatal care but is not a primary focus during the postpartum assessment.

Question 62: Correct Answer: A) Erythromycin ointment

Rationale: Erythromycin ointment is routinely applied to newborns' eyes to prevent ophthalmia neonatorum, a bacterial infection that can cause blindness. Acyclovir is an antiviral medication used to treat herpes infections, not for ophthalmia neonatorum prevention. Gentamicin is an antibiotic used for various infections but not specifically for ophthalmia neonatorum. Nystatin is an antifungal medication used for treating fungal infections,

not for preventing bacterial eye infections in newborns.
Question 63: Correct Answer: C) Pulse Oximetry
Rationale: Pulse oximetry is a non-invasive screening tool used to detect critical congenital heart defects in newborns. It measures the oxygen saturation levels in the blood, helping identify infants who may require further cardiac evaluation. The other options, such as the Denver Developmental Screening Test, Apgar Score, and Ballard Score, are not specific tools for CHD screening and serve different purposes in newborn assessment.
Question 64: Correct Answer: A) Post-term pregnancies are defined as those lasting beyond 42 weeks of gestation.
Rationale: Post-term pregnancies are defined as those lasting beyond 42 weeks of gestation, posing an increased risk of fetal complications such as macrosomia and meconium aspiration. Induction of labor is often recommended in post-term pregnancies to prevent adverse outcomes. Post-term pregnancies are actually associated with a higher incidence of meconium-stained amniotic fluid, indicating fetal distress.
Question 65: Correct Answer: B) Decreased oxygen saturation in the blood
Rationale: Cyanotic Heart Disease results in decreased oxygen saturation in the blood due to mixing of oxygenated and deoxygenated blood in the heart. Option A is incorrect as Cyanotic Heart Disease typically presents with decreased pulmonary blood flow. Option C is incorrect as an enlarged heart size is often seen on chest X-ray in Cyanotic Heart Disease. Option D is incorrect as tachycardia is more common than bradycardia in this condition.
Question 66: Correct Answer: D) Recommending the use of nipple shields
Rationale: In this scenario, the mother's engorged breasts and the baby's poor latch indicate latch-on problems. Recommending the use of nipple shields can help improve latch and alleviate discomfort for both the mother and the baby. Encouraging the mother to pump milk before feedings may exacerbate engorgement, switching to formula feeding is not necessary if latch issues can be resolved, and advising the mother to stop breastfeeding temporarily may hinder the establishment of breastfeeding.
Question 67: Correct Answer: C) Category III
Rationale: Category III fetal heart rate pattern is associated with fetal distress during labor, indicating the need for immediate intervention. This pattern includes absent variability, recurrent late decelerations, bradycardia, and sinusoidal heart rate pattern. Category I is considered normal, while Category II requires close monitoring but does not necessarily indicate distress. Category IV is not a recognized classification for fetal heart rate patterns.
Question 68: Correct Answer: B) Initiating broad-spectrum antibiotics
Rationale: In septic shock, the cornerstone of treatment is early administration of broad-spectrum antibiotics to target the underlying infection. While vasopressors may be needed to support blood pressure, addressing the infection is crucial. Encouraging ambulation and providing warm blankets are not priorities in the management of septic shock.
Question 69: Correct Answer: A) Decreased platelet count

Rationale: In DIC, there is widespread activation of the coagulation cascade leading to consumption of platelets and clotting factors, resulting in a decreased platelet count. Elevated blood pressure, increased fetal movements, and decreased uterine contractions are not typical findings of DIC.
Question 70: Correct Answer: B) Encouraging relaxation techniques before bedtime
Rationale: Encouraging relaxation techniques before bedtime, such as deep breathing exercises or mindfulness meditation, can help Ms. Smith manage her anxiety and improve her sleep quality. Prescribing sedative medications may not address the underlying cause of her sleep disturbances and can lead to dependency. Consuming caffeine in the evening can exacerbate sleep problems, and watching TV in bed can disrupt the sleep-wake cycle, making it harder for Ms. Smith to fall asleep.
Question 71: Correct Answer: B) Initiating phototherapy
Rationale: Phototherapy is the first-line treatment for hyperbilirubinemia in newborns. It helps convert unconjugated bilirubin into a form that can be excreted by the body. Encouraging breastfeeding is important, but in this scenario, phototherapy is the immediate intervention needed to lower John's bilirubin levels. Administering antibiotics and supplementing with iron drops are not indicated for hyperbilirubinemia.
Question 72: Correct Answer: C) Hypoxic-Ischemic Encephalopathy
Rationale: Hypoxic-Ischemic Encephalopathy (HIE) is a neurological condition in newborns caused by perinatal asphyxia. It results from oxygen deprivation and reduced blood flow to the brain, leading to brain injury. Meconium Aspiration Syndrome (MAS) is a respiratory complication, Necrotizing Enterocolitis (NEC) affects the gastrointestinal system, and Patent Ductus Arteriosus (PDA) is a cardiac issue. Therefore, option C is the correct answer as it specifically pertains to a neurological complication in newborns.
Question 73: Correct Answer: C) Oxytocin may cause hypotension as a side effect, so blood pressure should be monitored closely.
Rationale: Oxytocin is commonly used to prevent postpartum hemorrhage by promoting uterine contractions. However, one of the potential side effects of oxytocin is hypotension. Therefore, it is essential to monitor the patient's blood pressure closely during oxytocin administration to prevent complications. Intravenous administration is preferred over intramuscular injection for oxytocin to ensure rapid and consistent absorption, leading to effective uterine contractions.
Question 74: Correct Answer: C) Respiratory Distress Syndrome
Rationale: Baby James is displaying classic signs of Respiratory Distress Syndrome (RDS), a common condition in premature infants due to surfactant deficiency. While Transient Tachypnea of the Newborn, Meconium Aspiration Syndrome, and Pneumothorax can also cause respiratory distress, the symptoms described align more closely with RDS, especially in a preterm infant like Baby James.
Question 75: Correct Answer: C) Bringing a pacifier to soothe the baby after the procedure.
Rationale: Providing a pacifier can help soothe the baby and provide comfort after the circumcision procedure.

Feeding immediately before the procedure is not recommended to prevent aspiration during sedation. Aspirin is contraindicated in infants due to the risk of Reye's syndrome. Checking the circumcision site every hour may disrupt the healing process and increase the risk of i

nfection.
Question 76: Correct Answer: A) Previous cesarean section
Rationale: A previous cesarean section is a significant factor that may contraindicate a vaginal delivery due to the risk of uterine rupture. Maternal age over 35 years (option B) and gestational diabetes (option C) are not absolute contraindications for a vaginal delivery but may require closer monitoring. Maternal height less than 5 feet (option D) is not a contraindication for a vaginal delivery.
Question 77: Correct Answer: B) Progestin-only pills
Rationale: Progestin-only pills, also known as the mini-pill, are the preferred contraceptive option for breastfeeding mothers as they do not affect milk supply. Combined oral contraceptives containing estrogen are not recommended during breastfeeding due to potential adverse effects on milk production. Condoms are effective but may not be the most suitable option for Ms. Smith's current situation. While IUDs are highly effective, they are typically recommended after the postpartum period due to the risk of infection.
Question 78: Correct Answer: C) Using a mild, fragrance-free soap for bathing the preterm newborn.
Rationale: Preterm newborns have delicate skin that is more susceptible to damage. Using a mild, fragrance-free soap helps prevent irritation and maintains the skin's natural pH balance. Emollients or moisturizers may be necessary for preterm newborns to prevent dryness. Keeping the skin covered helps maintain warmth and prevent excessive moisture loss. Alcohol-based products can be too harsh and drying for preterm newborn skin.
Question 79: Correct Answer: C) Preeclampsia
Rationale: Mrs. Johnson's symptoms of lower back pain, contractions, fatigue, and swelling in hands and face are indicative of preeclampsia, a serious pregnancy complication characterized by high blood pressure and signs of damage to other organ systems. While gestational diabetes, preterm labor, and placenta previa are also significant birth risk factors, the constellation of symptoms described by Mrs. Johnson align more closely with preeclampsia, requiring prompt assessment and management to prevent adverse outcomes for both mother and baby.
Question 80: Correct Answer: B) Quetiapine
Rationale: Quetiapine, an atypical antipsychotic, is commonly used as a first-line treatment for postpartum psychosis due to its efficacy in managing psychotic symptoms. Fluoxetine is an SSRI used for depression, not psychosis. Alprazolam is a benzodiazepine for anxiety, and Bupropion is an antidepressant, not typically indicated for psychosis.
Question 81: Correct Answer: C) Providing oxygen therapy
Rationale: Respiratory distress in a newborn is a serious concern that requires prompt intervention. Providing oxygen therapy is crucial to ensure the baby receives adequate oxygenation. Administering oral glucose gel, placing the baby in a prone position, and offering a pacifier are not appropriate actions for managing respiratory distress and may delay necessary treatment.
Question 82: Correct Answer: B) Perinatal grief is a normal response to a significant loss during pregnancy or after birth.
Rationale: Perinatal grief is a complex emotional response experienced by both parents following a miscarriage, stillbirth, or neonatal death. It is a normal and individualized process that can vary in duration and intensity. This grief can be influenced by various factors including cultural, social, and psychological aspects, not solely biological factors. Understanding perinatal grief is crucial for healthcare providers to offer appropriate support and interventions to families experiencing such losses.
Question 83: Correct Answer: B) Induction of labor with prostaglandins
Rationale: Induction of labor with prostaglandins, especially in women attempting a VBAC, is associated with an increased risk of uterine rupture. Maternal age over 35 years, fetal macrosomia, and spontaneous onset of labor are not direct risk factors for uterine rupture during a VBAC. It is essential to carefully monitor women undergoing a VBAC, especially when labor is induced, to minimize the risk of complications.
Question 84: Correct Answer: A) Maternal hypertension
Rationale: Placental abruption, the premature separation of the placenta from the uterine wall, is associated with various risk factors. Maternal hypertension is a significant risk factor for placental abruption due to the increased vascular resistance and potential damage to the placental vessels. Prolonged rupture of membranes, fetal macrosomia, and maternal age under 20 years are not direct risk factors for placental abruption, although they may contribute to other complications during pregnancy and labor.
Question 85: Correct Answer: B) Intramuscular administration of Vitamin K is the preferred route for newborns.
Rationale: Intramuscular administration of Vitamin K is the recommended route for newborns to prevent Vitamin K deficiency bleeding. Oral and topical routes are not as effective in achieving adequate levels of Vitamin K in newborns. Breast milk alone does not provide sufficient Vitamin K to prevent bleeding disorders in newborns.
Question 86: Correct Answer: C) Pituitary gland
Rationale: The pituitary gland is responsible for producing oxytocin and vasopressin, crucial hormones during labor and lactation. Oxytocin stimulates uterine contractions during childbirth and promotes milk ejection during breastfeeding. Vasopressin helps regulate water balance in the body. The thyroid gland produces hormones that regulate metabolism, the adrenal gland secretes stress hormones, and the pancreas produces insulin for glucose regulation, making them incorrect choices in this context. Hence, the correct answer is the Pituitary gland.
Question 87: Correct Answer: C) Autonomy
Rationale: The new mother's desire to delay vaccinations for her newborn reflects the ethical principle of autonomy, as she is asserting her right to make decisions based on her values and beliefs. Fidelity pertains to keeping promises and being trustworthy, veracity to truthfulness in communication, and paternalism to making decisions in the best interest of the patient without their input. In this scenario, respecting

the mother's autonomy involves acknowledging her right to make informed choices regarding her child's healthcare, even if healthcare providers may recommend otherwise.

Question 88: Correct Answer: B) Distributive shock
Rationale: Amniotic fluid embolism can lead to distributive shock in the postpartum period. This type of shock is characterized by systemic vasodilation and maldistribution of blood flow, leading to decreased perfusion. Cardiogenic shock is related to heart failure, obstructive shock is caused by mechanical obstruction of blood flow, and hypovolemic shock is due to decreased intravascular volume. Therefore, distributive shock is the most common type associated with amniotic fluid embolism in the postpartum period.

Question 89: Correct Answer: D) Instrument-assisted delivery
Rationale: Instrument-assisted deliveries, such as forceps or vacuum extraction, increase the risk of hematoma formation due to the trauma caused to the birth canal tissues. Prolonged bed rest (Option A) is not a direct risk factor for hematoma. While cold packs (Option B) can help reduce swelling postpartum, they do not contribute to hematoma development. Adequate intake of vitamin C (Option C) promotes wound healing but is not specifically linked to hematoma formation. Nurses should be aware of the risk factors associated with hematoma to provide appropriate care and monitoring for postpartum mothers.

Question 90: Correct Answer: A) Milia
Rationale: Milia are small, white, pimple-like bumps that commonly appear on a newborn's face due to blocked oil glands. They are considered a normal variation and usually disappear on their own within a few weeks. Petechiae are tiny red or purple spots caused by broken blood vessels under the skin, not specific to the integumentary system. Jaundice is a yellow discoloration of the skin and eyes due to high bilirubin levels, while Mongolian spots are blue-gray patches often found on the lower back and buttocks, both requiring further evaluation and monitoring.

Question 91: Correct Answer: A) Encourage frequent breastfeeding sessions
Rationale: Breast engorgement is a common issue in the postpartum period characterized by swelling, warmth, and tenderness of the breasts. Encouraging frequent breastfeeding helps in relieving engorgement by effectively emptying the breasts and promoting milk flow. Ice packs can reduce swelling but may hinder milk flow if applied directly. Avoiding breastfeeding can lead to further engorgement and potential complications. Using a breast pump should be considered if the baby is unable to latch effectively.

Question 92: Correct Answer: C) To obtain cerebrospinal fluid for analysis
Rationale: The main purpose of performing a lumbar puncture in a newborn is to obtain cerebrospinal fluid for analysis, which can help in diagnosing various conditions such as infections or bleeding in the central nervous system. Administering intrathecal medications is a potential use of a lumbar puncture but not the primary purpose. Measuring intracranial pressure is typically done through other methods. Assessing spinal cord abnormalities would require different imaging techniques.

Question 93: Correct Answer: C) "Let your baby decide when they are hungry and feed on demand."
Rationale: Newborns should be fed on demand, as they will signal when they are hungry. Feeding schedules should be flexible and responsive to the baby's cues. Option A is too rigid and may not meet the baby's individual needs. Option B suggests frequent feeding intervals that may not be necessary. Option D provides a fixed schedule that may not align with the baby's hunger cues.

Question 94: Correct Answer: A) Encourage frequent voiding
Rationale: Following a UTI diagnosis, encouraging frequent voiding helps prevent stasis of urine in the bladder, which can contribute to UTI recurrence. While prophylactic antibiotics may be indicated in some cases, they are not routinely used for UTI prevention. Cranberry juice consumption may have some benefits in UTI prevention, but it is not considered a primary intervention. Educating on proper hand hygiene is important for overall infection prevention but is not specific to UTI recurrence.

Question 95: Correct Answer: A) Maternal hemorrhage
Rationale: Amniocentesis is associated with certain risks, including maternal hemorrhage, infection, and injury to the fetus. Maternal hemorrhage can occur due to inadvertent trauma to maternal blood vessels during the procedure. Fetal macrosomia, placental abruption, and polyhydramnios are not direct complications of amniocentesis. Fetal macrosomia refers to a large fetus, placental abruption is the separation of the placenta from the uterine wall, and polyhydramnios is an excess of amniotic fluid.

Question 96: Correct Answer: C) "Afterpains happen as a result of hormonal changes after childbirth."
Rationale: Afterpains are primarily caused by the release of the hormone oxytocin, which stimulates uterine contractions to control bleeding and help the uterus return to its pre-pregnancy size. The other options do not accurately explain the physiological basis of afterpains, making them incorrect choices.

Question 97: Correct Answer: A) Encouraging skin-to-skin contact between the mother and newborn
Rationale: Skin-to-skin contact immediately after birth promotes bonding, regulates the newborn's temperature, and facilitates breastfeeding initiation. Placing the newborn in a separate bassinet or allowing only brief contact can hinder bonding and breastfeeding. Initiating formula feeding is not recommended as the first feeding; breastfeeding or colostrum feeding is preferred for newborns.

Question 98: Correct Answer: C) Regular physical activity
Rationale: Regular physical activity during pregnancy is a protective antenatal factor against the development of gestational diabetes mellitus (GDM). Exercise helps in maintaining healthy blood sugar levels and improves insulin sensitivity. Family history of diabetes (option A) and previous history of GDM (option D) are risk factors for GDM. Obesity (option B) is also a risk factor for developing GDM due to insulin resistance. Regular physical activity stands out as the correct option due to its positive impact on glucose metabolism during pregnancy.

Question 99: Correct Answer: B) Mastitis
Rationale: Mastitis is a common postpartum infection affecting breastfeeding mothers. It is caused by milk stasis and bacterial growth in the breast tissue. The characteristic symptoms include red, tender, warm, and

swollen breasts, often accompanied by systemic symptoms like fever and chills. Endometritis is an infection of the uterine lining, while wound infection refers to infections at the site of a surgical incision. Urinary tract infection involves the urinary system. However, mastitis specifically targets the breast tissue due to milk duct obstruction, making it the correct answer in this scenario.

Question 100: Correct Answer: A) Encourage a high-fiber diet and adequate fluid intake
Rationale: Encouraging a high-fiber diet and adequate fluid intake helps prevent constipation, which can exacerbate hemorrhoids. Fiber softens the stool, making it easier to pass without straining, thus reducing the discomfort associated with hemorrhoids. Ice packs, stool softeners, and warm sitz baths can provide symptomatic relief but do not address the root cause of constipation.

Question 101: Correct Answer: D) Perform a blood patch procedure
Rationale: The described postural headache is characteristic of a spinal headache. The definitive treatment for a spinal headache is a blood patch procedure, where the patient's blood is injected into the epidural space to seal the leak and alleviate symptoms. Encouraging caffeine intake, administering muscle relaxants, or initiating IV fluids would not address the underlying cause of the spinal headache.

Question 102: Correct Answer: B) Apply lanolin cream to the nipples after each feeding
Rationale: Lanolin cream helps soothe and protect sore and cracked nipples, promoting healing and providing relief to the mother. Nipple shields may interfere with proper latch and milk transfer, worsening the issue. Using soap on the nipples can further dry out the skin, exacerbating the problem. Continuing to breastfeed through the pain can lead to further damage and may discourage the mother from breastfeeding altogether.

Question 103: Correct Answer: A) Respect for autonomy
Rationale: When educating a culturally diverse population in the postpartum period, respecting autonomy is crucial as it involves honoring individuals' rights to make decisions based on their own values and beliefs. Confidentiality (option B) is important but not specific to cultural diversity. Justice (option C) refers to fairness in resource allocation and is not directly related to cultural education. Beneficence (option D) focuses on doing good for the patient, which is important but not as central as respecting autonomy in a culturally diverse context.

Question 104: Correct Answer: B) History of infertility treatments
Rationale: Multiple gestation pregnancies are often a result of infertility treatments such as in vitro fertilization (IVF) which increase the chances of conceiving twins or higher-order multiples. Maternal age over 35 years is a risk factor for other pregnancy complications but not specifically for multiple gestation. Low pre-pregnancy BMI is not directly linked to multiple gestation. Having a history of previous uncomplicated singleton pregnancy does not increase the likelihood of having a multiple gestation.

Question 105: Correct Answer: A) A collection of blood outside blood vessels
Rationale: A hematoma is a localized collection of blood outside blood vessels, usually due to trauma during childbirth or a surgical procedure. It can lead to pain, swelling, and discoloration at the site. Options B, C, and D are incorrect as they do not accurately define a hematoma. Benign skin conditions, excessive hair loss, and bacterial infections are unrelated to hematoma formation. Understanding the definition of a hematoma is crucial for maternal newborn nurses to recognize and manage this postpartum complication effectively.

Question 106: Correct Answer: C) Nonmaleficence
Rationale: Nonmaleficence is the ethical principle that requires healthcare providers to prioritize the prevention of harm to patients. It underscores the importance of avoiding actions that may cause harm or risk to the patient's well-being. Autonomy pertains to respecting patients' rights to make decisions, beneficence involves promoting the patient's well-being, and justice relates to fairness in healthcare resource allocation. By adhering to the principle of nonmaleficence, healthcare providers prioritize patient safety and strive to minimize risks during care delivery.

Question 107: Correct Answer: D) Holding the baby in an upright position during feeding
Rationale: It is crucial to hold the baby in an upright position during bottle feeding to prevent choking and reduce the risk of ear infections. Holding the bottle parallel to the floor (option A) can cause the baby to swallow air, leading to discomfort. Using a fast-flow nipple (option B) can overwhelm the baby and increase the risk of overfeeding. Allowing the baby to feed while lying flat (option C) can also result in choking and is not recommended.

Question 108: Correct Answer: A) Autonomy
Rationale: In this scenario, the nurse should prioritize the ethical principle of autonomy, which respects the mother's right to make decisions regarding her child's healthcare. Autonomy emphasizes the individual's right to self-determination and informed consent. While beneficence (doing good), nonmaleficence (avoiding harm), and justice (fairness) are also important ethical principles in healthcare, in this case, respecting the mother's autonomy takes precedence over other considerations.

Question 109: Correct Answer: A) Apply warm compresses to the affected leg
Rationale: Superficial thrombophlebitis is the inflammation of a vein due to a blood clot formation. The initial management includes applying warm compresses to the affected area to promote vasodilation and relieve pain. Anticoagulant therapy is not indicated for superficial thrombophlebitis as it is primarily a self-limiting condition. Encouraging ambulation and leg elevation can help prevent complications but are not the primary interventions. Performing a venous Doppler ultrasound is usually reserved for deep vein thrombosis diagnosis.

Question 110: Correct Answer: D) Reduced blood volume
Rationale: During the postpartum period, there is a physiological decrease in blood volume due to the redistribution of fluids back to the intravascular space. This reduction in blood volume can lead to orthostatic hypotension, causing symptoms like lightheadedness and dizziness when standing up. Options A, B, and C are incorrect as increased blood pressure, decreased cardiac output, and elevated estrogen levels are not typically associated with the symptom described in the scenario.

Question 111: Correct Answer: A) Jaundice within 24 hours of birth
Rationale: A newborn with ABO incompatibility typically

presents with jaundice within the first 24 hours of life. This occurs due to the breakdown of red blood cells and subsequent release of bilirubin. Jaundice is the most common clinical manifestation of ABO incompatibility in newborns. While hypoglycemia, respiratory distress, and bradycardia can occur in newborns for various reasons, they are not specific to ABO incompatibility.

Question 112: Correct Answer: A) Advanced maternal age is defined as 35 years or older.
Rationale: Advanced maternal age is commonly defined as 35 years or older. Women of advanced maternal age are at increased risk for various pregnancy complications such as gestational diabetes, preeclampsia, and chromosomal abnormalities in the fetus. While 40 years or older is also considered an advanced maternal age, the standard definition is 35 years or older, making option A the correct answer.

Question 113: Correct Answer: C) Notify the healthcare provider immediately
Rationale: The described signs and symptoms indicate a possible wound infection at the episiotomy site. The priority nursing action would be to notify the healthcare provider immediately for further evaluation and appropriate treatment. Applying ice packs or sitz baths may not address the underlying infection, and administering pain medication alone does not address the infection.

Question 114: Correct Answer: D) These lacerations involve only the vaginal mucosa and do not extend into the underlying tissues.
Rationale: First-degree vaginal lacerations involve only the vaginal mucosa and do not extend into the underlying tissues. They are the least severe type of vaginal lacerations and typically do not require suturing in the operating room. Lacerations that involve the perineal muscles and extend into the anal sphincter are classified as second-degree lacerations, which are more extensive than first-degree lacerations.

Question 115: Correct Answer: C) Increased risk of gastrointestinal infections
Rationale: Early introduction of complementary feedings in newborns can increase the risk of gastrointestinal infections due to the immature digestive system of the newborn. The gut of a newborn is not fully developed to handle solid foods, which can lead to digestive issues and infections. It is important to follow recommended guidelines and wait until the appropriate age to introduce complementary feedings to minimize the risk of complications and ensure the optimal health and development of the newborn.

Question 116: Correct Answer: C) Monitor the baby closely and document findings
Rationale: It is normal for newborns to pass meconium within the first 24 hours after birth. However, a delay in passing meconium can sometimes indicate an underlying issue. The nurse should closely monitor the baby for signs of bowel movement, abdominal distension, and discomfort. Documenting findings will help in determining if further intervention is necessary. Encouraging breastfeeding, administering suppositories, or performing rectal stimulation without proper assessment can lead to unnecessary interventions and potential harm to the newborn.

Question 117: Correct Answer: B) Hypoxic-ischemic encephalopathy
Rationale: The correct answer is B) Hypoxic-ischemic encephalopathy. The symptoms of poor muscle tone, weak suck, and diminished reflexes in a newborn are indicative of neurological impairment, commonly seen in hypoxic-ischemic encephalopathy due to perinatal asphyxia. While Spina bifida, Intraventricular hemorrhage, and Kernicterus are also neurological conditions, they typically present with different clinical features, making them less likely in this scenario.

Question 118: Correct Answer: B) Notify the healthcare provider immediately
Rationale: The worsening respiratory distress, collapsed lung with mediastinal shift on chest X-ray, and the need for further intervention indicate a possible tension pneumothorax. In this critical situation, the priority nursing action is to notify the healthcare provider immediately for prompt intervention, which may include needle decompression or chest tube insertion. Increasing the oxygen flow rate may not alleviate the underlying cause. Chest physiotherapy is not indicated in the management of pneumothorax. Positioning the infant on the affected side can further compromise respiratory function in this scenario.

Question 119: Correct Answer: B) Assessing for signs of urinary tract infection (UTI)
Rationale: Pain and burning sensation during urination are common symptoms of UTI postpartum. It is crucial to assess for UTI promptly to initiate appropriate treatment. While other conditions like urinary retention, kidney stones, or pelvic organ prolapse can also cause similar symptoms, UTI is more common in the postpartum period and requires immediate attention to prevent complications.

Question 120: Correct Answer: A) HBIG is given to newborns within 12 hours of birth if the mother is HBsAg positive.
Rationale: HBIG is recommended for newborns born to HBsAg-positive mothers within 12 hours of birth to provide passive immunity against Hepatitis B. Administering HBIG later than 12 hours may not be as effective in preventing transmission. Options B, C, and D are incorrect as HBIG is not routinely given to all newborns, is not contraindicated based on birth weight, and is not administered orally due to poor absorption.

Question 121: Correct Answer: C) Maternal age <20 years
Rationale: Maternal age <20 years is not typically associated with an increased risk of shoulder dystocia. Advanced maternal age, maternal diabetes, and maternal obesity are known risk factors. Young maternal age is not a significant contributor to shoulder dystocia compared to the other options provided.

Question 122: Correct Answer: D) Infants of diabetic mothers may require surfactant replacement therapy to manage respiratory distress syndrome.
Rationale: Infants of diabetic mothers are at increased risk for respiratory distress syndrome due to delayed lung maturation. Despite advancements in neonatal care, some infants may still require surfactant replacement therapy to manage respiratory distress syndrome effectively. Maternal glycemic control plays a crucial role in reducing the risk of complications in infants of diabetic mothers, including respiratory distress syndrome.

Question 123: Correct Answer: D) Performing partial exchange transfusion
Rationale: In managing polycythemia/hyperviscosity in newborns, a partial exchange transfusion is a crucial

intervention to reduce the hematocrit level and prevent complications such as hyperviscosity syndrome. Encouraging increased fluid intake helps in hydration but does not directly address the high hematocrit levels. Administering iron supplements and initiating phototherapy are not primary interventions for polycythemia/hyperviscosity in newborns, making them incorrect choices.

Question 124: Correct Answer: A) "Acetaminophen is safe to use while breastfeeding."
Rationale: Acetaminophen is considered safe during breastfeeding as it is minimally excreted into breast milk. The nurse should reassure the mother that she can safely use acetaminophen while breastfeeding. Options B, C, and D are incorrect as they provide misleading information that may discourage the mother from using a safe medication while breastfeeding.

Question 125: Correct Answer: C) Within 2 weeks after birth
Rationale: The cord stump usually falls off within 1 to 2 weeks after birth. If it takes longer, it is important to consult a healthcare provider. Falling off within 24 hours is too soon and might indicate a potential issue. Waiting for 4 weeks for the cord to fall off is too long and could suggest delayed healing or infection.

Question 126: Correct Answer: D) Physiologic flexion contractures
Rationale: Physiologic flexion contractures are a common musculoskeletal finding in newborns characterized by a positional deformity due to intrauterine positioning. This condition typically resolves spontaneously within a few weeks after birth without any treatment. Polydactyly refers to extra fingers or toes, syndactyly is the fusion of digits, and talipes equinovarus is a congenital foot deformity known as clubfoot. Unlike physiologic flexion contractures, these conditions may require medical intervention for correction.

Question 127: Correct Answer: D) Protein
Rationale: During lactation, protein requirements increase to support milk production. Protein-rich foods such as lean meats, poultry, fish, eggs, dairy, legumes, and nuts are important for breastfeeding mothers. Iron is needed to prevent anemia, but the requirement does not significantly increase during lactation. Vitamin C aids in iron absorption but does not need to be consumed in increased amounts. Calcium is important for bone health but does not have a significantly increased requirement during lactation.

Question 128: Correct Answer: B) Providing supportive care and monitoring fetal ultrasound
Rationale: In the case of suspected Zika virus infection during pregnancy, there is no specific antiviral treatment available. Supportive care, rest, and monitoring fetal ultrasound for signs of congenital Zika syndrome are essential. Antibiotics are not effective against viral infections like Zika. Bed rest alone is not sufficient to manage the potential complications associated with Zika virus in pregnancy.

Question 129: Correct Answer: D) Applying breast milk to nipples after feeding
Rationale: Applying breast milk to cracked nipples after feeding can promote healing and prevent infection due to its antibacterial properties. Alcohol-based solutions can be drying and irritating. Air-drying nipples is beneficial but may not provide the same protective benefits as breast milk. Scented lotions can contain chemicals that may be harmful to the baby and should be avoided.

Question 130: Correct Answer: C) It analyzes fetal DNA circulating in the mother's blood
Rationale: Cell-free DNA testing is a non-invasive prenatal screening test that analyzes fetal DNA present in the mother's blood. It is primarily used to screen for common chromosomal conditions such as Down syndrome. Options A, B, and D are incorrect as cell-free DNA testing does not detect all birth defects, is not recommended for all pregnant women, and is a screening test, not a diagnostic test.

Question 131: Correct Answer: C) Meconium aspiration syndrome
Rationale: The presentation of respiratory distress, cyanosis, and coarse breath sounds in a newborn born through meconium-stained amniotic fluid is indicative of meconium aspiration syndrome. While transient tachypnea of the newborn, pneumothorax, and respiratory distress syndrome can also present with respiratory distress, the history of meconium-stained amniotic fluid points towards meconium aspiration syndrome as the likely diagnosis.

Question 132: Correct Answer: A) Breast engorgement
Rationale: Breast engorgement is a common issue in the postpartum period due to increased blood flow and milk production. Nursing interventions include warm compresses, proper positioning for breastfeeding, and encouraging frequent feeding. Delayed cord clamping, newborn jaundice, and maternal hypertension are important topics in maternal newborn nursing but are not directly related to breast engorgement.

Question 133: Correct Answer: D) Nasal flaring during breathing
Rationale: Nasal flaring during breathing (Option D) in a newborn is a concerning sign that indicates respiratory distress and requires immediate intervention. Milia on the nose (Option A) is a benign condition. The absence of a red reflex in the eyes (Option B) may indicate eye abnormalities but does not require immediate intervention. Slight ear asymmetry (Option C) is a common variation and does not typically necessitate urgent action.

Question 134: Correct Answer: D) Preparing for rapid delivery in a safe environment
Rationale: In the case of precipitous delivery, the key nursing intervention is to prepare for rapid delivery in a safe environment to ensure the safety of both the mother and the newborn. This includes having necessary equipment ready, ensuring a clear pathway for the baby's delivery, and being prepared to manage any potential complications that may arise. Encouraging slow breathing techniques (option A) may be helpful in managing pain during labor but is not the priority in a precipitous delivery situation. Administering oxytocin to speed up labor (option B) is contraindicated in precipitous delivery as it can further accelerate labor and increase the risk of complications. Supporting the perineum to prevent tearing (option C) is important in all deliveries but may be challenging in the rapid nature of precipitous delivery.

Question 135: Correct Answer: A) Iron-deficiency anemia
Rationale: Ms. Johnson's presentation of fatigue, weakness, and shortness of breath along with a low hemoglobin level of 9 g/dL at 32 weeks gestation is indicative of iron-deficiency anemia, which is common in

pregnancy due to increased iron requirements for fetal growth and maternal erythropoiesis. Folate and vitamin B12 deficiencies can present with similar symptoms but are less common causes of anemia in pregnancy. Hemolytic anemia is characterized by the premature destruction of red blood cells, which is not the primary concern in Ms. Johnson's case.

Question 136: Correct Answer: D) Premature rupture of membranes
Rationale: Premature rupture of membranes is a significant risk factor for cord prolapse as it can lead to the cord slipping through the cervix before the baby, increasing the chances of compression and compromising blood flow. Multiple gestation, post-term pregnancy, and maternal obesity are not direct risk factors for cord prolapse, although they may pose other complications during labor.

Question 137: Correct Answer: B) Provide Ms. Johnson with resources for mental health support
Rationale: Encouraging Ms. Johnson to seek mental health support is essential in promoting beneficence, which focuses on doing good for the patient. Providing resources for support demonstrates care and concern for her well-being. Disregarding her concerns or advising her to suppress her emotions would not align with beneficence as it does not prioritize her mental health needs.

Question 138: Correct Answer: D) Loperamide
Rationale: Loperamide is an antidiarrheal agent that can exacerbate constipation by slowing down GI motility. Bisacodyl and Psyllium are commonly used to treat constipation by promoting bowel movements. Docusate sodium is a stool softener that helps prevent constipation by facilitating easier passage of stool.

Question 139: Correct Answer: A) It assesses fetal heart rate in response to fetal movement.
Rationale: A Nonstress Test (NST) is a common antenatal test that assesses fetal well-being by monitoring the fetal heart rate in response to fetal movement. This test helps to evaluate the fetal central nervous system and oxygenation status. Options B, C, and D are incorrect as they do not accurately describe the purpose or procedure of a Nonstress Test.

Question 140: Correct Answer: B) Anti-A
Rationale: In ABO incompatibility, maternal antibodies against the ABO blood group antigens (anti-A or anti-B) can cross the placenta and attack the newborn's red blood cells, leading to hemolysis. These antibodies recognize the A or B antigens that the newborn expresses on their red blood cells, causing destruction and subsequent hemolytic anemia. Unlike Rh incompatibility, which involves the Rh(D) antigen, ABO incompatibility is primarily mediated by anti-A or anti-B antibodies targeting the newborn's red blood cells.

Question 141: Correct Answer: B) Digoxin
Rationale: Digoxin is commonly used in newborns with congenital heart defects to improve cardiac function by increasing the strength of the heart muscle contractions. Albuterol is a bronchodilator, ibuprofen is a nonsteroidal anti-inflammatory drug, and loratadine is an antihistamine, none of which are used to manage congenital heart defects in newborns.

Question 142: Correct Answer: C) Hemolytic anemia
Rationale: The newborn's presentation of pallor, jaundice, and hepatosplenomegaly along with a hemoglobin level of 10 g/dL is indicative of hemolytic anemia, which is commonly seen in hemolytic disease of the newborn due to ABO incompatibility. Iron-deficiency anemia is characterized by low iron levels, aplastic anemia by bone marrow suppression, and sickle cell anemia by abnormal hemoglobin production, none of which align with the newborn's presentation.

Question 143: Correct Answer: B) Heart rate of 180 bpm
Rationale: A heart rate of 180 bpm in a newborn is considered tachycardia and requires immediate intervention as it may indicate underlying cardiac issues or distress. Acrocyanosis is a common finding in newborns and does not require immediate intervention. A respiratory rate of 40 breaths per minute is within the normal range for a newborn. Caput succedaneum is swelling of the soft tissues of the scalp and typically resolves on its own without intervention.

Question 144: Correct Answer: B) Place a hat on the baby's head
Rationale: Placing a hat on the newborn's head helps prevent heat loss as the head has a large surface area for heat loss. Delaying drying or transferring to a radiant warmer can disrupt skin-to-skin contact, which is crucial for thermoregulation. While wrapping in a warm blanket can help, placing a hat is more effective in preventing heat loss from the head.

Question 145: Correct Answer: A) Assure the mother that changes in breast milk color are normal and can vary throughout the day.
Rationale: Breast milk can vary in color, consistency, and even taste based on the mother's diet, hydration level, and the time of day. Assuring the mother that these variations are normal can help alleviate her concerns. It is important to educate mothers that changes in breast milk color do not necessarily indicate spoilage, and it is safe for the baby to consume. Consuming adequate water is essential for milk production but may not directly impact the color consistency of breast milk. Switching to formula feeding is not necessary unless there are specific medical reasons to do so.

Question 146: Correct Answer: C) Chest CT angiography
Rationale: Chest CT angiography is the gold standard for diagnosing pulmonary embolism due to its high sensitivity and specificity. D-dimer assay is a screening test but not confirmatory. Pulmonary angiography is invasive and reserved for cases where CT is inconclusive. Ventilation-perfusion scan is less commonly used now due to lower sensitivity compared to CT angiography.

Question 147: Correct Answer: C) Folic Acid
Rationale: Folic acid is essential for the prevention of neural tube defects like spina bifida in the developing fetus. It plays a vital role in early pregnancy to support the rapid cell division and growth of the neural tube. Vitamin C is important for immune function and iron is necessary for oxygen transport, but they do not specifically prevent neural tube defects. Vitamin D is crucial for bone health but is not directly linked to neural tube defect prevention.

Question 148: Correct Answer: C) Hematocrit
Rationale: In the given scenario, the low blood pressure and hemoglobin level suggest a potential issue with blood volume or red blood cell concentration. Hematocrit measures the percentage of red blood cells in the blood and is likely to be decreased in cases of anemia, which can present with symptoms of lightheadedness and

dizziness. While Serum Calcium, Serum Potassium, and Platelet Count are important lab values, they are less likely to be directly related to the symptoms described in this context.

Question 149: Correct Answer: A) Acrocyanosis
Rationale: Acrocyanosis is a common finding in newborns characterized by a bluish discoloration of the hands and feet due to peripheral vasoconstriction. It is considered a normal variation and typically resolves on its own. Erythema toxicum presents as pink or red blotches with small white or yellow papules, Harlequin color change is a transient color change seen in some newborns, and Cutis marmorata is a mottled skin pattern that appears as a lacy red or blue pattern, all of which are different from the bluish discoloration associated with acrocyanosis.

Question 150: Correct Answer: A) Developmental Dysplasia of the Hip (DDH)
Rationale: Asymmetry in the gluteal skinfolds is a common sign of Developmental Dysplasia of the Hip (DDH) in newborns. DDH is characterized by abnormal development of the hip joint, leading to instability or dislocation. Clubfoot (Talipes Equinovarus) presents with inwardly twisted foot, Osteogenesis Imperfecta is a genetic disorder causing brittle bones, and Congenital Torticollis involves a tilted head due to muscle tightness.

RNC-MNN Practice Questions (SET 3)

Question 1: Mrs. Smith, a 32-year-old postpartum woman, presents with sudden onset shortness of breath, chest pain, and tachycardia. She is 3 days post vaginal delivery. On assessment, she is tachypneic and hypoxic. Her vital signs are: HR 110 bpm, RR 24/min, SpO2 88%. What is the priority nursing intervention for Mrs. Smith?
A) Administer oxygen therapy
B) Perform a chest X-ray
C) Start anticoagulant therapy
D) Encourage deep breathing exercises

Question 2: Which of the following is NOT a common feeding cue exhibited by a newborn indicating readiness to breastfeed?
A) Rooting reflex
B) Sucking on hands or fingers
C) Crying loudly
D) Turning head side to side with mouth open

Question 3: Which of the following is a common maternal postpartum complication characterized by excessive bleeding after childbirth?
A) Mastitis
B) Endometritis
C) Postpartum hemorrhage
D) Thromboembolism

Question 4: Which assessment finding is indicative of constipation in a postpartum woman?
A) Frequent loose stools
B) Abdominal cramping relieved by passing gas
C) Infrequent bowel movements
D) Increased appetite

Question 5: During a forceps-assisted delivery, the obstetrician encounters shoulder dystocia after delivering the fetal head. Which maneuver should the obstetrician perform next to resolve the shoulder dystocia?
A) McRoberts maneuver
B) Rubin maneuver
C) Woods' screw maneuver
D) Jacquemier maneuver

Question 6: Which medication is commonly used to prevent hemorrhagic disease of the newborn?
A) Vitamin K
B) Ibuprofen
C) Acetaminophen
D) Furosemide

Question 7: Which of the following statements regarding adoption in the context of maternal postpartum assessment is accurate?
A) Birth parents have no legal rights after the adoption is finalized.
B) Open adoption allows birth parents to have ongoing contact with the child.
C) Closed adoption involves sharing identifying information between birth parents and adoptive parents.
D) Semi-open adoption prohibits any form of communication between birth parents and adoptive parents.

Question 8: Which of the following is a characteristic feature of HELLP syndrome in the context of maternal postpartum complications?
A) Hypertension
B) Elevated liver enzymes
C) Thrombocytopenia
D) Normal urine protein

Question 9: Which of the following is a common barrier to parent/infant interactions in the postpartum period?
A) Skin-to-skin contact immediately after birth
B) Encouraging rooming-in for the mother and baby
C) Providing education on breastfeeding techniques
D) Separating the mother and baby for long periods

Question 10: Scenario: Mrs. Johnson, a first-time mother, asks the nurse about the care of her newborn son after circumcision. The nurse educates her on post-circumcision care. Which instruction should the nurse provide to Mrs. Johnson?
A) Apply petroleum jelly to the circumcision site at each diaper change.
B) Clean the circumcision site with alcohol wipes after each diaper change.
C) Avoid bathing the baby until the circumcision site is completely healed.
D) Use scented baby wipes to clean the circumcision site gently.

Question 11: At 34 weeks of gestation, Mrs. Johnson, a 25-year-old pregnant woman, complains of sudden severe abdominal pain and vaginal bleeding. On examination, her uterus is tender, and fetal distress is noted. Which antepartum complication is most likely presenting in Mrs. Johnson?
A) Ectopic pregnancy
B) Placental abruption
C) Oligohydramnios
D) Hyperemesis gravidarum

Question 12: Which maternal factor is NOT commonly associated with an increased risk of Intrauterine Growth Restriction (IUGR)?
A) Hypertension
B) Smoking
C) Multiparity
D) Diabetes

Question 13: Scenario: Emily, a 32-year-old postpartum mother, discloses to the nurse that her partner has been verbally abusive towards her since the birth of their baby. She expresses fear and uncertainty about her safety and the well-being of her child. What is the most appropriate nursing intervention in this situation?
A) Advise Emily to confront her partner about the abuse and seek couples counseling.
B) Provide Emily with resources on domestic violence

shelters and safety planning.
C) Suggest Emily to ignore the verbal abuse and focus on caring for her baby.
D) Encourage Emily to keep the abuse a secret to maintain family harmony.

Question 14: What is a crucial nursing intervention when caring for a postpartum patient receiving Methadone (Subutex) Sublingual Tablets?
A) Encouraging the patient to skip Methadone doses to prevent dependence.
B) Monitoring for signs of opioid withdrawal in the newborn.
C) Administering Methadone with other sedatives to enhance its effects.
D) Advising the patient to discontinue Methadone if they experience mild withdrawal symptoms.

Question 15: During the transition to extrauterine life, which of the following is a normal physiological change in a newborn within the first 4 hours after birth?
A) Respiratory rate of 60 breaths per minute
B) Heart rate of 180 beats per minute
C) Acrocyanosis in extremities
D) Blood pressure of 100/70 mmHg

Question 16: During a postpartum assessment, Nurse Jones observes that a mother is experiencing challenges with breastfeeding and is considering complementary feedings for her newborn. Which statement by the mother indicates a correct understanding of complementary feedings?
A) "I will introduce solid foods to my baby's diet starting at one month of age to ensure proper growth."
B) "I plan to offer complementary feedings such as iron-fortified cereals around six months of age while continuing to breastfeed."
C) "I will switch completely to formula feeding to avoid any breastfeeding challenges."
D) "I understand that introducing complementary feedings can replace breastfeeding entirely and is recommended for newborns."

Question 17: Mrs. Smith, a 32-year-old pregnant woman at 34 weeks gestation, presents to the labor and delivery unit with complaints of fluid leakage per vagina for the past 12 hours. On examination, pooling of amniotic fluid is noted. She denies any contractions or fever. Fetal heart rate monitoring shows reassuring patterns. What is the most appropriate initial nursing action for Mrs. Smith?
A) Administer tocolytic therapy
B) Perform a sterile speculum examination
C) Start intravenous antibiotics
D) Induce labor immediately

Question 18: Which of the following is a contraindication for a Vaginal Birth After Cesarean (VBAC)?
A) Previous classical cesarean incision
B) One prior low transverse cesarean incision
C) Gestational diabetes
D) Maternal age over 35 years

Question 19: Mrs. Smith, a postpartum patient, has developed a post-cesarean section wound infection. The healthcare provider prescribes an antimicrobial medication to treat the infection. Which of the following antimicrobials is commonly used for postpartum wound infections?
A) Acetaminophen
B) Cefazolin
C) Omeprazole
D) Metoclopramide

Question 20: Which cultural factor may affect family integration in the postpartum period?
A) Preference for extended family involvement
B) High socioeconomic status
C) Emphasis on individualism
D) Limited access to healthcare services

Question 21: During a postpartum education session, a new mother expresses concerns about her ability to bond with her baby due to feelings of inadequacy and self-doubt. Which action by the nurse best exemplifies the ethical principle of justice in this scenario?
A) Encouraging the new mother to seek professional counseling for her feelings
B) Providing the new mother with information on local parenting support groups
C) Dismissing the new mother's concerns as common postpartum emotions
D) Limiting the new mother's visitation hours with her baby in the hospital

Question 22: Which antiretroviral medication is commonly used for the prevention of mother-to-child transmission of HIV during pregnancy and delivery?
A) Acyclovir
B) Zidovudine
C) Metronidazole
D) Amoxicillin

Question 23: During a postpartum assessment, Nurse Jones notes that a new mother is experiencing symptoms of fatigue, weight gain, and cold intolerance. These symptoms are suggestive of:
A) Postpartum depression
B) Postpartum thyroiditis
C) Postpartum hemorrhage
D) Postpartum preeclampsia

Question 24: Scenario: Baby Emma, born at 37 weeks gestation, is showing signs of hypoglycemia, including jitteriness and poor feeding. The nurse should initiate which intervention first?
A) Offer a pacifier to soothe the baby.
B) Check the baby's temperature.
C) Initiate a heel stick for blood glucose monitoring.
D) Encourage breastfeeding or formula feeding.

Question 25: Scenario: Baby James, born prematurely at 32 weeks, is in the neonatal intensive care unit. He is receiving respiratory support with continuous positive airway pressure (CPAP). The nurse notices that James has developed bradycardia and cyanosis. What is the appropriate nursing action?
A) Increase the CPAP pressure

B) Administer a dose of surfactant
C) Perform chest physiotherapy
D) Provide tactile stimulation

Question 26: Scenario: Sarah, a newborn, is being assessed for Congenital Heart Disease (CHD). Which screening tool is commonly used to assess CHD in newborns?
A) Denver Developmental Screening Test
B) Apgar Score
C) Pulse Oximetry
D) Ballard Score

Question 27: Mrs. Johnson, a 32-year-old G2P1 woman, is scheduled to receive the Hepatitis B vaccine during her prenatal care visit. Which of the following statements regarding the Hepatitis B vaccine is accurate?
A) The Hepatitis B vaccine is contraindicated during pregnancy.
B) The Hepatitis B vaccine is administered intramuscularly in the deltoid muscle.
C) The Hepatitis B vaccine provides lifelong immunity after a single dose.
D) The Hepatitis B vaccine is only recommended for healthcare workers.

Question 28: Mrs. Smith, a 28-year-old primiparous woman, gave birth to a healthy baby girl two weeks ago. She has been experiencing persistent feelings of sadness, hopelessness, and worthlessness since delivery. She often cries for no apparent reason and struggles to bond with her baby. Which of the following is the most appropriate initial nursing intervention for Mrs. Smith?
A) Encourage her to get more rest and sleep when the baby sleeps.
B) Suggest she joins a new mothers' support group.
C) Advise her to increase her caffeine intake to boost energy levels.
D) Recommend immediate psychiatric hospitalization for safety concerns.

Question 29: Which type of insulin has the fastest onset of action?
A) Regular insulin
B) NPH insulin
C) Lispro insulin
D) Glargine insulin

Question 30: Scenario: Mrs. Smith has just given birth to a newborn baby girl. The baby is diagnosed with early-onset neonatal sepsis. Which of the following is the most common causative organism for early-onset neonatal sepsis?
A) Group B Streptococcus
B) Escherichia coli
C) Listeria monocytogenes
D) Staphylococcus aureus

Question 31: What is the appropriate nursing intervention for a newborn exhibiting jitteriness suspected to be due to hypoglycemia?
A) Administering oxygen therapy
B) Initiating enteral feedings
C) Placing the newborn in a cold environment
D) Administering a sedative medication

Question 32: Mrs. Smith, a 28-year-old postpartum mother, complains of shortness of breath and chest pain. On assessment, her vital signs are: heart rate 110 bpm, respiratory rate 24/min, blood pressure 130/80 mmHg, and oxygen saturation of 95%. Which of the following maternal postpartum conditions is most likely causing these symptoms?
A) Pulmonary embolism
B) Postpartum hemorrhage
C) Preeclampsia
D) Mastitis

Question 33: Mrs. Smith has just given birth to a full-term newborn baby boy. During the postpartum assessment, the nurse observes that the baby is experiencing jaundice. Which of the following interventions is most appropriate for managing neonatal jaundice?
A) Encouraging formula feeding
B) Initiating phototherapy
C) Administering iron supplements
D) Applying cold compresses to the baby's skin

Question 34: What is the normal range for pH in umbilical cord arterial blood gas analysis in a newborn?
A) 7.25 - 7.35
B) 7.10 - 7.20
C) 7.40 - 7.50
D) 6.90 - 7.00

Question 35: Which of the following is a risk factor for prolonged labor in maternal newborn nursing?
A) Maternal obesity
B) Normal fetal position
C) Adequate uterine contractions
D) Previous uncomplicated vaginal delivery

Question 36: Which of the following is a characteristic feature of inborn errors of metabolism in newborns?
A) Acquired during pregnancy
B) Presenting with symptoms later in childhood
C) Often result in metabolic crises
D) Can be cured with dietary modifications

Question 37: Mrs. Smith, a postpartum mother, is experiencing severe postpartum blues and is feeling overwhelmed with caring for her newborn. She expresses feelings of inadequacy and guilt. As a nurse providing care to Mrs. Smith, which action demonstrates the ethical principle of non-maleficence?
A) Encouraging Mrs. Smith to ignore her feelings and focus solely on caring for her baby.
B) Providing emotional support and reassurance to Mrs. Smith.
C) Dismissing Mrs. Smith's concerns as common postpartum emotions.
D) Prescribing medication without assessing Mrs. Smith's mental health status.

Question 38: During labor, a primigravida at 41 weeks gestation experiences prolonged and difficult

labor, resulting in fetal hypoxia and acidosis. Which of the following maternal conditions is most likely to contribute to this scenario?
A) Maternal obesity
B) Maternal age over 35
C) Maternal diabetes
D) Maternal hypothyroidism

Question 39: Which of the following is a characteristic feature of Disseminated Intravascular Coagulation (DIC) in the context of maternal postpartum complications?
A) Decreased platelet count
B) Elevated fibrinogen levels
C) Prolonged prothrombin time (PT)
D) Increased antithrombin III levels

Question 40: During a newborn assessment, the nurse notices that the baby has a high-pitched cry, poor muscle tone, and difficulty feeding. The nurse also observes that the baby's head appears larger in proportion to the rest of the body. Which condition should the nurse suspect in this newborn?
A) Down syndrome
B) Cerebral palsy
C) Hydrocephalus
D) Hypothyroidism

Question 41: Baby James, born at 36 weeks gestation, is admitted to the neonatal intensive care unit (NICU) for respiratory distress. During the assessment, the nurse observes abdominal distension and bilious vomiting. Which of the following conditions should the nurse suspect in this preterm newborn?
A) Malrotation with volvulus
B) Meconium ileus
C) Gastroesophageal reflux
D) Pyloric stenosis

Question 42: Mrs. Smith, a 28-year-old postpartum mother, presents with a fever of 101.5℉, uterine tenderness, and foul-smelling lochia four days after a cesarean section. Her vital signs are stable, and she reports feeling fatigued. What is the most likely cause of Mrs. Smith's symptoms?
A) Endometritis
B) Mastitis
C) Urinary tract infection
D) Wound infection

Question 43: Ms. Smith, a 2-day-old newborn, is diagnosed with a congenital heart defect. The nurse assesses the baby and notes cyanosis, tachypnea, and poor feeding. Which of the following conditions is most likely present in this newborn?
A) Patent Ductus Arteriosus
B) Tetralogy of Fallot
C) Atrial Septal Defect
D) Ventricular Septal Defect

Question 44: Which maternal factor is a contraindication for a vaginal birth after cesarean (VBAC)?
A) Previous cesarean section with a low transverse incision
B) Maternal desire for a trial of labor
C) Presence of cephalopelvic disproportion
D) History of uterine rupture

Question 45: What is a common barrier that may prevent women from disclosing intimate partner violence (IPV) during the postpartum period?
A) Fear of legal consequences for the partner
B) Lack of awareness about available support services
C) Feeling that IPV is a private matter and should not be discussed
D) Belief that healthcare providers are not equipped to help with IPV issues

Question 46: Mrs. Smith has just given birth to a healthy newborn. She is experiencing postpartum pain and requests pain relief medication. As the nurse caring for her, which analgesic would be most appropriate to administer considering the safety for the newborn if breastfeeding is planned?
A) Ibuprofen
B) Codeine
C) Morphine
D) Tramadol

Question 47: A 32-year-old G3P3 postpartum woman complains of lower abdominal pain, malaise, and chills on the fifth day after a vaginal delivery. On examination, her temperature is 39℃, heart rate is 110 bpm, and blood pressure is 130/80 mmHg. Which of the following is the most appropriate initial intervention?
A) Administering intravenous antibiotics
B) Ordering a pelvic ultrasound
C) Performing a complete blood count
D) Initiating antipyretic therapy

Question 48: During a postpartum assessment, a nurse observes that a new mother is making eye contact with her baby, talking softly, and gently stroking the infant's cheek. This behavior is indicative of:
A) Attachment bonding
B) Neglectful behavior
C) Postpartum depression
D) Infantile regression

Question 49: Mrs. Smith gave birth to a healthy baby boy yesterday. During the routine newborn assessment, the nurse notes that the baby's skin appears slightly yellow. The nurse suspects hyperbilirubinemia. Which of the following factors puts the newborn at higher risk for developing hyperbilirubinemia?
A) Term baby born at 39 weeks
B) Exclusive breastfeeding
C) ABO incompatibility
D) Maternal diabetes

Question 50: During a routine postpartum assessment, the nurse notes that a 32-year-old mother has developed pedal edema, crackles in the lungs, and a persistent cough. Which of the following conditions should the nurse suspect in this

postpartum patient?
A) Heart failure
B) Pulmonary edema
C) Deep vein thrombosis
D) Pneumonia

Question 51: Mrs. Johnson, a 28-year-old pregnant woman at 38 weeks gestation, is diagnosed with a transverse lie during a routine prenatal visit. The healthcare provider discusses the management options with Mrs. Johnson. Which intervention is contraindicated in the management of a transverse lie?
A) External cephalic version
B) Amnioinfusion
C) Oxytocin augmentation
D) Cesarean section

Question 52: Which of the following is a benefit of delayed cord clamping in newborns?
A) Increased risk of neonatal anemia
B) Decreased iron stores
C) Improved cardiovascular stability
D) Higher incidence of respiratory distress syndrome

Question 53: Mrs. Smith, a 28-year-old pregnant woman, admits to smoking a pack of cigarettes daily. She is currently in her second trimester. What is the most appropriate nursing intervention for Mrs. Smith regarding her smoking habit?
A) Encourage her to continue smoking as quitting abruptly may cause stress.
B) Provide education on the risks of smoking during pregnancy and offer smoking cessation resources.
C) Suggest she switches to a "light" cigarette brand to reduce harm.
D) Advise her to increase her daily cigarette intake to cope with pregnancy-related stress.

Question 54: Scenario: Baby James is born prematurely and requires resuscitation. The healthcare team is preparing to establish an airway. Which method is most appropriate for establishing an airway in a newborn during resuscitation?
A) Endotracheal intubation
B) Inserting a nasopharyngeal airway
C) Performing a jaw-thrust maneuver
D) Placing a laryngeal mask airway

Question 55: Scenario: Baby James, born to a mother with gestational diabetes, is at risk for hypoglycemia. What is a common symptom of hypoglycemia in newborns?
A) Hyperactivity and restlessness
B) Hypotonia and poor feeding
C) Hypertension and tachycardia
D) Hyperthermia and diaphoresis

Question 56: Scenario: Mrs. Smith, a 32-year-old pregnant woman at 38 weeks gestation, is admitted to the labor and delivery unit. Upon assessment, the fetal heart rate is noted to be consistently above 160 beats per minute. Mrs. Smith is experiencing contractions every 2 minutes. What fetal heart rate abnormality is most likely present in this scenario?
A) Bradycardia
B) Altered Variability
C) Tachycardia
D) Decelerations

Question 57: Mrs. Smith, a 32-year-old woman, gave birth to twins via cesarean section. The newborns are both healthy and thriving. During the postpartum assessment, which finding would be most concerning in this multiple birth scenario?
A) Engorged breasts
B) Uterine atony
C) Vaginal bleeding
D) Perineal pain

Question 58: During a postpartum education session, the nurse discusses the importance of nutrition for postpartum mothers with Ms. Johnson, a 30-year-old new mother. Which dietary advice is most appropriate for the nurse to provide regarding postpartum self-care?
A) "Limit your fluid intake to avoid water retention."
B) "Consume a diet high in processed foods for convenience."
C) "Include foods rich in iron and protein to support healing and energy levels."
D) "Avoid fruits and vegetables to prevent gas and bloating."

Question 59: Scenario: Baby James, born prematurely at 32 weeks, is admitted to the neonatal intensive care unit (NICU) for respiratory distress. On day 3 of life, he develops temperature instability, poor perfusion, and feeding intolerance. His blood culture is drawn, and sepsis is suspected. Which of the following clinical manifestations is most commonly associated with late-onset neonatal sepsis?
A) Apnea and bradycardia
B) Hyperbilirubinemia
C) Hypoglycemia
D) Temperature instability

Question 60: Which substance abuse during pregnancy is associated with an increased risk of fetal alcohol syndrome and neurodevelopmental disorders in the newborn?
A) Smoking
B) Drugs
C) Marijuana
D) Alcohol

Question 61: Which statement regarding Rh Immune Globulin (RhoGAM) administration is accurate for a postpartum client who is Rh-negative and has given birth to an Rh-positive baby?
A) RhoGAM should be administered within 72 hours postpartum.
B) RhoGAM is contraindicated if the mother has a history of Rh incompatibility.
C) RhoGAM is administered intramuscularly in the deltoid muscle.
D) RhoGAM is given only if the baby is Rh-negative.

Question 62: Baby James, a 1-week-old infant, is diagnosed with G6PD deficiency. His parents are concerned about managing his condition. Which of

the following statements best describes the management of G6PD deficiency in newborns?
A) Avoiding exposure to sunlight is the primary management strategy.
B) Providing a diet rich in iron supplements is essential to manage G6PD deficiency.
C) Educating parents about avoiding triggers such as certain foods and medications is crucial.
D) Administering blood transfusions regularly is necessary for newborns with G6PD deficiency.

Question 63: Which statement regarding apnea in newborns is true?
A) Apnea is defined as a pause in breathing lasting less than 10 seconds.
B) Central apnea is more common in preterm infants.
C) Apnea of prematurity typically resolves by term gestation.
D) Gastroesophageal reflux decreases the risk of apnea.

Question 64: Mrs. Smith, a postpartum patient, is prescribed a diuretic medication due to fluid retention following childbirth. Which nursing intervention is essential when administering diuretics to postpartum patients?
A) Encouraging increased sodium intake
B) Monitoring for signs of dehydration
C) Administering the medication with a full stomach
D) Limiting fluid intake to enhance diuretic effect

Question 65: Which respiratory condition in newborns is characterized by rapid breathing, grunting, nasal flaring, and chest retractions?
A) Transient tachypnea of the newborn
B) Bronchopulmonary dysplasia
C) Apnea of prematurity
D) Congenital diaphragmatic hernia

Question 66: Which medication is commonly used to promote GI motility in postpartum women experiencing constipation?
A) Ondansetron
B) Metoclopramide
C) Furosemide
D) Atenolol

Question 67: Ms. Smith has just given birth to a healthy newborn baby boy. During the initial assessment, the nurse emphasizes the importance of skin care for the newborn. Which of the following statements regarding newborn skin care is accurate?
A) It is recommended to bathe the newborn immediately after birth to remove any vernix.
B) Applying lotion or powder to the newborn's skin is essential to keep it moisturized.
C) Keeping the newborn's skin clean and dry helps prevent diaper rash.
D) Using scented baby wipes is preferred over plain wipes for newborn skin care.

Question 68: Mrs. Smith, a postpartum client, is experiencing bladder distention following a vaginal delivery. Which intervention should the nurse prioritize to promote bladder emptying and prevent urinary retention?
A) Encourage the client to drink plenty of fluids
B) Assist the client to the bathroom every 4 hours
C) Offer warm sitz baths to promote relaxation
D) Provide privacy and encourage the client to void every 2-3 hours

Question 69: During maternal postpartum assessment, which finding would require immediate intervention?
A) Engorged breasts
B) Lochia rubra with small clots
C) Fundus firm at the level of the umbilicus
D) Sudden onset of shortness of breath

Question 70: During a postpartum assessment, a new mother mentions using nicotine patches to quit smoking. What nursing intervention is most appropriate in this situation?
A) Encourage the mother to continue using nicotine patches as they are safe during the postpartum period.
B) Educate the mother on the potential risks of nicotine exposure to the newborn through breast milk.
C) Suggest increasing the nicotine patch dosage for better smoking cessation outcomes.
D) Advise the mother to apply the nicotine patches on the baby's clothing to prevent direct skin contact.

Question 71: What is the recommended treatment for hypoglycemia in newborns?
A) Intravenous glucose bolus
B) Continuous glucose monitoring
C) Early breastfeeding
D) Skin-to-skin contact

Question 72: During a postpartum education session, a new mother asks about the peak action time of NPH insulin. How should the nurse best respond?
A) 1-2 hours
B) 4-12 hours
C) 18-24 hours
D) 30 minutes

Question 73: Which of the following is a common congenital heart defect in newborns characterized by a hole in the septum between the heart's upper chambers?
A) Tetralogy of Fallot
B) Patent Ductus Arteriosus
C) Ventricular Septal Defect
D) Coarctation of the Aorta

Question 74: Which statement regarding hemorrhoids is accurate?
A) Hemorrhoids are varicose veins in the lower extremities.
B) Hemorrhoids are caused by a bacterial infection.
C) Hemorrhoids can be internal or external.
D) Hemorrhoids are typically not associated with pregnancy.

Question 75: Baby James, born at 36 weeks gestation, is admitted to the neonatal intensive care unit with signs of sepsis. Blood cultures reveal the presence of Gram-positive cocci in clusters. Which of the following bacterial pathogens is the most likely cause of Baby James' sepsis?

A) Staphylococcus aureus
B) Streptococcus pneumoniae
C) Enterococcus faecalis
D) Staphylococcus epidermidis

Question 76: Which of the following is a common early sign of neonatal sepsis?
A) Bradycardia
B) Hypothermia
C) Hyperglycemia
D) Jaundice

Question 77: What is a potential respiratory complication that can occur in infants of diabetic mothers?
A) Transient tachypnea of the newborn (TTN)
B) Bronchopulmonary dysplasia (BPD)
C) Meconium aspiration syndrome (MAS)
D) Persistent pulmonary hypertension of the newborn (PPHN)

Question 78: During a postpartum assessment, the nurse observes that a new mother is experiencing significant anxiety and requests that the baby be taken to the nursery for the night. What is the most appropriate nursing action in this situation?
A) Reassure the mother and encourage rooming-in for bonding.
B) Honor the mother's request and arrange for the baby to stay in the nursery.
C) Educate the mother on the benefits of rooming-in and offer support.
D) Inform the mother that separation is not recommended for newborns.

Question 79: During a routine newborn assessment, the nurse is preparing to administer eye prophylaxis to a newborn. Which action is essential before applying the medication?
A) Wiping the eyes with a dry cloth
B) Ensuring the infant is lying on their back
C) Cleaning the eyes with sterile saline
D) Checking the expiration date of the medication

Question 80: During the assessment of a patient in prolonged labor, the nurse notes persistent occiput posterior position of the fetus. Which maternal position is most beneficial to help rotate the fetus to the optimal position for delivery?
A) Supine position
B) Left lateral position
C) Semi-Fowler's position
D) Hands-and-knees position

Question 81: What is a potential complication for a pregnant woman who has undergone bariatric surgery?
A) Increased risk of preeclampsia
B) Decreased risk of gestational diabetes
C) Higher likelihood of post-term pregnancy
D) Lower incidence of cesarean section

Question 82: Which antimicrobial medication is contraindicated in pregnant women due to its potential to cause discoloration of fetal teeth and inhibition of bone growth?

A) Azithromycin
B) Doxycycline
C) Erythromycin
D) Penicillin

Question 83: Which statement regarding meconium-stained amniotic fluid is true?
A) Meconium-stained amniotic fluid is always a sign of fetal distress.
B) Meconium is the baby's first stool, typically greenish-black in color.
C) Meconium aspiration syndrome occurs when the baby inhales meconium into the lungs.
D) Meconium passage before birth is a normal occurrence.

Question 84: Scenario: Sarah, a 28-year-old postpartum mother, is experiencing symptoms of postpartum depression. The healthcare provider prescribes a psychotropic drug to help manage her condition. Which psychotropic drug is commonly used to treat postpartum depression?
A) Lorazepam
B) Sertraline
C) Methylphenidate
D) Haloperidol

Question 85: Which of the following is a common indication for administering Tylenol (acetaminophen) in the postpartum period?
A) Hypertension management
B) Prevention of blood clots
C) Pain relief
D) Treatment of urinary tract infections

Question 86: Which of the following is a potential maternal complication associated with cesarean delivery?
A) Decreased risk of infection
B) Increased risk of postpartum hemorrhage
C) Reduced risk of surgical complications
D) Lower risk of thromboembolism

Question 87: Which of the following is a potential antepartum risk factor for the development of oligohydramnios in pregnancy?
A) Maternal hypertension
B) Fetal macrosomia
C) Multiple gestation
D) Maternal age over 35 years

Question 88: Which psychotropic drug should be avoided during breastfeeding due to its potential adverse effects on the infant?
A) Fluoxetine
B) Paroxetine
C) Diazepam
D) Lithium

Question 89: Which hematologic condition in newborns is characterized by an abnormal increase in the number of red blood cells?
A) Thrombocytopenia
B) Hemolytic disease of the newborn
C) Polycythemia
D) Neutropenia

Question 90: During a newborn assessment, the nurse observes that the infant's eyes are not aligned and one eye appears to be deviated inward. The nurse suspects the presence of which condition?
A) Strabismus
B) Anisocoria
C) Nystagmus
D) Ptosis

Question 91: Mrs. Smith, a 32-year-old primiparous woman, gave birth to a healthy baby girl via vaginal delivery. During the postpartum assessment, she expresses feelings of overwhelming sadness, anxiety, and difficulty bonding with her newborn. Which of the following best describes the family dynamic being exhibited by Mrs. Smith?
A) Postpartum depression
B) Baby blues
C) Adjustment disorder
D) Postpartum psychosis

Question 92: Which of the following is a risk factor for developing chronic hypertension in pregnancy?
A) Age below 20 years
B) History of smoking
C) Normal body mass index (BMI)
D) Primigravida status

Question 93: During a postpartum assessment, the nurse observes a newborn demonstrating a disorganized suck-swallow pattern with frequent coughing and choking during breastfeeding. Which intervention would be most appropriate for the nurse to implement?
A) Suggest the mother use a faster flow nipple to reduce the baby's effort.
B) Encourage the mother to feed the baby in a quiet, dimly lit room.
C) Refer the newborn for a swallow study to assess for underlying issues.
D) Instruct the mother to switch to exclusively pumping and bottle feeding.

Question 94: During a prenatal visit, a pregnant woman at 28 weeks gestation expresses concerns about the risk of preterm labor and asks about medications that can help prevent early contractions. The healthcare provider explains the use of tocolytic agents in such situations. Which of the following medications is a beta-adrenergic receptor agonist commonly used as a tocolytic agent to delay preterm labor?
A) Nifedipine
B) Terbutaline
C) Indomethacin
D) Betamethasone

Question 95: During the postpartum period, which physiological change is expected in the reproductive system of a woman?
A) Increased estrogen levels
B) Decreased uterine size
C) Absence of Lochia discharge
D) Ovulation within the first week postpartum

Question 96: What is a common manifestation of perinatal grief that healthcare providers should be aware of?
A) Increased social support from family and friends.
B) Denial of the loss and avoidance of discussing the baby.
C) Rapid acceptance and quick return to normal activities.
D) Minimal impact on the parent's emotional well-being.

Question 97: Which of the following statements regarding gestational diabetes mellitus (GDM) is true?
A) GDM is a type of diabetes that occurs only during pregnancy.
B) GDM does not require monitoring of blood glucose levels.
C) GDM has no impact on the fetus or newborn.
D) GDM is not a risk factor for developing type 2 diabetes later in life.

Question 98: When assessing a postpartum woman's genitourinary system, which finding would require further evaluation by the healthcare provider?
A) Lochia rubra with small clots
B) Bladder distention
C) Perineal laceration healing without signs of infection
D) Engorged and tender breasts

Question 99: During the initial assessment of a newborn, which vital sign is crucial to determine the need for resuscitation?
A) Blood pressure
B) Heart rate
C) Temperature
D) Respiratory rate

Question 100: During the initial physiologic adaptations of a newborn, which of the following statements regarding the respiratory system is true?
A) Newborns have a higher respiratory rate compared to adults.
B) Newborns have fully developed alveoli at birth.
C) Newborns primarily rely on surfactant to maintain lung compliance.
D) Newborns have a decreased pulmonary blood flow after birth.

Question 101: At 41 weeks gestation, Mrs. Johnson, a primigravida, presents for a BPP due to post-term pregnancy. The ultrasound reveals absent fetal breathing movements, no gross body movements, and decreased amniotic fluid volume, while fetal tone is normal. The NST shows a non-reactive tracing. What is the appropriate management based on this BPP result?
A) Immediate induction of labor
B) Repeat BPP in 24 hours
C) Close monitoring with NST twice weekly
D) Emergency cesarean section

Question 102: Which hematologic disorder is characterized by a deficiency in clotting factors, leading to excessive bleeding in the postpartum period?
A) Thrombocytopenia

B) Disseminated Intravascular Coagulation (DIC)
C) Hemolytic Disease of the Newborn (HDN)
D) Von Willebrand Disease

Question 103: Mrs. Smith, a postpartum mother, is experiencing difficulty with breastfeeding her newborn. She mentions that her nipples are sore and cracked. What is the most appropriate nursing intervention to help alleviate Mrs. Smith's discomfort?
A) Encourage the use of a nipple shield
B) Recommend applying lanolin cream on the nipples
C) Suggest using a breast pump to express milk
D) Advise on proper latch technique and positioning during breastfeeding

Question 104: During a routine antenatal visit, Mrs. Johnson, a 28-year-old pregnant woman, mentions a history of gestational diabetes in her previous pregnancy. Which of the following assessments should the nurse prioritize based on this obstetrical history?
A) Fetal movement monitoring
B) Blood pressure monitoring
C) Glucose screening tests
D) Maternal weight gain

Question 105: Which anatomical structure in the breast is responsible for storing milk before it is released during breastfeeding?
A) Alveoli
B) Lactiferous ducts
C) Lactiferous sinuses
D) Areola

Question 106: Mrs. Smith, a 38-year-old pregnant woman, is scheduled for an amniocentesis procedure. Which of the following conditions is NOT a common indication for performing amniocentesis?
A) Advanced maternal age (35 years or older)
B) Family history of genetic disorders
C) Routine prenatal screening tests showing normal results
D) Abnormal ultrasound findings

Question 107: Which of the following is a risk factor for developing gestational hypertension during pregnancy?
A) Obesity
B) Regular exercise
C) Low salt intake
D) Non-smoker

Question 108: Mrs. Smith, a 28-year-old postpartum mother, is breastfeeding her newborn. She asks the nurse about the composition of breast milk. Which of the following components is NOT typically found in breast milk?
A) Lactose
B) Casein
C) Immunoglobulins
D) Hemoglobin

Question 109: Scenario: Sarah, a newborn, is being monitored for hypoglycemia. Which intervention is most appropriate for managing hypoglycemia in a newborn?
A) Delay feeding to prevent further decrease in blood sugar levels.
B) Administering a bolus of dextrose intravenously.
C) Encouraging breastfeeding or formula feeding every 2-3 hours.
D) Monitoring blood glucose levels once a day.

Question 110: Which of the following is a common symptom of breast engorgement in postpartum mothers?
A) Warm, red, and tender breasts
B) Cool, pale, and soft breasts
C) Nipple discharge
D) Breast asymmetry

Question 111: Which of the following is a risk factor for apnea in newborns?
A) Term gestation
B) Maternal smoking during pregnancy
C) Adequate oxygenation at birth
D) Birth weight above 2500 grams

Question 112: Which of the following maternal conditions is a significant risk factor for complications during labor and birth?
A) Hypothyroidism
B) Preeclampsia
C) Ovarian Cancer
D) Rheumatoid Arthritis

Question 113: Which blood type is considered the universal donor in the context of ABO incompatibility in newborns?
A) Type A
B) Type B
C) Type AB
D) Type O

Question 114: Mrs. Smith, a 28-year-old postpartum woman, presents with fever, uterine tenderness, and foul-smelling lochia on the third day after a cesarean section. Her vital signs are temperature 38.5蚓, pulse 100 bpm, and blood pressure 120/70 mmHg. What is the most likely diagnosis?
A) Mastitis
B) Endometritis
C) Urinary tract infection
D) Wound infection

Question 115: Which intervention is commonly used to manage prolonged labor in maternal newborn nursing?
A) Early epidural administration
B) Frequent position changes
C) Oxytocin augmentation
D) Immediate cesarean section

Question 116: Which statement regarding the administration of diuretics in the postpartum period is accurate?
A) Diuretics are contraindicated in postpartum women due to the risk of dehydration.
B) Diuretics are commonly used to prevent postpartum hemorrhage.

C) Diuretics may be prescribed to manage postpartum edema.
D) Diuretics are primarily given to increase breast milk production.

Question 117: During the administration of epidural anesthesia to a laboring woman, the nurse notes a decrease in the woman's blood pressure. Which of the following interventions is most appropriate in this situation?
A) Administering more epidural medication to enhance pain relief.
B) Placing the woman in a supine position.
C) Increasing the rate of intravenous fluids.
D) Encouraging the woman to push immediately.

Question 118: Mrs. Smith, a postpartum patient, is prescribed ibuprofen for pain relief after a cesarean section. Which of the following statements regarding ibuprofen administration is accurate?
A) Ibuprofen should be taken on an empty stomach to enhance absorption.
B) Ibuprofen can be safely taken with other NSAIDs for increased pain relief.
C) Ibuprofen should be avoided in the third trimester of pregnancy due to potential harm to the fetus.
D) Ibuprofen is safe to use in breastfeeding mothers without any precautions.

Question 119: Mrs. Smith, a 28-year-old postpartum mother, has been exhibiting symptoms of persistent sadness, loss of interest in activities, and feelings of worthlessness since giving birth to her baby three weeks ago. She also mentions having trouble sleeping and concentrating. Which of the following conditions is Mrs. Smith most likely experiencing?
A) Postpartum Depression
B) Postpartum Psychosis
C) Postpartum Anxiety
D) Postpartum Blues

Question 120: What is a potential complication of chronic hypertension in pregnancy?
A) Preterm birth
B) Low birth weight
C) Macrosomia
D) Preeclampsia

Question 121: Which antenatal factor is NOT associated with an increased risk of infertility?
A) Advanced maternal age
B) History of sexually transmitted infections (STIs)
C) Regular menstrual cycles
D) Polycystic ovary syndrome (PCOS)

Question 122: Ms. Johnson, a 35-year-old multiparous woman, is experiencing symptoms of postpartum depression, including persistent sadness and loss of interest in activities. Which intervention should the nurse prioritize for Ms. Johnson?
A) Encourage social isolation to prevent overwhelming feelings.
B) Refer Ms. Johnson to a support group for mothers with postpartum depression.
C) Minimize discussions about her feelings to avoid distress.
D) Prescribe antidepressant medication without further assessment.

Question 123: Mrs. Smith, a new mother, is holding her newborn baby skin-to-skin shortly after delivery. The infant is making sucking motions and turning towards the mother's breast. This behavior is an example of:
A) Rooting reflex
B) Moro reflex
C) Tonic neck reflex
D) Babinski reflex

Question 124: Ms. Smith, a 2-day-old newborn, presents with irritability, poor feeding, and high-pitched crying. Upon assessment, the nurse notes bulging fontanelles and increased head circumference. Which of the following is the most appropriate nursing intervention for this newborn?
A) Encourage frequent breastfeeding
B) Administer acetaminophen for pain relief
C) Place the newborn in a prone position
D) Notify the healthcare provider immediately

Question 125: Which maternal postpartum complication is commonly associated with substance use disorder during pregnancy?
A) Postpartum hemorrhage
B) Mastitis
C) Postpartum depression
D) Endometritis

Question 126: Mrs. Smith, a new mother, has decided to place her newborn for adoption. She expresses feelings of guilt and sadness during postpartum assessment. As a nurse providing care, which action is most appropriate?
A) Encourage Mrs. Smith to suppress her emotions and focus on her recovery.
B) Provide emotional support and offer resources for counseling.
C) Advise Mrs. Smith to avoid discussing her decision with anyone.
D) Suggest Mrs. Smith to keep her feelings to herself to avoid judgment.

Question 127: Emily, a 28-year-old woman, gave birth to a stillborn baby at 38 weeks gestation. She is experiencing intense grief and is struggling to cope with the loss. As a nurse caring for Emily, what is the most appropriate action to support her during this difficult time?
A) Avoid discussing the baby or the loss to prevent further emotional distress
B) Encourage Emily to quickly return to her normal routine to distract herself
C) Provide a safe and supportive environment for Emily to grieve openly
D) Minimize the significance of the loss and focus on the future

Question 128: During a postpartum assessment, a nurse suspects a new mother may be struggling with substance abuse. Which physical signs may indicate substance abuse in a postpartum mother?

A) Fatigue and irritability
B) Dilated pupils and slurred speech
C) Breast engorgement and nipple tenderness
D) Increased appetite and weight gain

Question 129: How long should a breastfeeding session typically last to ensure the newborn receives enough hindmilk for optimal nutrition?
A) 5-10 minutes per breast
B) 15-20 minutes per breast
C) 25-30 minutes per breast
D) 35-40 minutes per breast

Question 130: What is a common maternal postpartum complication associated with multiple births?
A) Hypertension
B) Gestational diabetes
C) Postpartum hemorrhage
D) Urinary tract infection

Question 131: Which bacterial infection is known to cause pneumonia, meningitis, and sepsis in newborns?
A) Streptococcus pneumoniae
B) Haemophilus influenzae type b (Hib)
C) Neisseria meningitidis
D) Streptococcus agalactiae

Question 132: Which type of anemia is commonly seen in pregnant women due to increased demand for iron during pregnancy?
A) Aplastic anemia
B) Hemolytic anemia
C) Thalassemia
D) Physiologic anemia of pregnancy

Question 133: A 28-year-old G2P1 woman at 39 weeks gestation is admitted to the labor and delivery unit with a temperature of 38.5℃ (101.3℉), tachycardia, and uterine tenderness. She reports a history of prolonged rupture of membranes for over 24 hours. Fetal heart rate monitoring shows late decelerations. What is the most likely diagnosis for this patient?
A) Preterm Premature Rupture of Membranes (PPROM)
B) Chorioamnionitis
C) Placental Abruption
D) Uterine Rupture

Question 134: Mrs. Smith, a postpartum mother, is experiencing nipple soreness while breastfeeding. Which breastfeeding device can help alleviate nipple soreness by ensuring proper latch and positioning?
A) Nipple shield
B) Breast pump
C) Nipple cream
D) Nursing bra

Question 135: Mrs. Smith has just given birth to a baby girl, and her 4-year-old son, Jake, is showing signs of jealousy and regression. He refuses to talk to his parents and has been throwing tantrums frequently. Which intervention by the nurse would be most appropriate to address Jake's behavior?

A) Encourage Mrs. Smith to spend more time with the baby
B) Provide Jake with a doll to care for like his mom cares for the baby
C) Ignore Jake's behavior to avoid reinforcing it
D) Tell Jake to stop misbehaving and act like a big brother

Question 136: During a postpartum assessment, a nurse observes a mother experiencing postpartum hemorrhage. Which intervention should the nurse prioritize in the management of this maternal complication?
A) Encouraging ambulation to prevent blood clots
B) Administering oxytocin to promote uterine contractions
C) Providing a warm blanket to maintain body temperature
D) Offering a high-protein diet to support recovery

Question 137: Which obstetrical history factor is associated with an increased risk of placental abnormalities and pregnancy complications?
A) History of placenta previa
B) Maternal smoking during pregnancy
C) History of post-term pregnancies
D) Previous cesarean section

Question 138: Which factor should be considered when administering analgesics to newborns?
A) Weight-based dosing
B) Frequency of maternal medication use
C) Gestational age at birth
D) Family history of allergies

Question 139: During the assessment of a pregnant woman with suspected placental abruption, which finding would be of most concern and require immediate intervention?
A) Maternal blood pressure of 140/90 mmHg
B) Fetal heart rate of 160 bpm
C) Vaginal bleeding with clots
D) Uterine tenderness and rigidity

Question 140: Which of the following maternal complications is a contraindication to breastfeeding?
A) Mastitis
B) Postpartum hemorrhage
C) Inverted nipples
D) Maternal HIV infection

Question 141: After assessing a postpartum patient with constipation, the nurse notes abdominal distention and discomfort. Which nursing intervention should be prioritized in this situation?
A) Encouraging the patient to increase physical activity
B) Administering a laxative to promote bowel movement
C) Providing a warm sitz bath to relieve abdominal discomfort
D) Notifying the healthcare provider for further evaluation

Question 142: Scenario: A newborn infant is brought to the nursery for assessment. The baby was born at 36 weeks gestation, weighs 2.5 kg, and has a length of 45 cm. On examination, the nurse notes that the baby has poor muscle tone, weak cry, and decreased activity. The skin appears pale, with jaundice noted

on the sclera. Which of the following assessments should the nurse prioritize for this newborn?
A) Blood pressure measurement
B) Capillary refill time assessment
C) Complete blood count (CBC)
D) Gestational age assessment

Question 143: When is amniocentesis typically performed during pregnancy?
A) First trimester
B) Second trimester
C) Third trimester
D) Anytime during pregnancy

Question 144: Which of the following is a characteristic feature of Transient Tachypnea of the Newborn (TTN)?
A) Onset typically occurs within the first few hours after birth.
B) It is a self-limiting condition that resolves within 24-72 hours.
C) TTN is commonly associated with prematurity.
D) Treatment includes administration of antibiotics.

Question 145: Which of the following is a common clinical manifestation of intestinal obstruction in newborns?
A) Constipation
B) Bilious vomiting
C) Normal bowel movements
D) Decreased abdominal distension

Question 146: Mrs. Smith, a 28-year-old postpartum mother, presents with symptoms of mastitis. Which of the following is a contraindication to breastfeeding in this scenario?
A) Engorgement
B) Cracked nipples
C) Mastitis
D) Breast abscess

Question 147: During a newborn assessment, the nurse observes a baby with abdominal distention, bloody stools, and signs of sepsis. Which gastrointestinal condition should be suspected?
A) Meconium ileus
B) Intussusception
C) Malrotation with volvulus
D) Necrotizing enterocolitis

Question 148: Which of the following is a neural tube defect characterized by the protrusion of the meninges and spinal cord through a vertebral defect?
A) Hydrocephalus
B) Spina Bifida
C) Anencephaly
D) Encephalocele

Question 149: What is a common recommendation for managing engorgement in a breastfeeding mother?
A) Limiting breastfeeding sessions to every 4 hours.
B) Applying cold packs to the breasts before feeding.
C) Massaging the breasts in a circular motion to express milk.
D) Avoiding warm showers or compresses.

Question 150: Mrs. Smith, a 32-year-old primigravida, experienced a late-term miscarriage at 24 weeks gestation. She is grieving the loss of her baby and expresses feelings of guilt and sadness. As a nurse providing care to Mrs. Smith, which intervention would be most appropriate in supporting her through perinatal grief?
A) Encouraging her to avoid talking about her feelings
B) Suggesting she should move on quickly and try for another pregnancy
C) Providing emotional support and encouraging her to express her feelings
D) Minimizing the significance of her loss and focusing on the future

ANSWERS WITH DETAILED EXPLANATION (SET 3)

Question 1: Correct Answer: A) Administer oxygen therapy
Rationale: Administering oxygen therapy is the priority intervention to improve Mrs. Smith's oxygenation status. Oxygen will help alleviate hypoxia and stabilize her condition. Chest X-ray may be done later to confirm the diagnosis of pulmonary embolus. Starting anticoagulant therapy is important but not the immediate priority. Deep breathing exercises are contraindicated in suspected pulmonary embolism as they can dislodge clots.

Question 2: Correct Answer: C) Crying loudly
Rationale: Crying loudly is a late feeding cue and often indicates that the newborn is already distressed or hungry. The other options, rooting reflex, sucking on hands or fingers, and turning head side to side with mouth open, are all early feeding cues that suggest the newborn is ready to breastfeed. It is crucial for nurses to recognize these early cues to facilitate successful breastfeeding initiation and bonding between the mother and newborn.

Question 3: Correct Answer: C) Postpartum hemorrhage
Rationale: Postpartum hemorrhage is a significant cause of maternal morbidity and mortality worldwide. It is defined as excessive bleeding of 500 ml or more after vaginal birth or 1000 ml or more after cesarean birth. Mastitis is inflammation of the breast tissue, endometritis is infection of the uterine lining, and thromboembolism is a blood clot that forms in a blood vessel.

Question 4: Correct Answer: C) Infrequent bowel movements
Rationale: Infrequent bowel movements are indicative of constipation in a postpartum woman. Constipation is characterized by difficulty passing stools and decreased frequency of bowel movements. Frequent loose stools are more indicative of diarrhea. Abdominal cramping relieved by passing gas is more suggestive of gas or bloating. Increased appetite is not a typical sign of constipation but may occur due to other factors.

Question 5: Correct Answer: A) McRoberts maneuver
Rationale: In cases of shoulder dystocia during forceps-assisted delivery, the McRoberts maneuver is the initial step to help dislodge the impacted shoulder. The Rubin maneuver involves rotating the fetus to dislodge the shoulder, Woods' screw maneuver is used in cases of breech delivery, and the Jacquemier maneuver is not a recognized obstetrical maneuver for shoulder dystocia.

Question 6: Correct Answer: A) Vitamin K
Rationale: Vitamin K is routinely administered to newborns to prevent hemorrhagic disease, a condition that can lead to bleeding issues in the first few days of life. It helps in the synthesis of clotting factors, reducing the risk of bleeding. Ibuprofen and acetaminophen are commonly used for pain relief and fever reduction in infants, not for preventing hemorrhagic disease. Furosemide is a diuretic medication used to treat conditions like edema and hypertension, not indicated for newborns in preventing hemorrhagic disease.

Question 7: Correct Answer: B) Open adoption allows birth parents to have ongoing contact with the child.
Rationale: Open adoption is a type of adoption where birth parents and adoptive parents have ongoing contact and share identifying information. This arrangement allows for communication and updates on the child's well-being. In contrast, closed adoption involves no contact or sharing of information, while semi-open adoption permits limited communication through a third party. Understanding the different types of adoption is crucial for maternal newborn nurses to provide comprehensive support and education to mothers considering adoption.

Question 8: Correct Answer: C) Thrombocytopenia
Rationale: HELLP syndrome is characterized by Hemolysis, Elevated Liver enzymes, and Low Platelet count. Thrombocytopenia is a hallmark feature of HELLP syndrome. Hypertension is common but not specific to HELLP. Elevated liver enzymes and proteinuria are also seen in HELLP syndrome, but thrombocytopenia is a distinguishing feature.

Question 9: Correct Answer: D) Separating the mother and baby for long periods
Rationale: Separating the mother and baby for extended periods can hinder the establishment of bonding and breastfeeding, leading to potential barriers in parent/infant interactions. This practice may disrupt the early initiation of breastfeeding, delay skin-to-skin contact, and impede the development of a secure attachment between the mother and baby. In contrast, options A, B, and C promote positive parent/infant interactions by facilitating immediate physical closeness, promoting rooming-in to enhance bonding, and providing essential education for successful breastfeeding.

Question 10: Correct Answer: A) Apply petroleum jelly to the circumcision site at each diaper change.
Rationale: Applying petroleum jelly to the circumcision site helps prevent the diaper from sticking to the area and promotes healing. Alcohol wipes can cause irritation and should be avoided. Bathing is allowed, but the circumcision site should be gently cleaned with warm water. Scented wipes may contain chemicals that can irritate the sensitive skin.

Question 11: Correct Answer: B) Placental abruption
Rationale: The sudden onset of severe abdominal pain, vaginal bleeding, uterine tenderness, and fetal distress are classic signs of placental abruption. This condition occurs when the placenta separates from the uterine wall before delivery. Ectopic pregnancy, oligohydramnios, and hyperemesis gravidarum are not typically associated with these symptoms and findings, making them less likely in this scenario.

Question 12: Correct Answer: C) Multiparity
Rationale: Multiparity, or having multiple previous pregnancies, is not a common maternal factor associated with an increased risk of IUGR. Hypertension, smoking, and diabetes are well-known risk factors for IUGR. Hypertension can lead to decreased blood flow to the placenta, affecting fetal growth. Smoking can restrict oxygen and nutrient supply to the fetus, impacting growth. Diabetes, especially uncontrolled, can result in macrosomia or IUGR due to abnormal glucose levels affecting fetal development.

Question 13: Correct Answer: B) Provide Emily with resources on domestic violence shelters and safety

planning.
Rationale: When a patient discloses intimate partner violence, the nurse's priority is to ensure the safety of the patient and her child. Providing resources on domestic violence shelters and safety planning empowers the patient to make informed decisions about her well-being. Encouraging secrecy or ignoring the abuse can further endanger the patient. Couples counseling is not recommended in cases of abuse as it can escalate the situation.

Question 14: Correct Answer: B) Monitoring for signs of opioid withdrawal in the newborn.
Rationale: Monitoring for signs of opioid withdrawal in the newborn is a critical nursing intervention when caring for a postpartum patient receiving Methadone. Methadone can cross the placenta and lead to neonatal abstinence syndrome (NAS) in the newborn. Encouraging the patient to skip doses or combining Methadone with other sedatives can be harmful and disrupt the treatment plan. Discontinuing Methadone abruptly can trigger withdrawal symptoms in the patient. Therefore, option B is the correct answer as it emphasizes the importance of vigilant monitoring for NAS signs in newborns exposed to Methadone during the postpartum period.

Question 15: Correct Answer: C) Acrocyanosis in extremities
Rationale: Acrocyanosis, a bluish discoloration of the hands and feet, is a common and normal finding in newborns during the first few hours after birth due to immature peripheral circulation. Respiratory rate typically ranges from 30-60 breaths per minute, heart rate averages 120-160 beats per minute, and blood pressure is around 60-80/40-50 mmHg in a term newborn. Therefore, acrocyanosis is the correct option as it aligns with the expected physiological changes during the transition to extrauterine life.

Question 16: Correct Answer: B) "I plan to offer complementary feedings such as iron-fortified cereals around six months of age while continuing to breastfeed."
Rationale: Option B reflects the correct understanding of complementary feedings, which should be introduced around six months of age while continuing breastfeeding. Options A, C, and D demonstrate misconceptions about the timing and purpose of complementary feedings, highlighting the importance of proper education and support for mothers considering this option.

Question 17: Correct Answer: B) Perform a sterile speculum examination
Rationale: In the scenario described, Mrs. Smith presents with signs and symptoms suggestive of premature rupture of membranes (PROM). The most appropriate initial nursing action is to perform a sterile speculum examination to confirm the presence of amniotic fluid leakage. This will help in assessing the color, odor, and amount of amniotic fluid, which is crucial in the management of PROM. Administering tocolytic therapy, starting intravenous antibiotics, or inducing labor immediately are not the initial actions indicated in this scenario.

Question 18: Correct Answer: A) Previous classical cesarean incision
Rationale: A previous classical cesarean incision is a contraindication for VBAC due to the increased risk of uterine rupture. This type of incision is associated with a higher risk of uterine rupture during a trial of labor. Options B, C, and D are not contraindications for VBAC. One prior low transverse cesarean incision is actually a favorable factor for VBAC, while gestational diabetes and maternal age over 35 years are not direct contraindications for VBAC.

Question 19: Correct Answer: B) Cefazolin
Rationale: Cefazolin is a first-line antibiotic commonly used to treat postpartum wound infections due to its effectiveness against a broad spectrum of bacteria commonly found in surgical site infections. Acetaminophen is a pain reliever, Omeprazole is a proton pump inhibitor used for gastric issues, and Metoclopramide is a gastrointestinal stimulant, none of which are indicated for wound infections.

Question 20: Correct Answer: A) Preference for extended family involvement
Rationale: In many cultures, there is a strong preference for extended family involvement in the postpartum period. This can impact family integration as the new mother may rely heavily on the support and guidance of her extended family members. Option B is incorrect as high socioeconomic status does not necessarily correlate with family integration. Option C is incorrect as cultures that emphasize individualism may actually hinder family integration. Option D is incorrect as limited access to healthcare services may affect health outcomes but not necessarily family integration.

Question 21: Correct Answer: B) Providing the new mother with information on local parenting support groups
Rationale: Option B aligns with the ethical principle of justice by ensuring that the new mother has access to community resources that can support her emotional well-being and bonding with her baby. Options A, C, and D do not uphold the principle of justice as they either suggest professional help without exploring community resources, dismiss the new mother's concerns, or restrict her access to bonding opportunities with her baby.

Question 22: Correct Answer: B) Zidovudine
Rationale: Zidovudine, also known as AZT, is a nucleoside reverse transcriptase inhibitor commonly used in pregnant women with HIV to reduce the risk of transmitting the virus to the baby. Acyclovir is an antiviral medication used to treat herpes infections, not HIV. Metronidazole is an antibiotic used for bacterial and parasitic infections, while Amoxicillin is a penicillin antibiotic, neither of which are used for HIV treatment or prevention.

Question 23: Correct Answer: B) Postpartum thyroiditis
Rationale: The symptoms described - fatigue, weight gain, and cold intolerance - are indicative of hypothyroidism, which can occur in postpartum thyroiditis. Postpartum depression (Option A) typically presents with mood disturbances. Postpartum hemorrhage (Option C) is characterized by excessive bleeding post-delivery. Postpartum preeclampsia (Option D) involves high blood pressure and protein in the urine. By comparing the symptoms presented in the question with the options provided, it is evident that the correct answer is postpartum thyroiditis.

Question 24: Correct Answer: C) Initiate a heel stick for blood glucose monitoring.
Rationale: Initiating a heel stick for blood glucose monitoring is the priority when a newborn shows signs of hypoglycemia. This will provide essential information to confirm hypoglycemia and guide further interventions.

Offering a pacifier, checking temperature, or encouraging feeding are important but should follow the confirmation of hypoglycemia through blood glucose monitoring to ensure appropriate management.

Question 25: Correct Answer: D) Provide tactile stimulation
Rationale: In a premature infant like James experiencing bradycardia and cyanosis, the appropriate nursing action is to provide tactile stimulation to stimulate the baby and improve heart rate. Increasing CPAP pressure may worsen the condition. Administering surfactant is not indicated in this situation. Chest physiotherapy is not appropriate for bradycardia and cyanosis but may be used for airway clearance in other conditions.

Question 26: Correct Answer: C) Pulse Oximetry
Rationale: Pulse oximetry is a non-invasive screening tool used to detect critical congenital heart defects in newborns. It measures the oxygen saturation levels in the blood, aiding in the early identification of CHD. The Denver Developmental Screening Test assesses a child's developmental progress, the Apgar Score evaluates a newborn's overall health at birth, and the Ballard Score is used to estimate gestational age.

Question 27: Correct Answer: B) The Hepatitis B vaccine is administered intramuscularly in the deltoid muscle.
Rationale: The correct answer is B) The Hepatitis B vaccine is administered intramuscularly in the deltoid muscle. The Hepatitis B vaccine is safe to administer during pregnancy and is recommended for all pregnant women, especially those at high risk. It is given in the deltoid muscle or anterolateral thigh. Option A is incorrect as the vaccine is safe during pregnancy. Option C is incorrect as multiple doses are required for long-term immunity. Option D is incorrect as the vaccine is recommended for various populations beyond healthcare workers.

Question 28: Correct Answer: B) Suggest she joins a new mothers' support group.
Rationale: Encouraging Mrs. Smith to join a new mothers' support group can provide her with emotional support, reassurance, and coping strategies from other women experiencing similar challenges. This intervention promotes social interaction, reduces isolation, and normalizes her feelings, which are essential in managing postpartum depression. Options A, C, and D are incorrect as rest alone, increased caffeine intake, and immediate hospitalization may not address the underlying emotional and psychological needs of Mrs. Smith.

Question 29: Correct Answer: C) Lispro insulin
Rationale: Lispro insulin is a rapid-acting insulin with the fastest onset of action, typically within 15 minutes. Regular insulin has a slower onset of action compared to Lispro. NPH insulin is an intermediate-acting insulin, and Glargine insulin is a long-acting insulin. Therefore, Lispro insulin is the correct option for the fastest onset of action.

Question 30: Correct Answer: A) Group B Streptococcus
Rationale: Group B Streptococcus (GBS) is the most common cause of early-onset neonatal sepsis. It is crucial to screen pregnant women for GBS colonization during pregnancy to prevent transmission to the newborn during delivery. Escherichia coli and other organisms can also cause neonatal sepsis, but GBS is the most prevalent in early-onset cases.

Question 31: Correct Answer: B) Initiating enteral feedings
Rationale: When jitteriness in a newborn is suspected to be due to hypoglycemia, the appropriate nursing intervention is to initiate enteral feedings to provide a source of glucose and raise the blood sugar levels. Enteral feedings can help stabilize the newborn's blood glucose levels and alleviate the symptoms of jitteriness. Administering oxygen therapy (Option A) is not indicated for jitteriness related to hypoglycemia. Placing the newborn in a cold environment (Option C) can exacerbate the issue. Administering a sedative medication (Option D) is not appropriate and can mask the underlying problem of hypoglycemia.

Question 32: Correct Answer: A) Pulmonary embolism
Rationale: Mrs. Smith's symptoms of shortness of breath and chest pain, along with tachycardia and tachypnea, are indicative of a pulmonary embolism, a serious complication in the postpartum period. Pulmonary embolism is a life-threatening condition that requires immediate medical intervention. Postpartum hemorrhage, preeclampsia, and mastitis do not typically present with these specific cardiopulmonary symptoms.

Question 33: Correct Answer: B) Initiating phototherapy
Rationale: Neonatal jaundice is a common condition in newborns caused by elevated bilirubin levels. Phototherapy is the standard treatment for neonatal jaundice as it helps to break down bilirubin in the baby's skin. Encouraging formula feeding, administering iron supplements, and applying cold compresses are not appropriate interventions for managing neonatal jaundice and can potentially worsen the condition.

Question 34: Correct Answer: A) 7.25 - 7.35
Rationale: The normal range for pH in umbilical cord arterial blood gas analysis in a newborn is typically between 7.25 - 7.35. This range indicates normal acid-base balance in the newborn and is crucial in assessing the baby's oxygenation status during labor and delivery. Options B, C, and D are outside the normal pH range for umbilical cord arterial blood gas analysis and would suggest acidosis or alkalosis, which could indicate fetal distress or other complications.

Question 35: Correct Answer: A) Maternal obesity
Rationale: Maternal obesity is a known risk factor for prolonged labor due to factors such as increased soft tissue, higher rates of induction, and augmented labor. Normal fetal position (Option B) and adequate uterine contractions (Option C) are actually favorable conditions for labor progression and not risk factors for prolonged labor. Previous uncomplicated vaginal delivery (Option D) is not a risk factor for prolonged labor as it is associated with efficient labor patterns.

Question 36: Correct Answer: C) Often result in metabolic crises
Rationale: Inborn errors of metabolism are genetic disorders that typically manifest in the neonatal period due to defects in enzymes or metabolic pathways. These conditions can lead to metabolic crises characterized by severe symptoms such as vomiting, lethargy, seizures, and metabolic acidosis. Unlike acquired conditions, these disorders are present from birth and require lifelong management. While dietary modifications may help manage some inborn errors of metabolism, they cannot be cured by such interventions. Symptoms usually appear early in life, not later in childhood.

Question 37: Correct Answer: B) Providing emotional support and reassurance to Mrs. Smith.

Rationale: Providing emotional support and reassurance to Mrs. Smith aligns with the ethical principle of non-maleficence by ensuring her emotional well-being and preventing harm. Option A could potentially harm Mrs. Smith by invalidating her feelings. Option C dismisses her concerns, which could lead to further distress. Option D without proper assessment may not address the root cause of her distress and could potentially cause harm by inappropriate medication use.

Question 38: Correct Answer: C) Maternal diabetes
Rationale: Maternal diabetes is a known risk factor for macrosomia (large birth weight), which can lead to prolonged and difficult labor, increasing the risk of fetal hypoxia and acidosis. While maternal obesity, advanced maternal age, and hypothyroidism can also impact labor, maternal diabetes has a direct association with fetal macrosomia and its related complications during labor. It is essential to monitor and manage maternal diabetes closely during pregnancy to prevent adverse outcomes for both the mother and the baby.

Question 39: Correct Answer: A) Decreased platelet count
Rationale: In DIC, there is consumption of platelets leading to decreased platelet count. Elevated fibrinogen levels are not seen in DIC; instead, there is a decrease. Prolonged PT is a feature of DIC due to impaired coagulation factors. Antithrombin III levels are decreased in DIC, not increased.

Question 40: Correct Answer: C) Hydrocephalus
Rationale: The symptoms described are indicative of hydrocephalus, a condition characterized by the accumulation of cerebrospinal fluid in the brain, leading to increased head size, poor muscle tone, and developmental delays. Down syndrome, cerebral palsy, and hypothyroidism may present with different clinical features and are not typically associated with the specific signs mentioned in the scenario.

Question 41: Correct Answer: A) Malrotation with volvulus
Rationale: Abdominal distension and bilious vomiting in a newborn, especially a preterm infant, are concerning for malrotation with volvulus, a surgical emergency where the bowel twists on itself. Meconium ileus is typically seen in newborns with cystic fibrosis, gastroesophageal reflux presents with spitting up, and pyloric stenosis manifests with non-bilious projectile vomiting.

Question 42: Correct Answer: A) Endometritis
Rationale: Mrs. Smith's presentation of fever, uterine tenderness, foul-smelling lochia, and fatigue is indicative of endometritis, which is an infection of the uterine lining commonly seen postpartum, especially after cesarean sections. Mastitis typically presents with breast tenderness, redness, and warmth. Urinary tract infections present with dysuria, frequency, and urgency. Wound infections are characterized by localized pain, redness, swelling, and purulent drainage.

Question 43: Correct Answer: B) Tetralogy of Fallot
Rationale: Tetralogy of Fallot is a congenital heart defect characterized by four abnormalities in the heart's structure, leading to cyanosis, tachypnea, and poor feeding. While Patent Ductus Arteriosus, Atrial Septal Defect, and Ventricular Septal Defect are also congenital heart defects, they do not typically present with the classic tetralogy of Fallot symptoms of cyanosis, tachypnea, and poor feeding.

Question 44: Correct Answer: D) History of uterine rupture
Rationale: A history of uterine rupture is a significant contraindication for VBAC due to the increased risk of uterine rupture recurring during a subsequent trial of labor. Uterine rupture can lead to life-threatening complications for both the mother and the baby, making it unsafe to attempt a vaginal birth after cesarean in this scenario. It is crucial to carefully assess maternal factors and previous obstetric history to determine the suitability of VBAC and minimize risks to maternal and fetal health.

Question 45: Correct Answer: C) Feeling that IPV is a private matter and should not be discussed
Rationale: Many women may feel that intimate partner violence (IPV) is a private matter and may be reluctant to disclose it due to shame, fear of judgment, or cultural beliefs. This perception can act as a significant barrier to seeking help and support. Healthcare providers need to create a safe and non-judgmental environment to encourage women to open up about IPV, provide appropriate support, and connect them with resources to ensure their safety and well-being.

Question 46: Correct Answer: A) Ibuprofen
Rationale: Ibuprofen is the preferred analgesic for postpartum pain in breastfeeding mothers due to its minimal excretion into breast milk and proven safety for newborns. Codeine, morphine, and tramadol are not recommended as they can lead to sedation, respiratory depression, and other adverse effects in newborns through breast milk transfer.

Question 47: Correct Answer: A) Administering intravenous antibiotics
Rationale: The clinical presentation of lower abdominal pain, malaise, chills, and fever on the fifth day post-vaginal delivery is concerning for endometritis. The most appropriate initial intervention is to administer intravenous antibiotics to cover likely pathogens. Ordering a pelvic ultrasound may be considered for further evaluation. Performing a complete blood count can help assess for leukocytosis. Initiating antipyretic therapy alone does not address the underlying infection.

Question 48: Correct Answer: A) Attachment bonding
Rationale: The described behavior of making eye contact, talking softly, and gentle touching indicates the process of attachment bonding between the mother and the infant. This bonding is crucial for the development of a secure attachment relationship. Neglectful behavior, postpartum depression, and infantile regression are not associated with positive parent/infant interactions and bonding.

Question 49: Correct Answer: C) ABO incompatibility
Rationale: ABO incompatibility is a risk factor for hyperbilirubinemia due to the breakdown of incompatible blood cells, leading to an increase in bilirubin levels. Term babies born at 39 weeks are at lower risk compared to preterm babies. Exclusive breastfeeding can contribute to jaundice but is not a direct risk factor. Maternal diabetes can lead to other complications but is not a primary risk factor for hyperbilirubinemia.

Question 50: Correct Answer: A) Heart failure
Rationale: The presence of pedal edema, crackles in the lungs, and a persistent cough in a postpartum mother is suggestive of heart failure. These symptoms indicate fluid overload and impaired cardiac function. Pulmonary edema, deep vein thrombosis, and pneumonia may present with some similar symptoms but do not encompass the combination of findings seen in heart

failure, making it the most likely diagnosis in this scenario.

Question 51: Correct Answer: C) Oxytocin augmentation
Rationale: Oxytocin augmentation is contraindicated in cases of transverse lie as it can increase the risk of cord prolapse. External cephalic version, amnioinfusion, and cesarean section are management options that may be considered depending on the clinical scenario. Oxytocin augmentation is not appropriate due to the risk of cord prolapse associated with transverse lie presentations.

Question 52: Correct Answer: C) Improved cardiovascular stability
Rationale: Delayed cord clamping allows for increased blood volume transfer from the placenta to the newborn, leading to improved cardiovascular stability. This process helps in the prevention of hypovolemia and promotes better perfusion to vital organs. Options A and B are incorrect as delayed cord clamping actually reduces the risk of neonatal anemia and enhances iron stores due to the additional blood volume received. Option D is incorrect as delayed cord clamping has been associated with a lower incidence of respiratory distress syndrome due to improved lung perfusion.

Question 53: Correct Answer: B) Provide education on the risks of smoking during pregnancy and offer smoking cessation resources.
Rationale: Smoking during pregnancy increases the risk of complications such as preterm birth, low birth weight, and birth defects. Providing education on these risks and offering smoking cessation resources is crucial to support Mrs. Smith in quitting smoking for the health of her and her baby. The other options are incorrect as they do not promote the best practice of smoking cessation during pregnancy.

Question 54: Correct Answer: A) Endotracheal intubation
Rationale: Endotracheal intubation is the most appropriate method for establishing an airway in a newborn during resuscitation as it allows for secure airway management and effective ventilation. Inserting a nasopharyngeal airway, performing a jaw-thrust maneuver, or placing a laryngeal mask airway may not provide the same level of airway protection and control as endotracheal intubation in a critical resuscitation scenario.

Question 55: Correct Answer: B) Hypotonia and poor feeding
Rationale: Hypotonia (weak muscle tone) and poor feeding are common symptoms of hypoglycemia in newborns. Option A is incorrect as hypoglycemic newborns typically display lethargy rather than hyperactivity. Option C and D are unrelated to hypoglycemia symptoms. Recognizing these signs promptly is crucial for early intervention and preventing complications associated with hypoglycemia in newborns.

Question 56: Correct Answer: C) Tachycardia
Rationale: In this scenario, the fetal heart rate is consistently above 160 beats per minute, indicating tachycardia. Tachycardia is defined as a baseline fetal heart rate greater than 160 beats per minute. Bradycardia refers to a baseline fetal heart rate less than 110 beats per minute, altered variability is a change in the normal beat-to-beat fluctuations, and decelerations are temporary decreases in the fetal heart rate.

Question 57: Correct Answer: B) Uterine atony

Rationale: In a multiple birth scenario, the mother is at higher risk for uterine atony due to the increased stretching of the uterus during pregnancy. This condition can lead to postpartum hemorrhage, making it a critical finding to monitor. Engorged breasts, vaginal bleeding, and perineal pain are common postpartum occurrences that do not pose immediate life-threatening risks in this context.

Question 58: Correct Answer: C) "Include foods rich in iron and protein to support healing and energy levels."
Rationale: Consuming foods rich in iron and protein is essential for postpartum mothers to support healing, replenish nutrient stores, and maintain energy levels. These nutrients are crucial for recovery and breastfeeding. Options A, B, and D are incorrect as they provide advice that is not conducive to optimal postpartum recovery and health.

Question 59: Correct Answer: D) Temperature instability
Rationale: Late-onset neonatal sepsis typically presents with non-specific symptoms such as temperature instability, poor feeding, lethargy, and respiratory distress. While apnea and bradycardia can occur in premature infants, they are more commonly associated with respiratory distress syndrome. Hyperbilirubinemia and hypoglycemia may be present in neonates for various reasons but are not specific to neonatal sepsis.

Question 60: Correct Answer: D) Alcohol
Rationale: Alcohol consumption during pregnancy is particularly harmful as it can result in fetal alcohol syndrome (FAS) characterized by physical, cognitive, and behavioral abnormalities in the newborn. Alcohol crosses the placenta and affects the developing fetus, leading to irreversible damage to the baby's brain and organs. While smoking, drug abuse, and marijuana use also have detrimental effects on pregnancy outcomes, alcohol is specifically known for causing FAS and neurodevelopmental disorders in infants. It is crucial for pregnant women to abstain from alcohol to prevent these serious complications.

Question 61: Correct Answer: A) RhoGAM should be administered within 72 hours postpartum.
Rationale: Rh-negative mothers who have given birth to Rh-positive babies should receive Rh Immune Globulin (RhoGAM) within 72 hours postpartum to prevent sensitization to Rh-positive blood cells. Administering RhoGAM within this timeframe helps to prevent the mother's immune system from producing antibodies against Rh-positive blood cells, which could affect future pregnancies. Options B, C, and D are incorrect as RhoGAM is not contraindicated in Rh incompatibility, is typically administered intramuscularly in the gluteal muscle, and is given regardless of the baby's Rh status.

Question 62: Correct Answer: C) Educating parents about avoiding triggers such as certain foods and medications is crucial.
Rationale: The management of G6PD deficiency in newborns primarily involves educating parents about avoiding triggers that can induce hemolysis, such as certain foods (e.g., fava beans) and medications (e.g., sulfa drugs). Sunlight exposure does not play a significant role in managing G6PD deficiency. Iron supplements are not specifically indicated for G6PD deficiency. Blood transfusions are reserved for severe cases of hemolytic anemia but are not a routine management strategy for G6PD deficiency. Therefore, option C is the correct answer as it highlights the

importance of trigger avoidance in managing G6PD deficiency in newborns.

Question 63: Correct Answer: C) Apnea of prematurity typically resolves by term gestation.
Rationale: Apnea of prematurity is a common condition in preterm infants characterized by pauses in breathing. It typically resolves by term gestation (Option C) as the central nervous system matures. Central apnea (Option B) is more common in full-term infants. Gastroesophageal reflux (Option D) can actually increase the risk of apnea by causing airway irritation. A pause in breathing lasting less than 10 seconds is considered normal, not apnea (Option A).

Question 64: Correct Answer: B) Monitoring for signs of dehydration
Rationale: When administering diuretics to postpartum patients, it is crucial to monitor for signs of dehydration as these medications can lead to fluid and electrolyte imbalances. Encouraging increased sodium intake (Option A) is not recommended as it can exacerbate fluid retention. Administering the medication with a full stomach (Option C) is not necessary for diuretics. Limiting fluid intake (Option D) can further contribute to dehydration and should be avoided.

Question 65: Correct Answer: A) Transient tachypnea of the newborn
Rationale: Transient tachypnea of the newborn (TTN) is a respiratory condition characterized by rapid breathing, grunting, nasal flaring, and chest retractions due to delayed clearance of fetal lung fluid. Bronchopulmonary dysplasia, apnea of prematurity, and congenital diaphragmatic hernia present with different clinical features and require distinct management strategies. Recognizing the signs and symptoms of TTN is essential for prompt intervention and improved outcomes in newborns.

Question 66: Correct Answer: B) Metoclopramide
Rationale: Metoclopramide is a prokinetic agent that enhances GI motility by increasing the frequency and strength of contractions in the stomach and small intestine. It is often prescribed to postpartum women to alleviate constipation. Ondansetron is an antiemetic used to treat nausea and vomiting, not constipation. Furosemide is a diuretic, and Atenolol is a beta-blocker, both unrelated to GI motility.

Question 67: Correct Answer: C) Keeping the newborn's skin clean and dry helps prevent diaper rash.
Rationale: Keeping the newborn's skin clean and dry is crucial in preventing diaper rash, as moisture and irritants can lead to skin breakdown. Bathing the newborn immediately after birth is not recommended as it can lead to heat loss. Lotions and powders are not necessary and may actually irritate the delicate newborn skin. Scented wipes can contain chemicals that may be harsh on the newborn's skin.

Question 68: Correct Answer: D) Provide privacy and encourage the client to void every 2-3 hours
Rationale: Encouraging the client to void every 2-3 hours is crucial in preventing urinary retention. Providing privacy can help the client relax and facilitate voiding. Options A and B do not address the frequency of voiding necessary to prevent retention. While warm sitz baths (Option C) can provide comfort, they do not directly address bladder emptying.

Question 69: Correct Answer: D) Sudden onset of shortness of breath

Rationale: Sudden onset of shortness of breath in the postpartum period could indicate a serious condition such as pulmonary embolism or heart failure, requiring immediate intervention. Engorged breasts, Lochia rubra with small clots, and a fundus firm at the level of the umbilicus are common postpartum findings that may not require immediate intervention but should be monitored closely. It is essential to recognize and respond promptly to signs of potential life-threatening complications to ensure the well-being of the mother.

Question 70: Correct Answer: B) Educate the mother on the potential risks of nicotine exposure to the newborn through breast milk.
Rationale: The most appropriate nursing intervention is to educate the mother on the risks of nicotine exposure to the newborn through breast milk. This empowers the mother to make informed decisions regarding smoking cessation methods that are safe for her and her baby. Options A, C, and D are incorrect as they promote unsafe practices and do not prioritize the well-being of the newborn.

Question 71: Correct Answer: A) Intravenous glucose bolus
Rationale: The recommended treatment for hypoglycemia in newborns is to administer an intravenous glucose bolus to rapidly increase blood sugar levels. Continuous glucose monitoring, early breastfeeding, and skin-to-skin contact are important interventions for maintaining blood sugar levels and promoting bonding but are not the primary treatment for acute hypoglycemia. In cases of severe hypoglycemia, prompt administration of glucose via IV is crucial to prevent neurological complications.

Question 72: Correct Answer: B) 4-12 hours
Rationale: NPH insulin has a peak action time ranging from 4 to 12 hours after administration. Options A, C, and D do not accurately reflect the peak action time of NPH insulin, which is crucial for determining the timing of meals and monitoring blood glucose levels to prevent hypoglycemia.

Question 73: Correct Answer: C) Ventricular Septal Defect
Rationale: A ventricular septal defect (VSD) is a common congenital heart defect in newborns where there is a hole in the septum separating the heart's lower chambers. This condition leads to abnormal blood flow between the ventricles, causing symptoms like heart murmur, poor feeding, and failure to thrive. Options A, B, and D are also congenital heart defects but are not characterized by a hole in the septum between the heart's upper chambers, making them incorrect choices for this question.

Question 74: Correct Answer: C) Hemorrhoids can be internal or external.
Rationale: Hemorrhoids can be classified as internal (inside the rectum) or external (under the skin around the anus). They are not varicose veins in the lower extremities, caused by a bacterial infection, or unrelated to pregnancy. Understanding the types of hemorrhoids is crucial for appropriate management and treatment strategies.

Question 75: Correct Answer: A) Staphylococcus aureus
Rationale: Staphylococcus aureus is a common cause of neonatal sepsis and is characterized by Gram-positive cocci in clusters. Streptococcus pneumoniae (option B) is more commonly associated with pneumonia and

meningitis. Enterococcus faecalis (option C) is a Gram-positive cocci in pairs or chains and is not typically associated with neonatal sepsis. Staphylococcus epidermidis (option D) is a common skin commensal and is often considered a contaminant in blood cultures rather than a pathogen causing sepsis in newborns.

Question 76: Correct Answer: B) Hypothermia
Rationale: Hypothermia is a common early sign of neonatal sepsis due to the body's response to infection. It is essential to monitor the newborn's temperature closely as hypothermia can be an indicator of underlying sepsis. Bradycardia, hyperglycemia, and jaundice can also occur in neonatal sepsis, but they are not typically early signs. Bradycardia may occur in later stages, hyperglycemia can be a result of stress response, and jaundice may be due to other causes such as physiological jaundice in newborns.

Question 77: Correct Answer: A) Transient tachypnea of the newborn (TTN)
Rationale: Infants of diabetic mothers are at increased risk of developing transient tachypnea of the newborn (TTN) due to delayed clearance of lung fluid. While bronchopulmonary dysplasia (BPD), meconium aspiration syndrome (MAS), and persistent pulmonary hypertension of the newborn (PPHN) are respiratory complications seen in neonates, they are not specifically associated with infants of diabetic mothers, making them incorrect choices.

Question 78: Correct Answer: B) Honor the mother's request and arrange for the baby to stay in the nursery.
Rationale: In cases where the mother expresses anxiety and requests separation, it is crucial to respect her feelings and support her emotional well-being. By honoring the mother's request to have the baby stay in the nursery, the nurse demonstrates empathy and patient-centered care, fostering a trusting relationship with the mother and promoting a positive postpartum experience.

Question 79: Correct Answer: D) Checking the expiration date of the medication
Rationale: Before administering eye prophylaxis, it is crucial to check the expiration date of the medication to ensure its efficacy and safety. Wiping the eyes with a dry cloth, ensuring the infant's position, or cleaning the eyes with sterile saline are not necessary steps before applying the medication for eye prophylaxis.

Question 80: Correct Answer: D) Hands-and-knees position
Rationale: The hands-and-knees position is most beneficial for rotating a fetus in occiput posterior position to occiput anterior, which is optimal for delivery. This position helps relieve pressure on the mother's back and pelvis, facilitating fetal rotation. Options A, B, and C do not provide the same advantages for fetal positioning and rotation during labor.

Question 81: Correct Answer: A) Increased risk of preeclampsia
Rationale: Women who have had bariatric surgery are at an increased risk of developing preeclampsia during pregnancy. This is due to the altered absorption of nutrients and changes in metabolism following the surgery. While bariatric surgery can reduce the risk of gestational diabetes, it does not eliminate it entirely. Post-term pregnancy is not a common complication associated with bariatric surgery. Additionally, the likelihood of cesarean section may be higher in these cases due to various factors related to the surgery. Therefore, the correct answer is A) Increased risk of preeclampsia.

Question 82: Correct Answer: B) Doxycycline
Rationale: Doxycycline is contraindicated in pregnant women as it can lead to discoloration of fetal teeth and inhibit bone growth. Azithromycin and erythromycin are safer alternatives for use during pregnancy. Penicillin is considered safe for use in pregnancy and is commonly used for various infections.

Question 83: Correct Answer: C) Meconium aspiration syndrome occurs when the baby inhales meconium into the lungs.
Rationale: Meconium-stained amniotic fluid does not always indicate fetal distress; it can be a normal occurrence. Meconium is indeed the baby's first stool, typically greenish-black in color. However, the critical complication associated with meconium-stained amniotic fluid is meconium aspiration syndrome, where the baby inhales meconium into the lungs, leading to respiratory issues. Therefore, option C is the correct answer as it highlights a significant complication related to meconium passage during labor.

Question 84: Correct Answer: B) Sertraline
Rationale: Sertraline is a selective serotonin reuptake inhibitor (SSRI) commonly used to treat postpartum depression due to its effectiveness in balancing neurotransmitters in the brain. Lorazepam is a benzodiazepine used for anxiety, not typically indicated for postpartum depression. Methylphenidate is a stimulant used for ADHD, and Haloperidol is an antipsychotic, not commonly used for postpartum depression.

Question 85: Correct Answer: C) Pain relief
Rationale: Tylenol (acetaminophen) is commonly used for pain relief in the postpartum period. It is a safe option for managing mild to moderate pain after childbirth. Options A, B, and D are not correct as Tylenol is not indicated for hypertension management, prevention of blood clots, or treatment of urinary tract infections postpartum. It is important to educate postpartum mothers on the appropriate use of Tylenol for pain relief and to watch for signs of overdose.

Question 86: Correct Answer: B) Increased risk of postpartum hemorrhage
Rationale: Cesarean delivery is associated with an increased risk of postpartum hemorrhage compared to vaginal delivery. While cesarean delivery may reduce the risk of infection in certain cases, it is also associated with an increased risk of surgical complications. Additionally, cesarean delivery poses a higher risk of thromboembolism compared to vaginal delivery.

Question 87: Correct Answer: A) Maternal hypertension
Rationale: Maternal hypertension is a known risk factor for oligohydramnios due to its impact on placental function and blood flow to the fetus. Hypertension can lead to decreased perfusion of the placenta, resulting in reduced amniotic fluid levels. Fetal macrosomia, multiple gestation, and maternal age over 35 years are not directly associated with oligohydramnios. While these factors may pose other risks in pregnancy, they are not specifically linked to the development of oligohydramnios.

Question 88: Correct Answer: D) Lithium
Rationale: Lithium is known to pass into breast milk and can have adverse effects on the infant, including

lethargy, hypotonia, and thyroid dysfunction. Fluoxetine and Paroxetine are SSRIs considered safe during breastfeeding with minimal infant exposure. Diazepam, a benzodiazepine, is also compatible with breastfeeding. However, lithium requires close monitoring and consideration of alternative medications to ensure the safety of the nursing infant.

Question 89: Correct Answer: C) Polycythemia
Rationale: Polycythemia is a hematologic condition in newborns where there is an abnormal increase in the number of red blood cells. This can lead to hyperviscosity and potential complications such as thrombosis. Thrombocytopenia (Option A) is a decrease in platelet count, hemolytic disease of the newborn (Option B) is caused by Rh or ABO blood group incompatibility, and neutropenia (Option D) is a decrease in neutrophils. These conditions are distinct from polycythemia, making it the correct answer.

Question 90: Correct Answer: A) Strabismus
Rationale: Strabismus, or crossed eyes, is a condition where the eyes are not aligned and one eye may turn in, out, up, or down. It is important to detect and treat strabismus early to prevent vision problems. Anisocoria is unequal pupil size, nystagmus is involuntary eye movement, and ptosis is drooping of the upper eyelid. These conditions are different from strabismus and require specific interventions.

Question 91: Correct Answer: A) Postpartum depression
Rationale: Postpartum depression is characterized by persistent feelings of sadness, anxiety, and difficulty bonding with the newborn. It is important to differentiate postpartum depression from baby blues, which are milder and resolve within a few weeks. Adjustment disorder may present with emotional distress but is usually in response to a specific stressor. Postpartum psychosis is a severe condition characterized by hallucinations, delusions, and disorganized thinking.

Question 92: Correct Answer: B) History of smoking
Rationale: Chronic hypertension in pregnancy is more likely to occur in women with a history of smoking. Smoking is a known risk factor for hypertension due to its vasoconstrictive effects. Options A, C, and D are not directly associated with an increased risk of chronic hypertension during pregnancy. Younger age, normal BMI, and being a first-time mother are not specific risk factors for chronic hypertension in pregnancy.

Question 93: Correct Answer: C) Refer the newborn for a swallow study to assess for underlying issues.
Rationale: A disorganized suck-swallow pattern with coughing and choking may indicate potential swallowing difficulties that require further evaluation. Referring the newborn for a swallow study (option C) can help identify any underlying issues and guide appropriate interventions. Using a faster flow nipple (option A) may overwhelm the baby and lead to more issues. Feeding in a quiet environment (option B) can be beneficial but may not address the root cause. Switching to exclusively pumping (option D) may not address the baby's specific feeding challenges.

Question 94: Correct Answer: B) Terbutaline
Rationale: Terbutaline is a beta-adrenergic receptor agonist that is commonly used as a tocolytic agent to delay preterm labor by relaxing the uterine smooth muscle. Nifedipine is a calcium channel blocker, Indomethacin is a nonsteroidal anti-inflammatory drug, and Betamethasone is a corticosteroid used for fetal lung maturation, but they are not typically used as tocolytics.

Question 95: Correct Answer: B) Decreased uterine size
Rationale: During the postpartum period, the uterus undergoes involution, which is the process of returning to its pre-pregnant size. This is a normal physiological change that occurs as the uterus sheds excess tissue and contracts back to its non-pregnant state. Increased estrogen levels are not expected immediately postpartum as they drop after delivery. Lochia discharge is a normal postpartum vaginal discharge consisting of blood and uterine tissue. Ovulation typically resumes around 6-8 weeks postpartum, not within the first week.

Question 96: Correct Answer: B) Denial of the loss and avoidance of discussing the baby.
Rationale: Denial and avoidance are common coping mechanisms in perinatal grief. Parents may find it challenging to acknowledge the loss and may avoid conversations related to the baby or the event. This behavior does not indicate a lack of grief but rather a way of managing the overwhelming emotions associated with the loss. Healthcare providers should be sensitive to these responses and provide a supportive environment for parents to express their feelings and work through their grief process.

Question 97: Correct Answer: A) GDM is a type of diabetes that occurs only during pregnancy.
Rationale: Gestational diabetes mellitus (GDM) is a type of diabetes that develops during pregnancy and usually resolves after delivery. It is essential to monitor blood glucose levels to ensure optimal management and prevent complications for both the mother and the baby. Untreated or poorly controlled GDM can lead to adverse outcomes such as macrosomia, neonatal hypoglycemia, and increased risk of developing type 2 diabetes for both the mother and the child later in life. Therefore, understanding the unique nature of GDM is crucial for providing appropriate care during pregnancy.

Question 98: Correct Answer: B) Bladder distention
Rationale: Bladder distention in a postpartum woman can indicate urinary retention, which can lead to complications such as urinary tract infections or bladder distention. Therefore, further evaluation by the healthcare provider is necessary to assess and address this issue. Options A, C, and D are normal findings in the postpartum period and do not require immediate intervention.

Question 99: Correct Answer: B) Heart rate
Rationale: Heart rate is a critical vital sign in assessing the need for resuscitation in a newborn. A low heart rate indicates the need for immediate intervention to support the newborn's cardiopulmonary function. Blood pressure, temperature, and respiratory rate are also important parameters in newborn assessment but are not as immediate in determining the need for resuscitation as the heart rate. Therefore, monitoring the heart rate is essential in identifying newborns who require prompt resuscitative measures.

Question 100: Correct Answer: C) Newborns primarily rely on surfactant to maintain lung compliance.
Rationale: Surfactant is crucial for reducing surface tension in the alveoli, preventing their collapse and aiding in lung expansion. Newborns have immature lungs at birth and surfactant production increases gradually. Options A, B, and D are incorrect as newborns have a faster respiratory rate, immature alveoli that continue to develop after birth, and an increased pulmonary blood

flow due to closure of fetal shunts, respectively.

Question 101: Correct Answer: D) Emergency cesarean section
Rationale: A BPP score of 0 in multiple parameters, along with a non-reactive NST, indicates fetal compromise and the need for prompt delivery. In this scenario, the absence of fetal breathing movements, gross body movements, and decreased amniotic fluid volume, coupled with a non-reactive NST, necessitates an emergency cesarean section to prevent adverse outcomes for the fetus.

Question 102: Correct Answer: B) Disseminated Intravascular Coagulation (DIC)
Rationale: Disseminated Intravascular Coagulation (DIC) is a serious condition where the body's clotting process is activated abnormally, leading to both clotting and bleeding simultaneously. In the postpartum period, DIC can be triggered by conditions such as sepsis, amniotic fluid embolism, or retained placental tissue. Thrombocytopenia (Option A) is a low platelet count, HDN (Option C) is caused by Rh or ABO incompatibility between mother and baby, and Von Willebrand Disease (Option D) is a genetic disorder affecting clotting factor levels, but they do not typically present with the same pattern of clotting and bleeding as seen in DIC.

Question 103: Correct Answer: D) Advise on proper latch technique and positioning during breastfeeding
Rationale: Proper latch technique and positioning are crucial for successful breastfeeding and can help prevent nipple soreness and cracking. Recommending a nipple shield (Option A) may not address the underlying issue and could potentially lead to further latch problems. Lanolin cream (Option B) can provide relief but does not address the root cause. Using a breast pump (Option C) may not be necessary if the issue can be resolved through proper latch and positioning techniques.

Question 104: Correct Answer: C) Glucose screening tests
Rationale: Given Mrs. Johnson's history of gestational diabetes, prioritizing glucose screening tests is essential to monitor and manage her blood sugar levels during the current pregnancy. While fetal movement monitoring, blood pressure monitoring, and maternal weight gain are important aspects of antenatal care, they may not be as directly impacted by the history of gestational diabetes as the need for glucose screening tests.

Question 105: Correct Answer: C) Lactiferous sinuses
Rationale: Lactiferous sinuses are small reservoirs located behind the areola where milk is stored before being released during breastfeeding. Alveoli are the milk-producing glands, while lactiferous ducts are the tubes that carry milk from the alveoli to the nipple. The areola is the pigmented area surrounding the nipple and does not play a direct role in milk storage.

Question 106: Correct Answer: C) Routine prenatal screening tests showing normal results
Rationale: Amniocentesis is typically recommended for pregnant women with advanced maternal age, a family history of genetic disorders, or abnormal ultrasound findings. It is not routinely performed when all prenatal screening tests show normal results, as the procedure carries a small risk of complications.

Question 107: Correct Answer: A) Obesity
Rationale: Obesity is a significant risk factor for developing gestational hypertension during pregnancy due to increased strain on the cardiovascular system. Regular exercise, low salt intake, and being a non-smoker are actually factors that can help reduce the risk of developing hypertension during pregnancy. Exercise promotes cardiovascular health, low salt intake can help regulate blood pressure, and not smoking reduces the risk of vascular complications.

Question 108: Correct Answer: D) Hemoglobin
Rationale: Breast milk does not contain hemoglobin. It is rich in lactose, a carbohydrate that provides energy; casein, a protein for growth; and immunoglobulins, which boost the baby's immune system. Hemoglobin is a protein found in red blood cells, not in breast milk. This distinction is crucial for understanding the nutritional value of breast milk for newborns.

Question 109: Correct Answer: C) Encouraging breastfeeding or formula feeding every 2-3 hours.
Rationale: Encouraging breastfeeding or formula feeding every 2-3 hours is the most appropriate intervention for managing hypoglycemia in a newborn. This helps maintain stable blood sugar levels and prevents further decrease. Option A is incorrect as delaying feeding can worsen hypoglycemia. Option B is not the first-line treatment and is usually reserved for severe cases. Option D is inadequate as frequent monitoring is essential in managing hypoglycemia effectively.

Question 110: Correct Answer: A) Warm, red, and tender breasts
Rationale: Breast engorgement is characterized by swelling, warmth, redness, and tenderness of the breasts due to an accumulation of milk. This can lead to discomfort and difficulty with breastfeeding. Options B, C, and D are not indicative of breast engorgement. Cool, pale, and soft breasts are not typical signs of engorgement but may indicate poor milk production or other issues. Nipple discharge could be a sign of infection or other conditions unrelated to engorgement. Breast asymmetry is a common occurrence and not specific to engorgement.

Question 111: Correct Answer: B) Maternal smoking during pregnancy
Rationale: Maternal smoking during pregnancy is a known risk factor for apnea in newborns due to the effects of nicotine and carbon monoxide on the respiratory centers in the brain. Term gestation (Option A) and birth weight above 2500 grams (Option D) are not risk factors for apnea. Adequate oxygenation at birth (Option C) is essential for preventing respiratory distress syndrome but is not directly linked to apnea.

Question 112: Correct Answer: B) Preeclampsia
Rationale: Preeclampsia is a serious condition characterized by high blood pressure and often the presence of protein in the urine after 20 weeks of pregnancy. It can lead to various complications during labor and delivery, affecting both the mother and the baby. Hypothyroidism, Ovarian Cancer, and Rheumatoid Arthritis are not typically considered direct risk factors for complications during labor and birth.

Question 113: Correct Answer: D) Type O
Rationale: In the context of ABO incompatibility in newborns, Type O blood is considered the universal donor because it lacks A or B antigens on the red blood cells. This absence of antigens reduces the risk of a hemolytic reaction when transfused to individuals with other blood types. Type O blood can be safely transfused to individuals with blood types A, B, AB, or O without causing an adverse reaction, making it crucial in

emergency situations.
Question 114: Correct Answer: B) Endometritis
Rationale: Endometritis is the inflammation of the endometrial lining of the uterus, commonly occurring after childbirth. The clinical presentation of fever, uterine tenderness, and foul-smelling lochia in the postpartum period is highly suggestive of endometritis. Mastitis presents with breast tenderness, erythema, and warmth. Urinary tract infection manifests with dysuria and frequency. Wound infection is characterized by localized pain, erythema, and purulent discharge.
Question 115: Correct Answer: C) Oxytocin augmentation
Rationale: Oxytocin augmentation is a common intervention used to manage prolonged labor by enhancing uterine contractions and promoting labor progression. Early epidural administration (Option A) may actually slow down labor in some cases. Frequent position changes (Option B) can help optimize fetal positioning but may not directly manage prolonged labor. Immediate cesarean section (Option D) is usually considered only in cases of fetal distress or other complications, not as a primary intervention for prolonged labor.
Question 116: Correct Answer: C) Diuretics may be prescribed to manage postpartum edema.
Rationale: Diuretics can be used in the postpartum period to help manage edema that may occur due to fluid shifts during pregnancy. They are not typically used to prevent postpartum hemorrhage, increase breast milk production, or as a routine measure due to the risk of dehydration. Postpartum edema can be uncomfortable for women, and diuretics may be prescribed in specific cases to alleviate this symptom.
Question 117: Correct Answer: C) Increasing the rate of intravenous fluids.
Rationale: A decrease in blood pressure is a common side effect of epidural anesthesia due to vasodilation. The most appropriate intervention is to increase the rate of intravenous fluids to help maintain adequate blood pressure and perfusion to the mother and baby. Administering more epidural medication can further lower blood pressure. Placing the woman in a supine position can worsen hypotension. Encouraging the woman to push immediately is not indicated until she is fully dilated.
Question 118: Correct Answer: C) Ibuprofen should be avoided in the third trimester of pregnancy due to potential harm to the fetus.
Rationale: Ibuprofen is contraindicated in the third trimester of pregnancy as it can cause premature closure of the ductus arteriosus in the fetus. It is important to educate pregnant patients about this risk and provide alternative pain relief options. While ibuprofen is generally considered safe during breastfeeding, caution should be exercised, especially in premature infants or those with specific medical conditions.
Question 119: Correct Answer: A) Postpartum Depression
Rationale: Postpartum depression is characterized by persistent feelings of sadness, loss of interest, sleep disturbances, and difficulty concentrating. It is a common mood disorder that affects many new mothers. Postpartum psychosis is a more severe condition characterized by hallucinations and delusions, while postpartum anxiety involves excessive worry and fear. Postpartum blues, also known as the "baby blues," are milder and shorter-lasting than postpartum depression.
Question 120: Correct Answer: D) Preeclampsia
Rationale: Preeclampsia is a potential complication of chronic hypertension in pregnancy, characterized by high blood pressure and damage to other organ systems, such as the liver and kidneys. Preterm birth, low birth weight, and macrosomia are more commonly associated with gestational hypertension rather than chronic hypertension. Preeclampsia is a serious condition that requires close monitoring and management to prevent adverse outcomes for both the mother and the baby.
Question 121: Correct Answer: C) Regular menstrual cycles
Rationale: Regular menstrual cycles are generally considered a positive factor for fertility, indicating ovulation and hormonal balance. Advanced maternal age, history of STIs, and PCOS are known risk factors for infertility. Advanced maternal age can lead to decreased ovarian reserve, STIs can cause tubal damage, and PCOS can disrupt ovulation, all contributing to infertility. Therefore, regular menstrual cycles do not pose a risk for infertility compared to the other options.
Question 122: Correct Answer: B) Refer Ms. Johnson to a support group for mothers with postpartum depression.
Rationale: Referring Ms. Johnson to a support group can provide her with a supportive environment and resources to cope with postpartum depression. Encouraging social isolation can worsen her symptoms. Minimizing discussions about her feelings may hinder her recovery process. Prescribing medication without further assessment is not recommended as a first-line intervention for postpartum depression.
Question 123: Correct Answer: A) Rooting reflex
Rationale: The rooting reflex is a normal infant reflex where the baby turns their head and opens their mouth in the direction of a touch on their cheek or mouth. This reflex helps the infant find the nipple for feeding. The Moro reflex is a startle reflex, the tonic neck reflex involves the baby turning their head to one side with the arm and leg on that side extended, and the Babinski reflex is a reflex where the baby's toes fan out when the sole of the foot is stroked.
Question 124: Correct Answer: D) Notify the healthcare provider immediately
Rationale: The presentation of irritability, poor feeding, high-pitched crying, bulging fontanelles, and increased head circumference in a newborn raises concern for intracranial hemorrhage. It is crucial to notify the healthcare provider promptly for further evaluation and management. Encouraging breastfeeding, administering acetaminophen, or placing the newborn in a prone position are not appropriate interventions for suspected intracranial hemorrhage and may delay necessary medical intervention.
Question 125: Correct Answer: C) Postpartum depression
Rationale: Substance use disorder during pregnancy is a risk factor for postpartum depression, a mood disorder that can significantly impact the mother's well-being and ability to care for her newborn. While postpartum hemorrhage, mastitis, and endometritis are also potential complications after childbirth, they are not directly linked to substance abuse during pregnancy. Identifying and addressing substance use disorders in the perinatal period is crucial to prevent adverse outcomes for both the mother and the newborn.

Question 126: Correct Answer: B) Provide emotional support and offer resources for counseling.
Rationale: It is crucial to offer emotional support and resources for counseling to a mother experiencing guilt and sadness after placing her newborn for adoption. Suppressing emotions or avoiding discussions can lead to further emotional distress. Providing a safe space for Mrs. Smith to express her feelings can facilitate healing and coping with the adoption decision.

Question 127: Correct Answer: C) Provide a safe and supportive environment for Emily to grieve openly
Rationale: Creating a safe space for Emily to grieve openly allows her to process her emotions and begin the healing process. Options A, B, and D are not recommended as they may invalidate Emily's feelings and hinder her grieving process.

Question 128: Correct Answer: B) Dilated pupils and slurred speech
Rationale: Dilated pupils and slurred speech are physical signs commonly associated with substance abuse. Fatigue and irritability can be non-specific symptoms, while breast engorgement and nipple tenderness are more related to breastfeeding challenges. Increased appetite and weight gain are not typical physical signs of substance abuse.

Question 129: Correct Answer: B) 15-20 minutes per breast
Rationale: A breastfeeding session should last approximately 15-20 minutes per breast to allow the newborn to access the hindmilk, which is rich in fat and essential for the baby's growth and development. Prolonged feedings can lead to nipple soreness and may not necessarily result in increased milk intake. Options A, C, and D are incorrect as they either suggest too short or too long feeding durations, which can impact the newborn's nutritional intake and breastfeeding effectiveness.

Question 130: Correct Answer: C) Postpartum hemorrhage
Rationale: Postpartum hemorrhage is a common maternal complication associated with multiple births due to the increased strain on the uterus from carrying multiple fetuses. The risk of postpartum hemorrhage is higher in women who have delivered twins or triplets compared to singleton births. Options A, B, and D are potential postpartum complications but are not specifically linked to multiple births. Hypertension may be associated with preeclampsia, gestational diabetes with abnormal glucose metabolism, and urinary tract infection with postpartum recovery, but postpartum hemorrhage is more prevalent in multiple births due to uterine overdistension.

Question 131: Correct Answer: D) Streptococcus agalactiae
Rationale: Streptococcus agalactiae, also known as Group B Streptococcus (GBS), can cause pneumonia, meningitis, and sepsis in newborns. While Streptococcus pneumoniae, Haemophilus influenzae type b (Hib), and Neisseria meningitidis are also bacterial pathogens that can cause serious infections, Streptococcus agalactiae is particularly associated with neonatal infections, making it a significant concern in maternal newborn nursing practice.

Question 132: Correct Answer: D) Physiologic anemia of pregnancy
Rationale: Physiologic anemia of pregnancy is a normal adaptation to the increased blood volume and demand for iron during pregnancy. Aplastic anemia (Option A) is a rare condition where the bone marrow does not produce enough blood cells, hemolytic anemia (Option B) is characterized by the premature destruction of red blood cells, and thalassemia (Option C) is a genetic disorder affecting hemoglobin production.

Question 133: Correct Answer: B) Chorioamnionitis
Rationale: The clinical presentation of a febrile patient with tachycardia, uterine tenderness, and fetal heart rate changes after prolonged rupture of membranes is highly suggestive of chorioamnionitis. Chorioamnionitis is an infection of the amniotic membranes and amniotic fluid, often associated with PROM. It can lead to serious maternal and fetal complications if not promptly diagnosed and treated. The other options, such as PPROM, placental abruption, or uterine rupture, do not align with the clinical presentation described in the scenario.

Question 134: Correct Answer: A) Nipple shield
Rationale: A nipple shield is a thin, flexible silicone cover that is placed over the nipple during breastfeeding to help with latch and positioning. It can alleviate nipple soreness by providing a barrier between the baby's mouth and the mother's nipple, allowing for more comfortable feeding. Breast pump, nipple cream, and nursing bra do not directly address latch and positioning issues associated with nipple soreness.

Question 135: Correct Answer: B) Provide Jake with a doll to care for like his mom cares for the baby
Rationale: Providing Jake with a doll to care for like his mom cares for the baby can help him express his feelings of jealousy and regression in a constructive way. This intervention promotes positive sibling bonding and allows Jake to imitate his mother's caregiving actions, fostering a sense of involvement and importance. Encouraging Mrs. Smith to spend more time with the baby may further exacerbate Jake's feelings of neglect. Ignoring Jake's behavior could lead to increased frustration, while telling him to stop misbehaving may invalidate his emotions and worsen the situation.

Question 136: Correct Answer: B) Administering oxytocin to promote uterine contractions
Rationale: In the case of postpartum hemorrhage, the priority intervention is administering oxytocin to promote uterine contractions and control bleeding. This helps prevent further blood loss and supports the uterus in contracting to reduce the risk of complications. While ambulation, maintaining body temperature, and a high-protein diet are important aspects of postpartum care, addressing the hemorrhage and stabilizing the mother's condition take precedence in this situation.

Question 137: Correct Answer: A) History of placenta previa
Rationale: A history of placenta previa is linked to an increased risk of placental abnormalities such as abnormal placental implantation and potential complications during pregnancy. Maternal smoking during pregnancy (option B) is a known risk factor for various adverse outcomes but is not directly related to placental abnormalities. History of post-term pregnancies (option C) may have its risks but does not specifically indicate placental issues. Previous cesarean section (option D) is a relevant obstetrical history factor but is not primarily associated with increased risk of placental abnormalities.

Question 138: Correct Answer: A) Weight-based dosing
Rationale: When administering analgesics to newborns, weight-based dosing is crucial to ensure appropriate medication dosages and minimize the risk of adverse effects. Newborns have unique pharmacokinetics that require careful consideration of their weight to determine the correct dosage. Factors such as maternal medication use, gestational age, and family history of allergies are important but do not directly impact the dosing of analgesics in newborns.

Question 139: Correct Answer: D) Uterine tenderness and rigidity
Rationale: Uterine tenderness and rigidity are concerning signs of placental abruption as they indicate ongoing bleeding and possible concealed hemorrhage. Maternal hypertension, fetal tachycardia, and vaginal bleeding are common findings in placental abruption but uterine tenderness and rigidity suggest a more severe and urgent situation requiring immediate intervention. Monitoring for signs of shock and preparing for emergent delivery are crucial in this scenario.

Question 140: Correct Answer: D) Maternal HIV infection
Rationale: Maternal HIV infection is a contraindication to breastfeeding due to the risk of vertical transmission of the virus to the infant. It is crucial to prevent the transmission of HIV from mother to child, and therefore, breastfeeding is not recommended in this situation. Mastitis, postpartum hemorrhage, and inverted nipples are not contraindications to breastfeeding. Mastitis is a breast infection that can be treated with antibiotics, postpartum hemorrhage is excessive bleeding after childbirth, and inverted nipples can often be managed with proper techniques and support.

Question 141: Correct Answer: D) Notifying the healthcare provider for further evaluation
Rationale: Abdominal distention and discomfort in a postpartum patient with constipation may indicate a more serious underlying issue such as an impacted bowel or bowel obstruction. Notifying the healthcare provider for further evaluation is crucial to rule out any complications and ensure appropriate management. While encouraging physical activity and providing comfort measures like sitz baths are important, they should not take precedence over addressing potential complications. Administering a laxative without further assessment could exacerbate the situation if there is an obstruction.

Question 142: Correct Answer: C) Complete blood count (CBC)
Rationale: In this case, the newborn is showing signs of possible anemia, which could be contributing to the poor muscle tone and pallor. A CBC would help in assessing the baby's hemoglobin levels and hematocrit, guiding further management. While monitoring blood pressure, assessing capillary refill time, and confirming gestational age are important aspects of newborn assessment, addressing the potential anemia takes precedence in this scenario.

Question 143: Correct Answer: B) Second trimester
Rationale: Amniocentesis is usually performed during the second trimester of pregnancy, between weeks 15 and 20. This timing allows for the collection of an adequate amount of amniotic fluid for testing while minimizing the risk to the fetus. Performing amniocentesis in the first trimester is associated with a higher risk of miscarriage. In the third trimester, the procedure becomes more challenging due to the larger size of the fetus and the reduced amount of amniotic fluid. Amniocentesis is not typically performed at any time during pregnancy but rather during the second trimester for optimal safety and accuracy.

Question 144: Correct Answer: B) It is a self-limiting condition that resolves within 24-72 hours.
Rationale: Transient Tachypnea of the Newborn (TTN) is characterized by tachypnea (rapid breathing) shortly after birth due to delayed clearance of fetal lung fluid. It usually presents within the first few hours after birth and resolves spontaneously within 24-72 hours without specific treatment. TTN is more common in term infants born via cesarean section and is not typically associated with prematurity. Antibiotics are not indicated in the treatment of TTN as it is a transient condition.

Question 145: Correct Answer: B) Bilious vomiting
Rationale: Bilious vomiting is a hallmark sign of intestinal obstruction in newborns. It indicates a distal obstruction, typically in the small intestine, causing bile to reflux back into the stomach and be vomited. Constipation (Option A) is more commonly associated with lower gastrointestinal issues. Normal bowel movements (Option C) would not be expected in the presence of an obstruction. Decreased abdominal distension (Option D) is not a typical finding in intestinal obstruction, as distension is more common due to gas and fluid accumulation proximal to the obstruction.

Question 146: Correct Answer: D) Breast abscess
Rationale: Breast abscess is a contraindication to breastfeeding as it can lead to contamination of breast milk with bacteria, potentially harming the infant. Engorgement, cracked nipples, and mastitis are common issues in breastfeeding mothers but are not contraindications to breastfeeding. It is important to address and treat breast abscess promptly to prevent complications and ensure the health of both the mother and the baby.

Question 147: Correct Answer: D) Necrotizing enterocolitis
Rationale: The symptoms described are indicative of necrotizing enterocolitis (NEC), a serious gastrointestinal emergency in newborns. NEC is characterized by abdominal distention, bloody stools, lethargy, and signs of sepsis. It is crucial to suspect NEC promptly and initiate treatment to prevent complications like bowel perforation. Meconium ileus, intussusception, and malrotation with volvulus present with different clinical features and are not associated with the specific symptoms mentioned in the scenario.

Question 148: Correct Answer: B) Spina Bifida
Rationale: Spina bifida is a neural tube defect where the spinal cord and meninges protrude through a vertebral defect, leading to varying degrees of paralysis and bowel/bladder dysfunction. Hydrocephalus is an abnormal accumulation of cerebrospinal fluid within the brain. Anencephaly is a neural tube defect where a major portion of the brain, skull, and scalp are absent. Encephalocele is a neural tube defect characterized by the protrusion of brain and meninges through a skull defect.

Question 149: Correct Answer: C) Massaging the breasts in a circular motion to express milk.
Rationale: Massaging the breasts in a circular motion can help to express milk and relieve engorgement. Limiting breastfeeding sessions can worsen

engorgement by reducing milk removal. Cold packs should be applied after feeding to reduce swelling. Warm showers or compresses can help with milk flow and comfort during breastfeeding, so they should not be avoided.

Question 150: Correct Answer: C) Providing emotional support and encouraging her to express her feelings

Rationale: Encouraging the patient to express her feelings and providing emotional support are essential in helping her navigate through the grieving process. Options A, B, and D are not appropriate as they may hinder the patient's ability to process her grief and may lead to further emotional dist

RNC-MNN Practice Questions (SET 4)

Question 1: Mrs. Smith gave birth to a healthy baby boy. The nurse educates her about the importance of vitamin K administration to prevent hemorrhagic disease of the newborn. Which statement by Mrs. Smith indicates a need for further teaching?
A) "I understand that vitamin K is essential for blood clotting."
B) "I will make sure my baby receives the vitamin K injection shortly after birth."
C) "I read that breast milk provides enough vitamin K, so I don't need to worry."
D) "I will follow up with the pediatrician to ensure my baby receives all necessary vaccinations."

Question 2: Which STI is known to cause ophthalmia neonatorum in newborns if not adequately treated?
A) Herpes simplex virus (HSV)
B) Human papillomavirus (HPV)
C) Human immunodeficiency virus (HIV)
D) Chlamydia trachomatis

Question 3: Ms. Smith brings her 2-day-old newborn to the clinic for a routine check-up. During the assessment, the nurse notices that the baby has not passed urine since birth. The nurse should suspect which of the following conditions?
A) Hypospadias
B) Posterior urethral valves
C) Cryptorchidism
D) Ureteropelvic junction obstruction

Question 4: During an antenatal visit, the obstetrician discusses the importance of kick counts with a pregnant woman at 28 weeks gestation. The obstetrician explains that kick counts involve monitoring fetal movements to assess fetal well-being. Which of the following statements regarding fetal kick counts is accurate?
A) Fetal movements should be counted for 30 minutes after each meal
B) A total of 10 fetal movements within 1 hour is considered normal
C) Fetal movements should only be counted in the morning
D) Decreased fetal movements are always a sign of fetal distress

Question 5: What is a common intervention to promote effective suck/swallow/sequence coordination in newborns during breastfeeding?
A) Using a nipple shield
B) Offering a pacifier before breastfeeding
C) Engaging in skin-to-skin contact
D) Supplementing with formula after breastfeeding

Question 6: Mrs. Smith has just given birth to a healthy newborn baby boy. The nurse is preparing to administer Vitamin K injection to the newborn. What is the primary purpose of administering Vitamin K to newborns?
A) To prevent hemorrhagic disease of the newborn
B) To boost the immune system
C) To promote weight gain
D) To prevent jaundice

Question 7: Scenario: Mrs. Smith gave birth to a full-term newborn baby boy. The baby is at risk for hypoglycemia due to maternal gestational diabetes. The nurse should prioritize which action to prevent hypoglycemia in the newborn?
A) Delay feeding until the baby shows signs of hunger.
B) Monitor the baby's blood glucose levels closely.
C) Administer IV fluids to maintain hydration.
D) Keep the baby warm with extra blankets.

Question 8: Which maternal postpartum complication is characterized by sudden chest pain, dyspnea, tachycardia, and hypotension, often accompanied by symptoms of anxiety and a feeling of impending doom?
A) Postpartum hemorrhage
B) Postpartum preeclampsia
C) Pulmonary embolism
D) Postpartum cardiomyopathy

Question 9: Ms. Johnson, a 28-year-old multipara, is in active labor at 41 weeks gestation. She has a history of two previous cesarean sections and is interested in attempting a vaginal birth after cesarean (VBAC). During labor, she experiences a uterine rupture. What is the most appropriate management for uterine rupture during a trial of labor after cesarean (TOLAC)?
A) Immediate cesarean section
B) Administer tocolytic medications
C) Increase oxytocin infusion rate
D) Continue with the trial of labor

Question 10: Mrs. Smith has just given birth to a full-term newborn baby boy. During the physical assessment, the nurse notes that the baby's skin appears yellow. The nurse also observes that the sclera of the baby's eyes is yellow. What condition should the nurse suspect in this newborn?
A) Physiological jaundice
B) Hypoglycemia
C) Hypothermia
D) Sepsis

Question 11: Ms. Smith, a new mother, is bottle-feeding her newborn baby. She asks the nurse about the proper positioning for bottle-feeding to prevent ear infections. What is the most appropriate response by the nurse?
A) Hold the baby in a semi-upright position during feeding.
B) Lay the baby flat on the back during feeding.
C) Hold the baby in a fully upright position during feeding.
D) Tilt the baby's head to one side during feeding.

Question 12: What is the maximum score a newborn can achieve on the Apgar score assessment?
A) 5
B) 10
C) 7
D) 15

Question 13: Sarah, a new mother, is prescribed methadone (Subutex) for opioid use disorder. She asks the nurse about breastfeeding while taking methadone. What is the nurse's best response?
A) "You should stop breastfeeding immediately."
B) "Breastfeeding is safe while taking methadone."
C) "Breastfeeding is safe only if you pump and discard the milk."
D) "Switch to formula feeding to avoid any risks."

Question 14: Which contraceptive method is most effective in preventing sexually transmitted infections (STIs) in addition to pregnancy?
A) Diaphragm
B) Birth control patch
C) Depo-Provera injection
D) Male and female condoms

Question 15: Which laboratory finding is characteristic of hemolytic anemia in newborns?
A) Low reticulocyte count
B) Elevated bilirubin levels
C) High iron levels
D) Normal hemoglobin levels

Question 16: What is the most common type of breech presentation?
A) Frank breech
B) Complete breech
C) Footling breech
D) Shoulder presentation

Question 17: During a postpartum assessment, the nurse notes that a mother has developed a fever, tachycardia, and uterine tenderness. Which condition should the nurse suspect?
A) Postpartum hemorrhage
B) Endometritis
C) Mastitis
D) Postpartum blues

Question 18: Ms. Johnson has just given birth to a full-term newborn. During the neurobehavioral assessment, the nurse observes the baby's response to stimuli. Which of the following behaviors would be considered normal for a newborn in response to a stimulus?
A) Grimacing and turning away
B) Cooing and smiling
C) Startling and crying
D) Staring blankly

Question 19: Which hormone is responsible for the let-down reflex during breastfeeding?
A) Estrogen
B) Progesterone
C) Oxytocin
D) Prolactin

Question 20: Which of the following is a normal finding during a newborn assessment of the head?
A) Fontanelles soft and flat
B) Fontanelles hard and bulging
C) Fontanelles sunken
D) Fontanelles pulsating

Question 21: In the context of maternal newborn nursing, which action best exemplifies the ethical principle of beneficence?
A) Providing pain relief medication to a postpartum mother as per her request.
B) Withholding necessary medical interventions due to personal beliefs.
C) Ignoring a newborn's feeding cues to stick to a rigid schedule.
D) Disregarding a mother's concerns about her newborn's health.

Question 22: Mrs. Smith, a 28-year-old postpartum mother, is experiencing excessive bleeding after giving birth. As the nurse, what is the priority action in managing this situation?
A) Encourage the mother to rest and elevate her legs
B) Administer oxytocin as prescribed
C) Apply ice packs to the perineum
D) Offer the mother pain medication for comfort

Question 23: Mrs. Smith, a 28-year-old postpartum mother, asks the nurse about the importance of postpartum self-care. Which of the following statements by the nurse is most appropriate regarding postpartum self-care?
A) "It is essential to resume your pre-pregnancy exercise routine immediately."
B) "You should avoid drinking plenty of water to prevent frequent urination."
C) "Getting enough rest and sleep is crucial for your recovery."
D) "Skipping meals is recommended to help with weight loss."

Question 24: During the process of 'Latch On' in breastfeeding, which action by the mother is crucial to ensure effective milk transfer to the infant?
A) Holding the baby's head too firmly
B) Allowing the baby to have only the nipple in the mouth
C) Ensuring the baby's mouth covers a large portion of the areola
D) Keeping the baby at a distance from the breast

Question 25: Which dietary recommendation is important for a pregnant woman with gestational diabetes?
A) High sugar intake
B) Low fiber intake
C) Regular carbohydrate consumption
D) High-fat diet

Question 26: Mrs. Smith, a postpartum mother, is diagnosed with iron-deficiency anemia. Which of the following statements regarding iron-deficiency anemia in the postpartum period is true?
A) Iron-deficiency anemia is a normal physiological change after childbirth.
B) Iron supplementation is not necessary for postpartum mothers with anemia.
C) Postpartum mothers with iron-deficiency anemia may experience fatigue and weakness.
D) Iron-rich foods should be avoided in the diet of postpartum mothers with anemia.

Question 27: Which of the following statements about Placenta Previa is true?
A) It is a condition where the placenta partially covers the cervix.
B) It is a condition where the placenta is located in the upper part of the uterus.
C) It is a condition where the placenta is implanted in the uterine wall.
D) It is a condition where the placenta is located on the anterior uterine wall.

Question 28: After giving birth, Mrs. Johnson, a 30-year-old mother, is experiencing afterpains during breastfeeding. Which of the following physiological changes contributes to the occurrence of afterpains in the postpartum period?
A) Decreased uterine contractions
B) Increased oxytocin levels
C) Low progesterone levels
D) Elevated white blood cell count

Question 29: What is a common latch-on problem that can occur during breastfeeding?
A) Engorgement
B) Mastitis
C) Nipple confusion
D) Plugged duct

Question 30: Which of the following statements regarding safe sleep practices for newborns is accurate?
A) Placing the newborn on their back to sleep is recommended to reduce the risk of Sudden Infant Death Syndrome (SIDS).
B) Placing the newborn on their stomach to sleep is the safest position.
C) Placing soft bedding, such as pillows and blankets, in the crib is encouraged for comfort.
D) Sharing a bed with the newborn is recommended to promote bonding.

Question 31: During a postpartum assessment, a nurse observes a newborn exhibiting symptoms of neonatal abstinence syndrome (NAS) such as irritability, poor feeding, and tremors. Which substance is most likely responsible for these symptoms if the mother has a history of substance abuse?
A) Alcohol
B) Benzodiazepines
C) Opioids
D) Amphetamines

Question 32: Which of the following is a contraindication to breastfeeding?
A) Maternal HIV infection
B) Maternal hypertension
C) Maternal diabetes
D) Maternal anemia

Question 33: Mrs. Smith, a postpartum mother, complains of constipation after giving birth. Which nursing intervention is most appropriate to promote bowel regularity in this patient?
A) Encouraging increased intake of high-fiber foods
B) Administering a stool softener as needed
C) Limiting fluid intake to avoid exacerbating constipation
D) Encouraging prolonged bed rest to conserve energy

Question 34: During a prenatal visit, a 20-year-old pregnant woman expresses concerns about being too young to have a healthy pregnancy. Which of the following statements regarding maternal age and pregnancy risks is accurate for younger mothers?
A) Younger mothers are at higher risk for gestational diabetes.
B) Younger mothers are at lower risk for preterm birth.
C) Younger mothers are at higher risk for chromosomal abnormalities in the fetus.
D) Younger mothers are at lower risk for pregnancy-induced hypertension.

Question 35: Which behavior is an example of a normal characteristic of parent/infant interactions in the postpartum period?
A) The parent shows disinterest in holding or feeding the infant.
B) The parent responds promptly to the infant's cues for feeding and comfort.
C) The parent expresses frustration and anger towards the infant.
D) The parent avoids making eye contact with the infant.

Question 36: During a routine newborn assessment, the nurse notes that Baby James has not received his Vitamin K injection yet. The parents express concerns about the necessity of this injection. Which of the following information should the nurse provide to educate the parents about the importance of Vitamin K administration in newborns?
A) Vitamin K injection is only necessary for premature infants.
B) Vitamin K helps in the absorption of calcium in newborns.
C) Newborns have low levels of Vitamin K at birth due to the sterile gut.
D) Vitamin K injection can be delayed until the baby is older.

Question 37: Baby Emma, born at 38 weeks, is diagnosed with hyperbilirubinemia. The healthcare provider recommends phototherapy. Which statement regarding phototherapy is accurate?
A) Phototherapy increases the production of bilirubin in the body.
B) Eye protection is not necessary during phototherapy.
C) Breastfeeding should be interrupted during phototherapy.
D) Monitor for signs of dehydration during phototherapy.

Question 38: When bottle feeding a newborn, it is important to:
A) Force the baby to finish the entire bottle at each feeding
B) Warm the formula in the microwave for quick heating
C) Burp the baby halfway through and after feeding
D) Use honey or corn syrup to sweeten the formula

Question 39: Which of the following is NOT a common cause of insufficient milk supply in breastfeeding mothers?
A) Maternal obesity

B) Maternal age over 30 years
C) Frequent breastfeeding
D) Maternal smoking

Question 40: During a postpartum education session, the nurse is discussing the importance of skin-to-skin contact between the mother and newborn. Which statement by the nurse best explains the benefits of this practice?
A) "Skin-to-skin contact helps regulate the baby's body temperature and promotes bonding between you and your newborn."
B) "It is unnecessary to have skin-to-skin contact with your baby; placing them in a crib is sufficient."
C) "Skin-to-skin contact can lead to infections in the newborn and should be avoided."
D) "Bonding with your baby can be achieved through other activities; skin-to-skin contact is not essential."

Question 41: Scenario: Baby James is born at 36 weeks gestation and is experiencing mild hypothermia. Which intervention should the nurse prioritize to help James maintain his body temperature?
A) Increasing the room temperature
B) Placing James under a radiant warmer
C) Encouraging skin-to-skin contact with the mother
D) Administering warm intravenous fluids

Question 42: Which vaccine is recommended for pregnant women to protect against influenza?
A) MMR vaccine
B) Varicella vaccine
C) Inactivated influenza vaccine
D) Rotavirus vaccine

Question 43: Ms. Johnson, a 32-year-old pregnant woman at 39 weeks gestation, arrives at the labor and delivery unit experiencing regular contractions every 5 minutes lasting 45 seconds. On examination, her cervix is dilated 4 cm. The fetal heart rate is reassuring. What is the most appropriate nursing intervention at this time?
A) Encourage the patient to walk around to help progress labor.
B) Administer oxytocin to augment labor.
C) Offer the patient pain medication to relieve discomfort.
D) Prepare the patient for immediate cesarean section.

Question 44: Mrs. Smith, a 32-year-old postpartum mother, presents with severe perineal pain and swelling after a vaginal delivery. On examination, a bluish, tender, and firm mass is noted in the perineal area. What is the most likely diagnosis?
A) Uterine Atony
B) Hematoma
C) Mastitis
D) Endometritis

Question 45: During a home visit, the nurse notices that the parents of a newborn have placed a space heater in the baby's room to keep the temperature warm. What action should the nurse take to address this safety concern?
A) Recommend the parents to keep the space heater on at all times

B) Advise the parents to place the space heater near the baby's crib
C) Educate the parents on safe sleep practices and recommend using sleep sacks for warmth
D) Suggest the parents use additional blankets to keep the baby warm

Question 46: Which of the following is a risk factor for neonatal thrombocytopenia?
A) Maternal preeclampsia
B) Neonatal jaundice
C) Maternal diabetes
D) Neonatal hypoglycemia

Question 47: Ms. Johnson, a 28-year-old postpartum mother, is diagnosed with deep vein thrombosis (DVT) in her left leg. What is the priority nursing action for Ms. Johnson?
A) Apply cold compresses to the affected leg
B) Administer anticoagulant therapy
C) Instruct the client to avoid leg elevation
D) Encourage prolonged bed rest

Question 48: Which symptom is commonly associated with a urinary tract infection (UTI) in the postpartum period?
A) Hypotension
B) Bradycardia
C) Dysuria
D) Hyperglycemia

Question 49: Which pattern of inheritance is characterized by the presence of a disease in each generation, affecting males and females equally, with no male-to-male transmission?
A) Autosomal Recessive
B) Autosomal Dominant
C) X-Linked Recessive
D) X-Linked Dominant

Question 50: In the care of newborns from a multiple birth, which intervention is crucial to prevent nipple confusion in breastfeeding?
A) Introducing pacifiers in the first week
B) Delaying breastfeeding until the newborns are more alert
C) Using nipple shields during breastfeeding
D) Initiating skin-to-skin contact and breastfeeding within the first hour

Question 51: Mrs. Smith, a 32-year-old pregnant woman at 36 weeks gestation, presents to the antenatal clinic for a routine check-up. During fetal assessment, the nurse-midwife performs a non-stress test (NST) to evaluate the fetal heart rate in response to fetal movement. Which of the following findings would be considered reassuring on the NST?
A) Fetal heart rate accelerations with fetal movement
B) Fetal heart rate decelerations with fetal movement
C) Absence of fetal heart rate variability
D) Baseline fetal heart rate of 90 bpm

Question 52: Which intervention is appropriate when managing a newborn with seizures?
A) Administering phenobarbital

B) Increasing environmental stimuli
C) Feeding the newborn immediately
D) Placing the newborn in a dark room

Question 53: During a routine antenatal visit, Mrs. Johnson, a 28-year-old pregnant woman at 30 weeks gestation, is diagnosed with polyhydramnios. Which fetal anomaly should be considered as a potential cause of polyhydramnios in this case?
A) Esophageal atresia
B) Patent ductus arteriosus
C) Clubfoot
D) Cleft lip

Question 54: Baby Emma is born at 38 weeks gestation and is experiencing mild respiratory distress shortly after birth. She has nasal flaring, grunting, and a respiratory rate of 60 breaths per minute. What is the priority nursing intervention for Baby Emma during the transition to extrauterine life?
A) Administer surfactant therapy
B) Provide continuous positive airway pressure (CPAP)
C) Initiate bag-mask ventilation
D) Encourage skin-to-skin contact with the mother

Question 55: Which medication is administered to newborns to prevent ophthalmia neonatorum, an eye infection caused by Neisseria gonorrhoeae or Chlamydia trachomatis?
A) Vitamin K
B) Erythromycin
C) Naloxone
D) Ibuprofen

Question 56: Which gastrointestinal complication in newborns is characterized by abdominal distension, bloody stools, and systemic signs of sepsis?
A) Hirschsprung's Disease
B) Gastroesophageal Reflux
C) Intussusception
D) Necrotizing Enterocolitis

Question 57: Mrs. Smith, a postpartum mother, complains of severe breast pain and swelling. She mentions that her breasts feel warm to touch and appear red. She is experiencing difficulty breastfeeding due to the pain. What is the most appropriate nursing intervention for Mrs. Smith's condition?
A) Encourage frequent breastfeeding sessions
B) Apply ice packs to the breasts
C) Advise Mrs. Smith to avoid breastfeeding until the pain subsides
D) Suggest using tight bras to reduce swelling

Question 58: Which of the following is a potential consequence of Vitamin K deficiency in newborns?
A) Hemolytic anemia
B) Hypocalcemia
C) Intracranial hemorrhage
D) Respiratory distress syndrome

Question 59: Which type of hyperbilirubinemia is characterized by unconjugated bilirubin levels exceeding 17 mg/dL in a term newborn?
A) Physiological jaundice
B) Breastfeeding jaundice
C) Pathological jaundice
D) Breast milk jaundice

Question 60: Which antihypertensive medication should be avoided in pregnant women due to its teratogenic effects?
A) Nifedipine
B) Hydralazine
C) Enalapril
D) Labetalol

Question 61: Which Apgar score component assesses the newborn's muscle tone?
A) Heart rate
B) Respiratory effort
C) Muscle tone
D) Reflex irritability

Question 62: Which antenatal factor is crucial for fetal assessment in determining the risk of birth complications?
A) Maternal age
B) Maternal height
C) Maternal occupation
D) Maternal hair color

Question 63: Scenario: Baby Liam, a 1-week-old neonate, is brought to the clinic for evaluation. His CBC shows a white blood cell count of 8,000/mm3 with a left shift. The differential count reveals 50% neutrophils, 40% lymphocytes, 5% monocytes, and 5% eosinophils. What condition is most likely present in this neonate?
A) Physiological leukopenia
B) Neonatal sepsis
C) Neonatal hyperbilirubinemia
D) Neonatal hypoglycemia

Question 64: Which of the following neural tube defects results in the absence of a major portion of the brain, skull, and scalp?
A) Hydrocephalus
B) Spina Bifida
C) Anencephaly
D) Encephalocele

Question 65: Which metabolic disorder in newborns results from a deficiency of the enzyme phenylalanine hydroxylase?
A) Galactosemia
B) Maple syrup urine disease
C) Phenylketonuria (PKU)
D) Homocystinuria

Question 66: What is a crucial aspect of maternal postpartum assessment in a mother with a history of substance abuse?
A) Monitoring the baby's weight gain
B) Assessing the mother's mental health
C) Encouraging immediate breastfeeding
D) Administering pain medications

Question 67: During a postpartum assessment, a nurse observes a new mother struggling with breastfeeding due to nipple soreness and poor latch.

Which of the following interventions would be most appropriate to improve positioning and latch?
A) Using a nipple shield
B) Applying lanolin cream on the nipples
C) Re-positioning the baby for a deeper latch
D) Supplementing with formula

Question 68: In the context of maternal postpartum care, which ethical principle emphasizes fairness and equality in the distribution of healthcare resources?
A) Autonomy
B) Beneficence
C) Non-maleficence
D) Justice

Question 69: Ms. Rodriguez, a 32-year-old pregnant woman, expresses concerns about her ability to balance work, pregnancy, and caring for her toddler. She reports feeling overwhelmed and anxious. Which intervention by the nurse is most appropriate to address Ms. Rodriguez's psychosocial needs?
A) Provide information on stress management techniques.
B) Suggest she quit her job to reduce stress.
C) Advise her to stop caring for her toddler until after the baby is born.
D) Recommend medication for anxiety relief.

Question 70: Which of the following is a common breastfeeding position that can help ensure proper latch and milk transfer?
A) Supine position
B) Side-lying position
C) Standing position
D) Reclining position

Question 71: Ms. Johnson, a 2-day-old newborn, is scheduled for a lumbar puncture to rule out meningitis. Which position should the nurse place the newborn in for the procedure?
A) Supine position
B) Prone position
C) Side-lying position
D) Flexed sitting position

Question 72: What is the primary advantage of Cell-Free DNA testing over traditional Quad Screen testing in prenatal screening?
A) Cell-Free DNA testing can detect neural tube defects.
B) Cell-Free DNA testing is less expensive than Quad Screen testing.
C) Cell-Free DNA testing has a higher detection rate for Down syndrome.
D) Cell-Free DNA testing can be performed earlier in pregnancy.

Question 73: Which substance is commonly associated with neonatal abstinence syndrome (NAS) in newborns of mothers with substance use disorder?
A) Cocaine
B) Marijuana
C) Heroin
D) Methamphetamine

Question 74: During a shoulder dystocia emergency, the healthcare provider successfully performs the McRoberts maneuver and applies suprapubic pressure without resolving the situation. Which of the following maneuvers should be attempted next?
A) Rubin maneuver
B) Woods' screw maneuver
C) Gaskin maneuver
D) Reverse Woods' screw maneuver

Question 75: Ms. Johnson, a 32-year-old pregnant woman, had a previous cesarean section due to breech presentation. She is now considering a Vaginal Birth After Cesarean (VBAC). Which of the following is a contraindication for VBAC?
A) Previous low transverse uterine incision
B) Two previous cesarean deliveries
C) Unknown previous uterine scar
D) Gestational diabetes

Question 76: Mrs. Patel, a postpartum mother from India, expresses concerns about following her cultural practices during her stay in the hospital. She requests to have her mother stay with her to assist with newborn care. What is the most appropriate action by the nurse?
A) Allow Mrs. Patel's mother to stay with her in accordance with her cultural beliefs.
B) Inform Mrs. Patel that hospital policy does not permit extended family to stay overnight.
C) Suggest Mrs. Patel adapt to the hospital routines and not have her mother stay.
D) Arrange for a hospital volunteer to assist Mrs. Patel instead of her mother.

Question 77: Baby James, born at 36 weeks gestation, is exhibiting signs of respiratory distress shortly after birth. The nurse observes nasal flaring, grunting, and chest retractions. What is the priority intervention for the nurse to implement?
A) Initiate continuous positive airway pressure (CPAP)
B) Administer surfactant via endotracheal tube
C) Provide oxygen therapy via face mask
D) Place the baby in a prone position

Question 78: After giving birth, Mrs. Johnson, a 32-year-old multiparous woman, expresses concerns about balancing her career with motherhood. She is unsure about returning to work and feels conflicted. What is the most suitable nursing intervention to assist Mrs. Johnson in her maternal role transition?
A) Suggesting Mrs. Johnson quit her job to focus on motherhood
B) Providing Mrs. Johnson with resources on childcare options and flexible work arrangements
C) Encouraging Mrs. Johnson to ignore her concerns and focus solely on her baby
D) Advising Mrs. Johnson to seek counseling for her conflicting emotions

Question 79: Which screening tool is commonly used to assess for Congenital Heart Defects (CHD) in newborns?
A) Ballard Score
B) Apgar Score
C) Pulse Oximetry

D) Capillary Refill Test

Question 80: A newborn infant is born to a mother who tested positive for hepatitis B surface antigen (HBsAg) during pregnancy. What is the most appropriate nursing action for the newborn?
A) Administering the hepatitis B vaccine and hepatitis B immune globulin (HBIG) within 12 hours of birth
B) Initiating antiretroviral therapy
C) Isolating the newborn from other infants
D) Delaying breastfeeding until the mother's HBsAg test results are confirmed

Question 81: During a routine prenatal visit, a pregnant woman at 36 weeks gestation expresses concern about the risk of cord prolapse during labor. Which maternal factor increases the risk of cord prolapse?
A) Polyhydramnios
B) Maternal age over 35 years
C) Multiparity
D) Maternal obesity

Question 82: During a routine antenatal visit, a pregnant woman in her second trimester mentions that she works in a daycare center and is concerned about the risk of contracting infections. Which of the following bacterial infections poses the highest risk to pregnant women and their newborns in this setting?
A) Streptococcus pneumoniae
B) Listeria monocytogenes
C) Chlamydia trachomatis
D) Bordetella pertussis

Question 83: When should eye prophylaxis be administered to a newborn to prevent ophthalmia neonatorum?
A) Within 24 hours of birth
B) Within 48 hours of birth
C) Within 72 hours of birth
D) Within 1 week of birth

Question 84: During an antepartum visit, Mrs. Johnson, a pregnant woman with gestational diabetes, asks about dietary recommendations to manage her condition. What advice should the nurse provide?
A) Mrs. Johnson should consume a high-carbohydrate diet to meet the increased energy demands of pregnancy.
B) Mrs. Johnson should avoid monitoring her blood glucose levels regularly to reduce stress.
C) Mrs. Johnson should include a balance of complex carbohydrates, lean proteins, and healthy fats in her meals.
D) Mrs. Johnson should skip meals to prevent postprandial hyperglycemia.

Question 85: During a postpartum assessment, Nurse Jones notes that Mrs. Johnson has a low platelet count. Which of the following conditions is associated with low platelet count in the postpartum period?
A) Gestational diabetes
B) Preeclampsia
C) Hyperthyroidism
D) Urinary tract infection

Question 86: At what time interval after birth is delayed cord clamping typically performed?
A) Immediately after birth
B) 30 seconds after birth
C) 1 minute after birth
D) 3 minutes after birth

Question 87: During a postpartum education session, a new mother asks the nurse about the Tdap vaccine. Which information should the nurse include when discussing the Tdap vaccine with postpartum mothers?
A) "The Tdap vaccine is not necessary for postpartum mothers."
B) "Postpartum mothers should receive the Tdap vaccine to protect their newborns from pertussis."
C) "Postpartum mothers should avoid the Tdap vaccine if they are breastfeeding."
D) "The Tdap vaccine is only recommended for postpartum mothers with a history of allergies."

Question 88: Which assessment finding is characteristic of superficial thrombophlebitis in postpartum women?
A) Warmth and erythema along the course of a superficial vein
B) Sudden onset of dyspnea and chest pain
C) Unilateral leg swelling with pain on palpation
D) Decreased pedal pulses and cool extremities

Question 89: Which congenital heart defect is commonly associated with Acyanotic Heart Disease in newborns?
A) Tetralogy of Fallot
B) Transposition of the great arteries
C) Ventricular septal defect
D) Tricuspid atresia

Question 90: During the postpartum period, a new mother is experiencing feelings of sadness, anxiety, and irritability. Which of the following actions by the nurse would be most appropriate in supporting the mother's maternal role transition?
A) Encouraging the mother to ignore her feelings and focus solely on caring for the baby.
B) Providing education on postpartum depression and available support resources.
C) Minimizing the mother's emotions as a normal part of the postpartum period.
D) Advising the mother to avoid seeking help and manage her emotions independently.

Question 91: During a postpartum assessment, you find that a new mother is experiencing hemorrhoids. She asks about over-the-counter (OTC) medications for relief. Which OTC medication would be most appropriate for managing hemorrhoids in this patient?
A) Topical corticosteroid cream
B) Oral nonsteroidal anti-inflammatory drug (NSAID)
C) Oral stool softener
D) Topical anesthetic cream

Question 92: Scenario: Baby Emma, a newborn, is brought to the hospital due to poor feeding, lethargy, and seizures. Upon assessment, she is found to have a musty odor to her skin and urine. Bloodwork reveals elevated phenylalanine levels. What inborn error of metabolism is most likely affecting Baby Emma?
A) Galactosemia
B) Maple syrup urine disease
C) Phenylketonuria
D) Homocystinuria

Question 93: Which postpartum self-care measure is essential to prevent constipation in the mother?
A) Avoiding fluid intake
B) Limiting fiber-rich foods
C) Engaging in regular physical activity
D) Ignoring the urge to defecate

Question 94: What is the recommended treatment for hypoglycemia in newborns?
A) Immediate feeding with formula
B) Intravenous glucose infusion
C) Skin-to-skin contact with the mother
D) Observation without intervention

Question 95: Which medication is commonly used in newborn resuscitation for its vasopressor effects to increase blood pressure and improve perfusion?
A) Furosemide
B) Dopamine
C) Acetaminophen
D) Oxytocin

Question 96: During a postpartum assessment, Nurse Jane observes a newborn turning head side to side with mouth open and searching for the breast. What feeding cue is the newborn displaying?
A) Hiccuping
B) Spitting up
C) Burping
D) Rooting

Question 97: Which of the following statements regarding the use of supplementary/complementary feedings in newborns is accurate?
A) Complementary feedings should be introduced within the first week of life.
B) Supplementary feedings are recommended as the primary source of nutrition for newborns.
C) Breastfeeding should be established before introducing any supplementary feedings.
D) Complementary feedings can replace breastfeeding entirely.

Question 98: Mrs. Smith has just given birth to a full-term newborn baby boy. During the initial assessment, the nurse notes that the baby's respiratory rate is 60 breaths per minute, heart rate is 140 beats per minute, and temperature is 36.8℃. The baby is crying softly and has pink skin color. Which of the following statements regarding the newborn's physiologic adaptations is accurate?
A) The baby's respiratory rate is within the normal range for a newborn.
B) The baby's heart rate is lower than expected for a newborn.
C) The baby's temperature is higher than the normal range for a newborn.
D) The baby's skin color indicates hypoxia.

Question 99: Which of the following is a risk factor for the development of hyperbilirubinemia in newborns?
A) Exclusive breastfeeding
B) Term gestation
C) ABO incompatibility
D) Maternal diabetes

Question 100: Which comfort measure is most appropriate for promoting newborn relaxation and sleep in the hospital setting?
A) Dimming the lights and reducing noise levels
B) Providing continuous loud white noise
C) Keeping the room brightly lit
D) Using strong scented candles for aromatherapy

Question 101: Ms. Smith, a 32-year-old G2P1 at 38 weeks gestation, presents to the labor and delivery unit with sudden and intense contractions. She reports a history of rapid labor with her first child. On examination, the fetal head is crowning. What is the priority nursing action in this situation?
A) Instruct the patient to push with contractions
B) Prepare for imminent delivery
C) Perform a vaginal exam to assess cervical dilation
D) Administer intravenous pain medication

Question 102: Which obstetrical history factor is considered a significant antenatal risk factor for adverse pregnancy outcomes?
A) Previous preterm birth
B) Maternal age over 35 years
C) History of gestational diabetes
D) Multiparity (having multiple children)

Question 103: During a postpartum assessment, a nurse notes that a patient is experiencing adverse effects of a diuretic medication. Which finding would indicate a potential complication related to diuretic therapy?
A) Decreased blood pressure
B) Hypokalemia
C) Increased urinary output
D) Swelling in the lower extremities

Question 104: Which hematologic condition in the postpartum period is characterized by a decrease in red blood cells, hemoglobin, and hematocrit levels, leading to fatigue and weakness?
A) Thrombocytopenia
B) Polycythemia
C) Anemia
D) Hemophilia

Question 105: Mrs. Smith, a 28-year-old G2P2 postpartum mother, is being assessed during her hospital stay. During the comprehensive postpartum health assessment, the nurse notes that Mrs. Smith's blood pressure is 150/90 mmHg. Which of the following actions should the nurse prioritize based on this finding?

A) Reassure Mrs. Smith that this is a normal postpartum blood pressure.
B) Notify the healthcare provider immediately.
C) Encourage Mrs. Smith to increase her fluid intake.
D) Document the finding and continue to monitor Mrs. Smith's blood pressure.

Question 106: Which fetal assessment method is commonly used to monitor fetal well-being during pregnancy?
A) Ultrasound
B) Blood pressure measurement
C) Urine analysis
D) Weight measurement

Question 107: Mrs. Smith, a 26-year-old pregnant woman at 36 weeks gestation, presents with new-onset hypertension and proteinuria. She is diagnosed with gestational hypertension. Which of the following statements regarding gestational hypertension is true?
A) Gestational hypertension typically resolves within 12 weeks postpartum.
B) Gestational hypertension is defined as hypertension that was present before pregnancy.
C) Gestational hypertension is not associated with an increased risk of adverse maternal outcomes.
D) Gestational hypertension may progress to preeclampsia if proteinuria is detected.

Question 108: Ms. Johnson, a 28-year-old HIV-positive pregnant woman, is prescribed antiretroviral therapy to prevent mother-to-child transmission. Which antiretroviral medication is commonly used during pregnancy due to its safety profile and effectiveness in reducing viral load?
A) Zidovudine (AZT)
B) Efavirenz (EFV)
C) Ritonavir (RTV)
D) Darunavir (DRV)

Question 109: During a lactation consultation, a mother asks about using a breast pump to increase milk supply. Which breastfeeding device can help stimulate milk production by mimicking a baby's sucking pattern?
A) Nipple shield
B) Supplemental nursing system
C) Manual breast pump
D) Electric breast pump

Question 110: Which of the following is a potential indication for an operative vaginal delivery using forceps or vacuum extraction?
A) Maternal exhaustion
B) Fetal macrosomia
C) Prolonged second stage of labor
D) Maternal request for a quick delivery

Question 111: During a routine antepartum assessment, a pregnant woman with a known cardiac condition complains of increasing shortness of breath and fatigue. Which of the following signs should alert the nurse to the possibility of cardiac decompensation in this patient?
A) Leg cramps
B) Decreased urinary frequency
C) Weight gain of 1 kg in a week
D) Back pain

Question 112: Which of the following is a recommended practice for cord care in newborns?
A) Cleaning the cord stump with alcohol swabs after every diaper change
B) Keeping the cord stump clean and dry
C) Applying powders and lotions to the cord stump
D) Immersing the baby in water before the cord stump falls off

Question 113: During the early postpartum period, how often should a newborn be breastfed to establish a good milk supply and promote bonding?
A) Every 2-3 hours
B) Every 4-5 hours
C) Every 6-7 hours
D) Every 8-9 hours

Question 114: Mrs. Smith, a 32-year-old primigravida at 41 weeks gestation, is admitted to the labor and delivery unit with signs of prolonged labor. Which of the following findings is consistent with prolonged labor?
A) Cervical dilation of 1 cm per hour
B) Fetal descent of 1 cm per hour
C) Inadequate uterine contractions
D) Maternal exhaustion and fatigue

Question 115: Which lab value is expected to decrease during pregnancy due to hemodilution?
A) Hemoglobin
B) Platelet count
C) Blood glucose
D) Serum creatinine

Question 116: A mother presents with symptoms of mastitis, which nipple problem is most likely associated with this condition?
A) Nipple blanching
B) Nipple bleb
C) Nipple vasospasm
D) Nipple fissures

Question 117: Which of the following is a correct guideline for bottle feeding a newborn?
A) Prop the bottle to allow the milk to flow faster
B) Hold the baby in a semi-upright position during feeding
C) Use a bottle nipple with a small hole to slow down feeding
D) Allow the baby to feed at their own pace

Question 118: During a postpartum education session, a new mother asks about hand expression of breast milk. Which of the following statements accurately describes the benefits of hand expression?
A) Hand expression is less efficient than using a breast pump
B) Hand expression can help stimulate milk production and maintain milk supply
C) Hand expression is only recommended for mothers with inverted nipples

D) Hand expression should be avoided as it can cause breast engorgement

Question 119: During a postpartum assessment, the nurse observes that a breastfeeding mother, Mrs. Johnson, has cracked nipples. Which intervention should the nurse suggest to promote healing and prevent further complications?
A) Continuing to breastfeed on the affected side
B) Applying soap to clean the nipples before each feeding
C) Using a lanolin-based nipple cream after each feeding
D) Switching to formula feeding temporarily

Question 120: Which medication used in labor is a uterotonic agent commonly administered to prevent postpartum hemorrhage by promoting uterine contractions?
A) Oxytocin
B) Magnesium sulfate
C) Misoprostol
D) Carboprost

Question 121: During a newborn assessment, which finding would require immediate intervention related to the genitourinary system?
A) Labial adhesions in a female newborn
B) Presence of vernix caseosa in the genital area
C) Absence of a urethral meatus in a male newborn
D) Physiologic jaundice on the abdomen

Question 122: Which of the following is a common indication for the use of oral sucrose in newborn care?
A) Pain relief during circumcision
B) Treatment of jaundice
C) Prevention of hypoglycemia
D) Promotion of weight gain

Question 123: Which of the following is a common symptom of Cyanotic Heart Disease in newborns?
A) Hypertension
B) Tachypnea
C) Hyperoxemia
D) Hypoglycemia

Question 124: Which maternal postpartum assessment finding would warrant immediate medical attention related to the reproductive system?
A) Lochia rubra on day 2 postpartum
B) Fundus firm and midline at the level of the umbilicus
C) Perineal laceration with minimal bleeding
D) Foul-smelling vaginal discharge

Question 125: Mrs. Smith, a 32-year-old pregnant woman at 28 weeks gestation, presents with symptoms of fever, malaise, and a sore throat. On examination, she has enlarged cervical lymph nodes. Her blood work shows leukocytosis. Which of the following viral infections is most likely causing her symptoms?
A) Cytomegalovirus (CMV)
B) Herpes Simplex Virus (HSV)
C) Epstein-Barr Virus (EBV)
D) Rubella Virus

Question 126: Which action by the nurse ensures newborn safety during transport within the healthcare facility?
A) Placing the newborn in a prone position
B) Using a properly secured infant car seat
C) Carrying the newborn in the nurse's arms
D) Leaving the newborn unattended on a flat surface

Question 127: Which bacterial infection is commonly associated with early-onset neonatal sepsis?
A) Group B Streptococcus (GBS)
B) Escherichia coli (E. coli)
C) Listeria monocytogenes
D) Staphylococcus aureus

Question 128: During a postnatal visit, the nurse observes that the baby's umbilical cord stump appears moist and has a foul odor. What action should the nurse take?
A) Instruct the mother to clean the cord stump more frequently with soap and water.
B) Apply hydrogen peroxide to the cord stump to help dry it out.
C) Assess for signs of infection and consult the healthcare provider.
D) Advise the mother to cover the cord stump with a sterile gauze pad.

Question 129: Which dietary recommendation is important for a breastfeeding mother to ensure an adequate milk supply?
A) Limiting fluid intake
B) Consuming caffeine in moderation
C) Avoiding carbohydrates
D) Eating a balanced diet rich in calories

Question 130: Scenario: Emily, a 2-day-old newborn, is diagnosed with cyanotic heart disease. She presents with cyanosis, tachypnea, and poor feeding. On assessment, a loud single second heart sound (S2) is heard. Which of the following congenital heart defects is most likely causing Emily's symptoms?
A) Atrial Septal Defect (ASD)
B) Tetralogy of Fallot (TOF)
C) Ventricular Septal Defect (VSD)
D) Patent Ductus Arteriosus (PDA)

Question 131: Which formula is recommended for infants with cow's milk protein allergy?
A) Similac Advance
B) Enfamil Gentlease
C) Nutramigen
D) Gerber Good Start

Question 132: When educating parents about tummy time for newborns, which information is essential to include?
A) Tummy time helps prevent flat spots on the baby's head.
B) Tummy time should be done immediately after feeding.
C) Tummy time is not necessary for newborns.
D) Tummy time should be done on a soft surface like a bed.

Question 133: Mrs. Smith, a 32-year-old primigravida at 38 weeks gestation, requests pain relief during labor. The healthcare provider decides to administer an opioid analgesic. Which of the following is a common opioid analgesic used in labor for its rapid onset and short duration of action?
A) Morphine
B) Fentanyl
C) Codeine
D) Tramadol

Question 134: Which contraceptive method is most suitable for a breastfeeding mother in the immediate postpartum period?
A) Combined oral contraceptives
B) Intrauterine device (IUD)
C) Condoms
D) Progestin-only pills

Question 135: Mrs. Smith has just given birth to a healthy baby boy. As part of the newborn care, which medication is commonly used for eye prophylaxis to prevent ophthalmia neonatorum?
A) Tetracycline ointment
B) Erythromycin ointment
C) Gentamicin drops
D) Ciprofloxacin ointment

Question 136: After assessing a postpartum mother with perineal edema and pain, the nurse notes signs of infection. Which action is the priority in this situation?
A) Initiating antibiotic therapy
B) Notifying the healthcare provider
C) Increasing the frequency of perineal care
D) Applying a warm compress to the perineum

Question 137: Which of the following statements regarding breastfeeding in the immediate postpartum period is true?
A) Colostrum is low in nutrients and antibodies.
B) Breastfeeding should be initiated within 1-2 hours after birth.
C) Newborns should be fed with formula until the mother's milk supply increases.
D) Breastfeeding is contraindicated if the mother is experiencing nipple soreness.

Question 138: Mrs. Smith, a postpartum patient, is experiencing constipation after delivery. The healthcare provider prescribes a GI motility drug to help improve bowel movements. Which of the following medications is commonly used for this purpose?
A) Ondansetron
B) Metoclopramide
C) Pantoprazole
D) Furosemide

Question 139: Which of the following is a common cause of sleep disturbances in postpartum women?
A) Decreased anxiety levels
B) Increased social support
C) Hormonal changes
D) Regular exercise

Question 140: Ms. Smith, a 32-year-old pregnant woman at 20 weeks gestation, presents for a routine ultrasound. The ultrasound report indicates an amniotic fluid index (AFI) of 5 cm. What does this finding suggest?
A) Normal amniotic fluid volume
B) Oligohydramnios
C) Polyhydramnios
D) Borderline amniotic fluid volume

Question 141: Mrs. Smith, a postpartum mother, is concerned about her newborn's breastfeeding pattern. She reports that her baby seems to be sucking weakly and often falls asleep at the breast. Which of the following actions by the nurse would be most appropriate in this situation?
A) Encourage the mother to switch to bottle feeding for better control.
B) Suggest using a nipple shield to enhance the baby's latch.
C) Teach the mother breast compression techniques to help stimulate milk flow.
D) Advise the mother to limit breastfeeding sessions to avoid exhaustion.

Question 142: What is a recommended nursing intervention for managing breast engorgement in postpartum mothers?
A) Encouraging frequent breastfeeding or pumping
B) Applying ice packs to the breasts
C) Avoiding any breast stimulation
D) Wearing tight-fitting bras

Question 143: Mrs. Smith, a 32-year-old pregnant woman, presents to the antenatal clinic for her routine check-up at 28 weeks of gestation. During the assessment, the nurse notes that Mrs. Smith has a history of gestational diabetes in her previous pregnancy. Which of the following antenatal factors should the nurse prioritize monitoring in Mrs. Smith's current pregnancy?
A) Blood pressure
B) Fetal movements
C) Blood glucose levels
D) Maternal weight gain

Question 144: During a newborn assessment, the nurse observes a newborn's hands with clenched fists and overlapping fingers. Which musculoskeletal condition is most likely present in this newborn?
A) Polydactyly
B) Syndactyly
C) Arthrogryposis Multiplex Congenita
D) Brachial Plexus Injury

Question 145: During a delivery, cord gases are obtained from a newborn. The results show a pH of 7.35, pO2 of 65 mmHg, pCO2 of 50 mmHg, and HCO3 of 22 mEq/L. What do these cord gas values indicate?
A) Normal
B) Respiratory alkalosis
C) Metabolic acidosis
D) Mixed acidosis

Question 146: When considering psychosocial and ethical issues in maternal newborn nursing, which concept involves treating individuals with respect and dignity, regardless of their personal beliefs or values?
A) Confidentiality
B) Cultural competence
C) Informed consent
D) Respect for persons

Question 147: Which nutrient is particularly important for lactating mothers to ensure an adequate milk supply for their newborn?
A) Vitamin C
B) Iron
C) Calcium
D) Protein

Question 148: Ms. Johnson, a 28-year-old pregnant woman, has a history of Rh incompatibility with her first pregnancy. She is now 32 weeks pregnant with her second child. Which of the following interventions is essential to prevent hemolytic disease in the newborn?
A) Administering Rh immunoglobulin (RhIg) at 28 weeks gestation
B) Delaying administration of RhIg until after delivery
C) Monitoring the newborn for signs of hemolytic disease without intervention
D) Administering RhIg only if the newborn tests positive for Rh incompatibility

Question 149: During pregnancy, which of the following physiological changes is associated with an increase in plasma volume?
A) Decreased heart rate
B) Decreased red blood cell production
C) Decreased blood pressure
D) Increased renal blood flow

Question 150: Which of the following is a risk factor for developing hemolytic disease of the newborn (HDN)?
A) Maternal O positive blood type
B) Rh-negative mother with Rh-positive fetus
C) Maternal antibodies against fetal platelets
D) Premature birth

ANSWERS WITH DETAILED EXPLANATION (SET 4)

Question 1: Correct Answer: C) "I read that breast milk provides enough vitamin K, so I don't need to worry."
Rationale: Mrs. Smith's statement indicating that breast milk provides enough vitamin K is incorrect. Breast milk is low in vitamin K, putting newborns at risk for deficiency. It is crucial for newborns to receive a vitamin K injection shortly after birth to prevent hemorrhagic disease of the newborn. The other options demonstrate understanding of the importance of vitamin K administration and appropriate follow-up care.

Question 2: Correct Answer: D) Chlamydia trachomatis
Rationale: Chlamydia trachomatis is known to cause ophthalmia neonatorum in newborns if not adequately treated. Ophthalmia neonatorum is a severe eye infection that can lead to blindness if left untreated. HSV, HPV, and HIV can also be transmitted from mother to newborn but are not specifically associated with causing ophthalmia neonatorum. Prompt screening, diagnosis, and treatment of chlamydia in pregnant women can help prevent this serious complication in newborns.

Question 3: Correct Answer: B) Posterior urethral valves
Rationale: Posterior urethral valves are a congenital condition in male infants that obstruct the flow of urine, leading to urinary retention. This can present with symptoms such as oliguria or anuria. Hypospadias is a condition where the urethral opening is on the underside of the penis, not related to urinary retention. Cryptorchidism refers to undescended testes, and ureteropelvic junction obstruction involves a blockage at the junction of the ureter and the kidney, both of which do not typically present with urinary retention in the newborn.

Question 4: Correct Answer: B) A total of 10 fetal movements within 1 hour is considered normal
Rationale: Fetal kick counts involve monitoring the number of fetal movements within a specific time frame, typically 1 hour. A total of 10 fetal movements within 1 hour is considered normal. Counting fetal movements after meals, throughout the day, and especially in the evening when fetal activity tends to increase, is recommended. Decreased fetal movements can indicate fetal distress, but it is not always the case as fetal activity patterns can vary.

Question 5: Correct Answer: C) Engaging in skin-to-skin contact
Rationale: Engaging in skin-to-skin contact is a common intervention to promote effective suck/swallow/sequence coordination in newborns during breastfeeding. This practice helps newborns regulate their breathing, heart rate, and temperature, leading to improved feeding outcomes. Using a nipple shield (Option A) may interfere with proper latch and milk transfer. Offering a pacifier before breastfeeding (Option B) can confuse the newborn's suckling reflex. Supplementing with formula after breastfeeding (Option D) may reduce the newborn's motivation to breastfeed effectively. Therefore, the correct answer is C as it supports optimal breastfeeding initiation and coordination.

Question 6: Correct Answer: A) To prevent hemorrhagic disease of the newborn
Rationale: Administering Vitamin K to newborns is crucial as it helps prevent hemorrhagic disease of the newborn, a condition where babies have low levels of clotting factors, putting them at risk of bleeding. The other options, such as boosting the immune system, promoting weight gain, and preventing jaundice, are not the primary purposes of administering Vitamin K to newborns.

Question 7: Correct Answer: B) Monitor the baby's blood glucose levels closely.
Rationale: Monitoring the baby's blood glucose levels closely is crucial in preventing and managing hypoglycemia in newborns at risk, especially those born to mothers with gestational diabetes. This allows for early detection and intervention if hypoglycemia occurs. Delaying feeding, administering IV fluids, or keeping the baby warm, although important, are not the primary interventions for preventing hypoglycemia in this scenario.

Question 8: Correct Answer: C) Pulmonary embolism
Rationale: Pulmonary embolism is a life-threatening condition in which a blood clot travels to the lungs, causing symptoms like chest pain, shortness of breath, rapid heart rate, and low blood pressure. It is crucial to differentiate pulmonary embolism from other postpartum complications like postpartum hemorrhage, preeclampsia, and cardiomyopathy. Postpartum hemorrhage presents with excessive bleeding, preeclampsia with hypertension and proteinuria, and cardiomyopathy with heart failure symptoms. Prompt recognition and treatment of pulmonary embolism are vital to prevent serious consequences.

Question 9: Correct Answer: A) Immediate cesarean section
Rationale: In the case of uterine rupture during a trial of labor after cesarean, the most appropriate management is an immediate cesarean section. Uterine rupture is a serious complication that can lead to fetal and maternal morbidity and mortality. Immediate delivery is crucial to prevent further harm to both the mother and the baby. Administering tocolytic medications, increasing oxytocin infusion rate, or continuing with the trial of labor are not appropriate actions in the presence of uterine rupture, as they can exacerbate the situation and increase the risk of adverse outcomes.

Question 10: Correct Answer: A) Physiological jaundice
Rationale: Physiological jaundice is common in newborns due to the immature liver's inability to effectively process bilirubin. This type of jaundice typically appears after the first 24 hours of life and resolves on its own without treatment. Hypoglycemia, hypothermia, and sepsis are also important conditions to consider in newborns but are not typically associated with yellow discoloration of the skin and sclera.

Question 11: Correct Answer: A) Hold the baby in a semi-upright position during feeding.
Rationale: Holding the baby in a semi-upright position during bottle-feeding helps prevent ear infections by allowing the milk to flow smoothly and reducing the risk of milk entering the Eustachian tube. This position also helps in reducing the chances of choking and aspiration. Option B is incorrect as laying the baby flat on the back during feeding can increase the risk of ear infections. Option C is incorrect as holding the baby in a fully upright position may cause the baby to gulp air along with milk, leading to gas and discomfort. Option D is incorrect as

tilting the baby's head to one side during feeding can also increase the risk of ear infections.

Question 12: Correct Answer: B) 10
Rationale: The Apgar score is a quick assessment tool used to evaluate a newborn's physical condition at one minute and five minutes after birth. It consists of five components: heart rate, respiratory effort, muscle tone, reflex irritability, and color. Each component is scored from 0 to 2, with a maximum total score of 10. A score of 7 or above is generally considered normal, while a score below 7 may indicate the need for medical intervention. Therefore, the correct answer is B) 10, as it represents the highest achievable score on the Apgar assessment.

Question 13: Correct Answer: B) "Breastfeeding is safe while taking methadone."
Rationale: Methadone is considered compatible with breastfeeding as long as the mother is stable on her dose. The benefits of breastfeeding usually outweigh the risks of exposing the infant to methadone through breast milk. Stopping breastfeeding abruptly or switching to formula can have negative consequences for both the mother and the baby. Pumping and discarding breast milk is not necessary unless advised by a healthcare provider.

Question 14: Correct Answer: D) Male and female condoms
Rationale: Male and female condoms are the most effective contraceptive methods in preventing both pregnancy and sexually transmitted infections (STIs). Condoms act as a barrier method, reducing the risk of STI transmission during sexual intercourse. Diaphragms, birth control patches, and Depo-Provera injections primarily focus on preventing pregnancy and do not provide protection against STIs. Therefore, for individuals seeking dual protection, the consistent and correct use of male or female condoms is recommended.

Question 15: Correct Answer: B) Elevated bilirubin levels
Rationale: Hemolytic anemia in newborns is characterized by an increased breakdown of red blood cells, leading to elevated bilirubin levels. This can result in jaundice, pale stools, and dark urine. A low reticulocyte count indicates decreased red blood cell production. High iron levels are not typically associated with hemolytic anemia. Normal hemoglobin levels may be seen in some cases of hemolytic anemia, but the key characteristic is the elevated bilirubin due to increased red blood cell breakdown.

Question 16: Correct Answer: A) Frank breech
Rationale: Frank breech presentation is the most common type of breech presentation, where the baby's buttocks present first with the legs flexed at the hips and extended at the knees. In complete breech, the baby's hips and knees are flexed, while in footling breech, one or both feet present first. Shoulder presentation is a transverse lie, not a breech presentation.

Question 17: Correct Answer: B) Endometritis
Rationale: The symptoms of fever, tachycardia, and uterine tenderness are indicative of endometritis, which is an infection of the uterine lining. This condition requires prompt treatment with antibiotics to prevent further complications. Options A, C, and D are incorrect as they do not align with the symptoms described and are unrelated to the clinical presentation of endometritis.

Question 18: Correct Answer: C) Startling and crying
Rationale: Newborns typically startle and cry in response to stimuli as their sensory systems are still developing. Grimacing and turning away may indicate discomfort or pain. Cooing and smiling usually develop later in the first few weeks of life. Staring blankly may suggest a lack of visual focus or attention.

Question 19: Correct Answer: C) Oxytocin
Rationale: Oxytocin is the hormone responsible for the let-down reflex during breastfeeding. It causes the muscles around the milk-producing cells to contract, pushing milk into the ducts. Estrogen and progesterone play a role in preparing the breasts for lactation during pregnancy but are not directly involved in the let-down reflex. Prolactin is responsible for milk production but not for the let-down reflex.

Question 20: Correct Answer: A) Fontanelles soft and flat
Rationale: During a newborn assessment, it is essential to evaluate the fontanelles on the infant's head. A normal finding would be soft and flat fontanelles, indicating proper skull development and hydration status. Hard and bulging fontanelles (Option B) may suggest increased intracranial pressure, while sunken fontanelles (Option C) can indicate dehydration. Pulsating fontanelles (Option D) are not a typical finding and could be a sign of abnormality.

Question 21: Correct Answer: A) Providing pain relief medication to a postpartum mother as per her request.
Rationale: Beneficence in maternal newborn nursing emphasizes the obligation to act in the best interest of the mother and newborn. Providing pain relief medication as requested by the postpartum mother aligns with this principle by addressing her needs and promoting her well-being. Options B, C, and D go against beneficence by either withholding necessary care, disregarding newborn cues, or ignoring maternal concerns, which can compromise the health and safety of the mother and newborn.

Question 22: Correct Answer: B) Administer oxytocin as prescribed
Rationale: Administering oxytocin is the priority action in managing postpartum bleeding as it helps the uterus contract, reducing the risk of hemorrhage. Resting and elevating legs, applying ice packs, and offering pain medication are important interventions but not the priority in this situation. Oxytocin helps prevent and treat postpartum hemorrhage by promoting uterine contractions, which is crucial in controlling bleeding.

Question 23: Correct Answer: C) "Getting enough rest and sleep is crucial for your recovery."
Rationale: Adequate rest and sleep are vital for postpartum recovery as they help the body heal, restore energy levels, and promote emotional well-being. Encouraging the new mother to prioritize rest can prevent exhaustion and support her overall health. Options A, B, and D are incorrect as they provide inaccurate information that could potentially harm the mother's recovery process.

Question 24: Correct Answer: C) Ensuring the baby's mouth covers a large portion of the areola
Rationale: During breastfeeding, it is essential for the baby's mouth to cover a significant portion of the areola along with the nipple to facilitate proper latch and effective milk transfer. This technique helps prevent nipple soreness and ensures that the baby can extract milk efficiently. Options A, B, and D are incorrect as holding the baby's head too firmly can be uncomfortable,

allowing only the nipple in the mouth leads to poor latch and potential nipple damage, and keeping the baby at a distance from the breast hinders effective milk transfer.

Question 25: Correct Answer: C) Regular carbohydrate consumption
Rationale: Pregnant women with gestational diabetes should focus on consuming carbohydrates regularly throughout the day to help maintain stable blood sugar levels. High sugar intake can spike blood glucose levels, low fiber intake can affect digestion and blood sugar control, and a high-fat diet may lead to weight gain and insulin resistance. Regular carbohydrate consumption, when balanced with protein and healthy fats, can help manage gestational diabetes effectively.

Question 26: Correct Answer: C) Postpartum mothers with iron-deficiency anemia may experience fatigue and weakness.
Rationale: Iron-deficiency anemia is a common condition in the postpartum period due to blood loss during childbirth. Symptoms include fatigue, weakness, pale skin, and shortness of breath. Iron supplementation is often necessary to replenish iron stores. Avoiding iron-rich foods would be counterproductive in managing this condition.

Question 27: Correct Answer: A) It is a condition where the placenta partially covers the cervix.
Rationale: Placenta Previa is a condition where the placenta partially or completely covers the cervix, leading to potential complications during labor and delivery. Option B is incorrect as the placenta should ideally be located in the upper part of the uterus. Option C describes Placenta Accreta, where the placenta is deeply implanted in the uterine wall. Option D refers to Anterior Placenta, which is a normal variation in placental placement.

Question 28: Correct Answer: B) Increased oxytocin levels
Rationale: Afterpains, or uterine cramping, are common in the postpartum period and are caused by increased oxytocin levels. Oxytocin helps the uterus contract and return to its pre-pregnancy size. Options A, C, and D are incorrect as decreased uterine contractions, low progesterone levels, and elevated white blood cell count are not directly related to the occurrence of afterpains in the postpartum period.

Question 29: Correct Answer: C) Nipple confusion
Rationale: Nipple confusion is a common latch-on problem where the baby has difficulty latching onto the breast properly, often due to the use of artificial nipples such as pacifiers or bottles. This can lead to breastfeeding difficulties and inadequate milk transfer. Engorgement, mastitis, and plugged ducts are issues related to milk supply and breast health, not specifically latch-on problems. Nipple confusion can be addressed through proper positioning, support, and avoiding the use of artificial nipples in the early stages of breastfeeding.

Question 30: Correct Answer: A) Placing the newborn on their back to sleep is recommended to reduce the risk of Sudden Infant Death Syndrome (SIDS).
Rationale: Placing the newborn on their back to sleep is the safest sleep position as recommended by the American Academy of Pediatrics to reduce the risk of SIDS. Placing the newborn on their stomach increases the risk of SIDS. Soft bedding in the crib can pose a suffocation hazard, and bed-sharing increases the risk of accidental suffocation or strangulation. Therefore, option A is the correct choice for safe sleep practices.

Question 31: Correct Answer: C) Opioids
Rationale: Symptoms of NAS, such as irritability, poor feeding, and tremors, are commonly seen in newborns exposed to opioids in utero. While alcohol, benzodiazepines, and amphetamines can also cause adverse effects on the newborn, opioids are most commonly associated with NAS due to withdrawal effects.

Question 32: Correct Answer: A) Maternal HIV infection
Rationale: Maternal HIV infection is a contraindication to breastfeeding due to the risk of transmission of the virus to the infant through breast milk. It is essential to prevent the vertical transmission of HIV from mother to child. Maternal hypertension, diabetes, and anemia are not contraindications to breastfeeding. In fact, breastfeeding is encouraged for mothers with these conditions as it provides numerous benefits for both the mother and the baby.

Question 33: Correct Answer: A) Encouraging increased intake of high-fiber foods
Rationale: Encouraging increased intake of high-fiber foods helps prevent and alleviate constipation by promoting bowel regularity. Fiber adds bulk to the stool, making it easier to pass. Administering a stool softener may be necessary in some cases, but dietary modifications should be the first-line intervention. Limiting fluid intake can worsen constipation, as hydration is essential for bowel function. Prolonged bed rest can contribute to constipation by reducing physical activity and slowing down bowel motility.

Question 34: Correct Answer: B) Younger mothers are at lower risk for preterm birth.
Rationale: Younger mothers, typically defined as those under 20 years of age, are generally at lower risk for preterm birth compared to older mothers. While younger mothers may face challenges related to social support and financial stability, they are less likely to experience complications such as gestational diabetes or pregnancy-induced hypertension. Therefore, option B is the correct answer as it accurately reflects the lower risk of preterm birth in younger mothers.

Question 35: Correct Answer: B) The parent responds promptly to the infant's cues for feeding and comfort.
Rationale: In the postpartum period, a normal characteristic of parent/infant interactions includes the parent responding promptly to the infant's cues for feeding and comfort. This behavior fosters bonding and attachment between the parent and infant. Options A, C, and D are incorrect as they describe behaviors that are not indicative of healthy parent/infant interactions. Disinterest, frustration, anger, and avoidance of eye contact are not typical or desirable responses from a parent towards their newborn. It is essential for parents to engage positively and responsively with their infants to promote healthy development and bonding.

Question 36: Correct Answer: C) Newborns have low levels of Vitamin K at birth due to the sterile gut.
Rationale: Newborns have low levels of Vitamin K at birth because they do not have the gut bacteria necessary for its synthesis. Administering Vitamin K injection to newborns helps prevent Vitamin K deficiency bleeding, a serious condition that can lead to life-threatening bleeding. Delaying the injection can put the baby at risk for this potentially fatal condition.

Question 37: Correct Answer: D) Monitor for signs of

dehydration during phototherapy.
Rationale: Phototherapy helps in the breakdown of bilirubin and its excretion from the body, reducing levels. Eye protection is essential to prevent eye damage from the lights. Breastfeeding should continue during phototherapy to prevent dehydration. Monitoring for signs of dehydration, such as decreased urine output, is crucial as phototherapy can increase insensible water loss.

Question 38: Correct Answer: C) Burp the baby halfway through and after feeding
Rationale: Burping the baby halfway through and after feeding helps release any swallowed air, reducing the risk of colic and discomfort. Option A is incorrect as forcing the baby to finish the entire bottle can lead to overfeeding and digestive issues. Option B is incorrect as microwaving formula can create hot spots that may burn the baby's mouth; it is safer to warm the formula in a bowl of warm water. Option D is incorrect as honey and corn syrup should never be given to infants due to the risk of botulism.

Question 39: Correct Answer: C) Frequent breastfeeding
Rationale: Frequent breastfeeding is actually essential for establishing and maintaining an adequate milk supply. Maternal obesity, advanced maternal age, and maternal smoking are known risk factors for insufficient milk supply. Maternal obesity can affect hormone levels necessary for milk production, advanced maternal age may impact milk production capacity, and smoking can reduce milk production and alter the composition of breast milk.

Question 40: Correct Answer: A) "Skin-to-skin contact helps regulate the baby's body temperature and promotes bonding between you and your newborn."
Rationale: Skin-to-skin contact between the mother and newborn helps regulate the baby's body temperature, promotes bonding, and supports breastfeeding initiation. Option B is incorrect as skin-to-skin contact is a beneficial practice for newborns. Option C is incorrect as proper hygiene practices can prevent infections during skin-to-skin contact. Option D is incorrect as skin-to-skin contact is a crucial aspect of early bonding and attachment between the mother and newborn.

Question 41: Correct Answer: C) Encouraging skin-to-skin contact with the mother
Rationale: Skin-to-skin contact with the mother is the most effective way to help a newborn maintain body temperature. It provides natural warmth and helps regulate the baby's temperature. Increasing room temperature or using a radiant warmer can be helpful but may not be as effective as skin-to-skin contact. Administering warm intravenous fluids is not a standard practice for managing mild hypothermia in newborns.

Question 42: Correct Answer: C) Inactivated influenza vaccine
Rationale: The correct option is C) Inactivated influenza vaccine. This vaccine is recommended for pregnant women to protect both themselves and their newborns from influenza. The other options, A) MMR vaccine, B) Varicella vaccine, and D) Rotavirus vaccine, are not typically administered during pregnancy due to potential risks to the fetus. Influenza vaccination during pregnancy has been shown to be safe and effective in preventing serious complications from influenza for both the mother and the baby.

Question 43: Correct Answer: A) Encourage the patient to walk around to help progress labor.
Rationale: Encouraging the patient to walk around can help facilitate the descent of the fetus and progress labor in cases of early labor. Administering oxytocin or offering pain medication may not be necessary at this stage. Immediate cesarean section is not indicated based on the information provided.

Question 44: Correct Answer: B) Hematoma
Rationale: A hematoma is a collection of blood outside of blood vessels. In the postpartum period, hematomas can occur in the perineal area due to trauma during delivery. The characteristic features include pain, swelling, and a bluish discoloration. It is important to differentiate hematomas from other postpartum complications like uterine atony, mastitis, and endometritis. Uterine atony is characterized by excessive uterine relaxation leading to postpartum hemorrhage. Mastitis is inflammation of the breast tissue, and endometritis is infection of the uterine lining. Therefore, in this scenario, the most likely diagnosis based on the symptoms described is a hematoma.

Question 45: Correct Answer: C) Educate the parents on safe sleep practices and recommend using sleep sacks for warmth
Rationale: Placing a space heater near the baby's crib can pose a fire hazard and increase the risk of burns. Safe sleep practices include keeping the sleep environment free of hazards like heaters and using sleep sacks or appropriate clothing for warmth. Keeping the space heater on at all times or using additional blankets can lead to overheating and increase the risk of SIDS, making options A and D incorrect.

Question 46: Correct Answer: A) Maternal preeclampsia
Rationale: Maternal preeclampsia is a known risk factor for neonatal thrombocytopenia due to the potential transfer of maternal antibodies that can affect the newborn's platelet count. Neonatal jaundice, maternal diabetes, and neonatal hypoglycemia are not directly linked to neonatal thrombocytopenia. While neonatal jaundice and hypoglycemia are common newborn complications, they do not have a direct association with thrombocytopenia. Maternal diabetes, although it can lead to other neonatal complications, is not a primary risk factor for thrombocytopenia in newborns.

Question 47: Correct Answer: B) Administer anticoagulant therapy
Rationale: Deep vein thrombosis is a serious condition that requires immediate anticoagulant therapy to prevent the clot from dislodging and causing a pulmonary embolism. Applying cold compresses can worsen the condition by promoting vasoconstriction. Leg elevation is essential to reduce swelling and improve venous return. Prolonged bed rest can increase the risk of clot propagation and pulmonary embolism, so early mobilization is encouraged.

Question 48: Correct Answer: C) Dysuria
Rationale: Dysuria, or painful urination, is a common symptom of UTIs in the postpartum period. It is often accompanied by a frequent urge to urinate and lower abdominal discomfort. Hypotension and bradycardia are not typical symptoms of UTIs but may indicate other medical conditions. Hyperglycemia is associated with high blood sugar levels and is not a direct symptom of UTIs.

Question 49: Correct Answer: B) Autosomal Dominant
Rationale: Autosomal Dominant inheritance pattern

manifests in each generation, affecting both males and females equally. There is no skipping of generations, and affected individuals have a 50% chance of passing the trait to their offspring. In contrast, Autosomal Recessive conditions often skip generations and require both parents to be carriers. X-Linked Recessive disorders predominantly affect males and can skip generations, while X-Linked Dominant disorders do not skip generations and affect both males and females.

Question 50: Correct Answer: D) Initiating skin-to-skin contact and breastfeeding within the first hour
Rationale: Initiating skin-to-skin contact and breastfeeding within the first hour after birth is crucial in promoting successful breastfeeding and preventing nipple confusion in newborns from multiple births. This practice helps establish bonding, regulates the newborns' body temperature, and stimulates breastfeeding. Options A, B, and C are not recommended as they may interfere with the establishment of breastfeeding and increase the risk of nipple confusion, leading to breastfeeding difficulties in newborns from multiple births.

Question 51: Correct Answer: A) Fetal heart rate accelerations with fetal movement
Rationale: In a non-stress test (NST), reassuring findings include fetal heart rate accelerations with fetal movement, indicating a healthy response of the fetal heart rate to fetal activity. Fetal heart rate decelerations with movement, absence of fetal heart rate variability, and a baseline fetal heart rate of 90 bpm are concerning findings that may indicate fetal distress or compromise.

Question 52: Correct Answer: A) Administering phenobarbital
Rationale: Administering phenobarbital is a common intervention in managing seizures in newborns as it is an anticonvulsant medication. Increasing environmental stimuli, feeding the newborn immediately, and placing the newborn in a dark room are not appropriate interventions for managing seizures in newborns and may exacerbate the condition. Phenobarbital helps control seizures by acting on the central nervous system.

Question 53: Correct Answer: A) Esophageal atresia
Rationale: Esophageal atresia, a congenital anomaly where the esophagus does not connect to the stomach, can lead to polyhydramnios due to the inability of the fetus to swallow amniotic fluid. Patent ductus arteriosus, clubfoot, and cleft lip are not typically associated with polyhydramnios.

Question 54: Correct Answer: B) Provide continuous positive airway pressure (CPAP)
Rationale: In a newborn experiencing mild respiratory distress, providing continuous positive airway pressure (CPAP) helps maintain lung volume and improve oxygenation. Administering surfactant therapy, initiating bag-mask ventilation, or encouraging skin-to-skin contact with the mother may not be the priority interventions for mild respiratory distress in the immediate transition period.

Question 55: Correct Answer: B) Erythromycin
Rationale: Erythromycin is administered to newborns to prevent ophthalmia neonatorum, an eye infection caused by Neisseria gonorrhoeae or Chlamydia trachomatis. Vitamin K is given to newborns to prevent hemorrhagic disease of the newborn. Naloxone is used to reverse opioid overdose. Ibuprofen is a nonsteroidal anti-inflammatory drug used for pain relief and fever reduction, not for preventing eye infections in newborns.

Question 56: Correct Answer: D) Necrotizing Enterocolitis
Rationale: Necrotizing Enterocolitis (NEC) is a serious gastrointestinal emergency in newborns, presenting with abdominal distension, bloody stools, and signs of sepsis. Hirschsprung's Disease is a congenital disorder affecting the colon, Gastroesophageal Reflux is the regurgitation of stomach contents, and Intussusception is the telescoping of one part of the intestine into another. Among the options provided, NEC is the correct answer due to its specific symptoms and association with gastrointestinal complications in newborns.

Question 57: Correct Answer: A) Encourage frequent breastfeeding sessions
Rationale: Breast engorgement is a common issue in postpartum mothers, characterized by swelling, pain, and redness of the breasts. Encouraging frequent breastfeeding sessions helps relieve engorgement by emptying the breasts regularly, reducing pain and swelling. Ice packs can constrict blood vessels and decrease milk supply, so they are not recommended. Avoiding breastfeeding can lead to further complications like mastitis. Tight bras can worsen engorgement by putting pressure on the breasts.

Question 58: Correct Answer: C) Intracranial hemorrhage
Rationale: Vitamin K deficiency in newborns can lead to impaired blood clotting, resulting in a serious complication known as intracranial hemorrhage. This condition occurs due to the inadequate production of clotting factors, putting the newborn at risk for bleeding within the skull. Hemolytic anemia (Option A) is not directly associated with Vitamin K deficiency. Hypocalcemia (Option B) is related to calcium levels and not Vitamin K. Respiratory distress syndrome (Option D) is primarily a lung disorder in premature infants and not linked to Vitamin K deficiency.

Question 59: Correct Answer: C) Pathological jaundice
Rationale: Pathological jaundice is defined as unconjugated bilirubin levels exceeding 17 mg/dL in a term newborn. This type of hyperbilirubinemia is often caused by underlying conditions such as hemolytic disease, sepsis, or enzyme deficiencies. Physiological jaundice, breastfeeding jaundice, and breast milk jaundice typically present with lower bilirubin levels and are usually transient and benign conditions in newborns.

Question 60: Correct Answer: C) Enalapril
Rationale: Enalapril (C) is contraindicated in pregnancy as it is associated with teratogenic effects, particularly in the second and third trimesters. Nifedipine (A) and Labetalol (D) are commonly used antihypertensives in pregnancy due to their safety profiles. Hydralazine (B) is also considered safe for use in pregnancy and is often used for hypertensive emergencies.

Question 61: Correct Answer: C) Muscle tone
Rationale: Muscle tone is one of the five components evaluated in the Apgar score assessment. It refers to the newborn's overall muscle strength and activity level. A score of 0 is given if the newborn is limp and floppy, 1 if there is some flexion of the arms and legs, and 2 if the newborn displays active movement and resistance to extension. Assessing muscle tone helps healthcare providers determine the newborn's neurological status and overall well-being. Therefore, the correct answer is C) Muscle tone, as it specifically relates to this aspect of the Apgar score assessment.

Question 62: Correct Answer: A) Maternal age
Rationale: Maternal age plays a significant role in fetal assessment as advanced maternal age (over 35 years) is associated with increased risks such as chromosomal abnormalities and pregnancy complications. Maternal height and occupation do not directly impact fetal assessment or birth risk factors. Maternal hair color is a genetic trait and does not influence fetal assessment or pregnancy outcomes.

Question 63: Correct Answer: B) Neonatal sepsis
Rationale: The white blood cell count of 8,000/mm3 with a left shift and increased neutrophils suggest an inflammatory response, which is commonly seen in neonatal sepsis. Physiological leukopenia is not a typical finding in neonates. Neonatal hyperbilirubinemia is characterized by elevated bilirubin levels, not by changes in the CBC. Neonatal hypoglycemia is related to low blood sugar levels, not to the CBC findings described.

Question 64: Correct Answer: C) Anencephaly
Rationale: Anencephaly is a severe neural tube defect where the brain, skull, and scalp do not form properly, leading to stillbirth or neonatal death. Hydrocephalus is the abnormal accumulation of cerebrospinal fluid within the brain. Spina bifida is a defect where the spinal cord and meninges protrude through a vertebral defect. Encephalocele is a defect characterized by the protrusion of brain and meninges through a skull defect.

Question 65: Correct Answer: C) Phenylketonuria (PKU)
Rationale: Phenylketonuria (PKU) is a metabolic disorder caused by a deficiency of the enzyme phenylalanine hydroxylase, leading to the accumulation of phenylalanine in the body. Galactosemia results from the inability to metabolize galactose, Maple syrup urine disease involves the inability to break down certain amino acids, and Homocystinuria is caused by a defect in the metabolism of the amino acid methionine, not phenylalanine.

Question 66: Correct Answer: B) Assessing the mother's mental health
Rationale: Assessing the mother's mental health is crucial in postpartum care for mothers with substance abuse history to identify any signs of postpartum depression or anxiety, which can impact both the mother and the newborn. Monitoring the baby's weight gain is important but not specific to substance abuse cases. Encouraging immediate breastfeeding may not be suitable depending on the substances used. Administering pain medications should be done judiciously considering the mother's history of substance abuse.

Question 67: Correct Answer: C) Re-positioning the baby for a deeper latch
Rationale: When a mother experiences nipple soreness and poor latch during breastfeeding, re-positioning the baby for a deeper latch is the most appropriate intervention. This helps ensure proper alignment of the baby's mouth to the breast, leading to effective milk transfer and reduced nipple pain. Using a nipple shield or applying lanolin cream may provide temporary relief but do not address the root cause of the issue. Supplementing with formula should only be considered after exhausting all efforts to improve breastfeeding success.

Question 68: Correct Answer: D) Justice
Rationale: Justice in maternal postpartum care ensures that all women receive fair and equal access to healthcare resources, regardless of their background or socioeconomic status. This principle promotes equity in the distribution of services, such as postpartum assessments, management, and education, to ensure that every mother receives the care she needs. Autonomy relates to respecting a patient's right to make decisions, beneficence focuses on doing good for the patient, and non-maleficence emphasizes avoiding harm. However, in the context of maternal postpartum care, the principle of justice specifically addresses the fair allocation of resources.

Question 69: Correct Answer: A) Provide information on stress management techniques.
Rationale: Providing information on stress management techniques is the most appropriate intervention to address Ms. Rodriguez's psychosocial needs. This option promotes empowerment and equips her with tools to cope with stress effectively. Suggesting she quit her job or stop caring for her toddler may not be feasible solutions and could add to her stress. Recommending medication should be considered only after non-pharmacological interventions have been explored.

Question 70: Correct Answer: B) Side-lying position
Rationale: The side-lying position is a common breastfeeding position that can help ensure proper latch and milk transfer. This position allows the mother and baby to be in a comfortable and relaxed posture, promoting effective breastfeeding. The supine, standing, and reclining positions may not provide optimal support for the baby to latch correctly and transfer milk efficiently. Therefore, the correct answer is the side-lying position for promoting successful breastfeeding.

Question 71: Correct Answer: C) Side-lying position
Rationale: The correct position for a lumbar puncture in a newborn is the side-lying position. This position allows for proper alignment of the spine and facilitates easier access to the lumbar area. Placing the newborn in the supine, prone, or flexed sitting position would not provide the optimal alignment needed for a successful lumbar puncture procedure.

Question 72: Correct Answer: C) Cell-Free DNA testing has a higher detection rate for Down syndrome.
Rationale: Cell-Free DNA testing, also known as Non-Invasive Prenatal Testing (NIPT), offers a higher detection rate for Down syndrome compared to Quad Screen testing. NIPT analyzes fetal DNA fragments present in the mother's blood and can detect chromosomal abnormalities with a high degree of accuracy. While Quad Screen testing is typically performed between 15-20 weeks of gestation, NIPT can be done as early as 10 weeks. However, it is important to note that Cell-Free DNA testing does not screen for neural tube defects, which is a limitation compared to Quad Screen testing.

Question 73: Correct Answer: C) Heroin
Rationale: Heroin is a potent opioid that can cross the placenta and lead to physical dependence in the fetus, resulting in NAS after birth. Cocaine, marijuana, and methamphetamine do not typically cause NAS as frequently as heroin due to their different mechanisms of action and effects on the developing fetus. Heroin use during pregnancy poses significant risks to both the mother and the newborn, highlighting the importance of early identification and intervention in pregnant women with substance use disorders.

Question 74: Correct Answer: B) Woods' screw

maneuver
Rationale: If the McRoberts maneuver and suprapubic pressure are unsuccessful, the Woods' screw maneuver is the next step. This maneuver involves rotating the posterior shoulder internally to dislodge it from behind the pubic bone. The Rubin maneuver (A) involves rotating the anterior shoulder externally to dislodge it. The Gaskin maneuver (C) involves positioning the mother on hands and knees. The Reverse Woods' screw maneuver (D) is not a recognized technique for managing shoulder dystocia.

Question 75: Correct Answer: B) Two previous cesarean deliveries
Rationale: VBAC is generally considered safe for women with one previous cesarean delivery with a low transverse uterine incision. However, having had two or more previous cesarean deliveries increases the risk of uterine rupture, making it a contraindication for VBAC. Options A, C, and D are not contraindications for VBAC and may still allow for a trial of labor after cesarean (TOLAC).

Question 76: Correct Answer: A) Allow Mrs. Patel's mother to stay with her in accordance with her cultural beliefs.
Rationale: It is essential to respect and accommodate cultural practices that support family integration. Allowing Mrs. Patel's mother to stay will enhance her comfort, facilitate communication, and promote bonding. This approach aligns with patient-centered care and acknowledges the significance of cultural considerations in maternal postpartum care.

Question 77: Correct Answer: A) Initiate continuous positive airway pressure (CPAP)
Rationale: In a preterm newborn with respiratory distress, the priority intervention is to initiate CPAP to support the baby's breathing and improve oxygenation. Nasal flaring, grunting, and chest retractions are signs of respiratory distress that require prompt intervention. Administering surfactant, providing oxygen therapy via face mask, and placing the baby in a prone position may be considered based on the assessment findings, but CPAP is the initial priority to stabilize the baby's respiratory status.

Question 78: Correct Answer: B) Providing Mrs. Johnson with resources on childcare options and flexible work arrangements
Rationale: Supporting Mrs. Johnson in exploring childcare options and work-life balance is essential. Option A may not align with Mrs. Johnson's career aspirations. Option C disregards Mrs. Johnson's valid concerns, and option D should be considered if Mrs. Johnson continues to struggle emotionally.

Question 79: Correct Answer: C) Pulse Oximetry
Rationale: Pulse oximetry is a non-invasive screening tool used to detect critical congenital heart defects in newborns. It measures the oxygen saturation levels in the blood, helping identify infants who may require further cardiac evaluation. The other options, Ballard Score, Apgar Score, and Capillary Refill Test, are assessments used for different purposes such as gestational age assessment, immediate newborn assessment, and circulatory status evaluation, respectively, but they are not specific for CHD screening.

Question 80: Correct Answer: A) Administering the hepatitis B vaccine and hepatitis B immune globulin (HBIG) within 12 hours of birth
Rationale: The newborn infant of a mother who is HBsAg positive should receive the hepatitis B vaccine and HBIG within 12 hours of birth to prevent perinatal transmission. Antiretroviral therapy is used for HIV, not hepatitis B. Isolating the newborn is not necessary for hepatitis B transmission prevention. Breastfeeding is safe in the context of hepatitis B, and delaying it is not indicated.

Question 81: Correct Answer: A) Polyhydramnios
Rationale: Polyhydramnios, an excess of amniotic fluid, is a significant risk factor for cord prolapse as the increased volume of amniotic fluid allows more room for the cord to descend alongside or in front of the presenting part. Maternal age over 35 years, multiparity, and maternal obesity are not direct risk factors for cord prolapse. It is essential to monitor and manage polyhydramnios closely during labor to prevent complications such as cord prolapse.

Question 82: Correct Answer: B) Listeria monocytogenes
Rationale: Listeria monocytogenes is a foodborne bacterium that can cause serious infections in pregnant women, leading to adverse outcomes such as miscarriage, stillbirth, or neonatal sepsis. Working in a daycare center may increase the risk of exposure to Listeria through contaminated food sources. While Streptococcus pneumoniae, Chlamydia trachomatis, and Bordetella pertussis are also concerning infections, Listeria poses the highest risk in this scenario due to its association with foodborne transmission and adverse pregnancy outcomes.

Question 83: Correct Answer: A) Within 24 hours of birth
Rationale: Eye prophylaxis with erythromycin ointment should be administered to newborns in the first 24 hours of birth to effectively prevent ophthalmia neonatorum. Delaying the administration beyond this timeframe increases the risk of infection transmission from the mother to the newborn during delivery. Administering eye prophylaxis within 48 hours, 72 hours, or 1 week of birth may not provide adequate protection against ophthalmia neonatorum.

Question 84: Correct Answer: C) Mrs. Johnson should include a balance of complex carbohydrates, lean proteins, and healthy fats in her meals.
Rationale: A balanced diet consisting of complex carbohydrates, lean proteins, and healthy fats can help Mrs. Johnson manage her gestational diabetes by promoting stable blood glucose levels. Option A is incorrect as a high-carbohydrate diet can lead to spikes in blood sugar levels. Option B is incorrect as regular blood glucose monitoring is essential for managing gestational diabetes. Option D is incorrect as skipping meals can result in hypoglycemia and is not recommended for women with gestational diabetes.

Question 85: Correct Answer: B) Preeclampsia
Rationale: Low platelet count in the postpartum period is commonly associated with preeclampsia, a hypertensive disorder of pregnancy. Preeclampsia can lead to HELLP syndrome, characterized by hemolysis, elevated liver enzymes, and low platelet count. Monitoring platelet levels is crucial in postpartum care for women with a history of preeclampsia to prevent complications such as bleeding disorders and organ damage. Gestational diabetes, hyperthyroidism, and urinary tract infections are not typically linked to low platelet count in the postpartum period.

Question 86: Correct Answer: D) 3 minutes after birth
Rationale: Delayed cord clamping involves waiting for at least 3 minutes after birth before clamping and cutting the umbilical cord. This delay allows for the transfer of additional blood from the placenta to the newborn, providing numerous benefits such as improved iron stores, cardiovascular stability, and neurodevelopment. Options A, B, and C are incorrect as they do not adhere to the recommended time interval for delayed cord clamping, which is at least 3 minutes after birth to maximize the advantages for the newborn.

Question 87: Correct Answer: B) "Postpartum mothers should receive the Tdap vaccine to protect their newborns from pertussis."
Rationale: Postpartum mothers should receive the Tdap vaccine to provide protection against pertussis for their newborns. Option A is incorrect as the Tdap vaccine is recommended for postpartum mothers. Option C is incorrect as postpartum mothers can safely receive the Tdap vaccine while breastfeeding. Option D is incorrect as allergies alone do not determine Tdap vaccine eligibility.

Question 88: Correct Answer: A) Warmth and erythema along the course of a superficial vein
Rationale: Superficial thrombophlebitis presents with warmth and erythema along the course of a superficial vein, indicating inflammation. Sudden onset of dyspnea and chest pain (Option B) are more indicative of pulmonary embolism. Unilateral leg swelling with pain on palpation (Option C) is characteristic of deep vein thrombosis. Decreased pedal pulses and cool extremities (Option D) are signs of arterial insufficiency, not thrombophlebitis.

Question 89: Correct Answer: C) Ventricular septal defect
Rationale: Ventricular septal defect is a common congenital heart defect associated with Acyanotic Heart Disease in newborns. It results in a left-to-right shunt, leading to increased pulmonary blood flow and eventual right-sided heart enlargement. Options A, B, and D are incorrect as they are typically associated with Cyanotic Heart Disease. Tetralogy of Fallot, Transposition of the great arteries, and Tricuspid atresia are characterized by cyanosis and do not fall under the category of Acyanotic Heart Disease.

Question 90: Correct Answer: B) Providing education on postpartum depression and available support resources.
Rationale: It is crucial for the nurse to recognize and address the mother's feelings of sadness, anxiety, and irritability during the postpartum period. By providing education on postpartum depression and available support resources, the nurse can empower the mother to seek help and access the necessary support. This approach promotes the mother's well-being, facilitates a smoother maternal role transition, and ensures early intervention if postpartum depression is present. Options A, C, and D are incorrect as they do not prioritize the mother's mental health and well-being, which are essential aspects of maternal role transition.

Question 91: Correct Answer: D) Topical anesthetic cream
Rationale: Topical anesthetic creams provide local pain relief and can help alleviate discomfort associated with hemorrhoids. While oral stool softeners may be beneficial in preventing constipation, topical treatments are more effective for symptomatic relief of hemorrhoids. Topical corticosteroid creams are used for inflammation, and oral NSAIDs are not typically recommended for hemorrhoid management.

Question 92: Correct Answer: C) Phenylketonuria
Rationale: Phenylketonuria (PKU) is an inborn error of metabolism where there is a deficiency of the enzyme phenylalanine hydroxylase, leading to the accumulation of phenylalanine in the blood and tissues. This results in symptoms like poor feeding, lethargy, seizures, and a musty odor to the skin and urine. Galactosemia, Maple syrup urine disease, and Homocystinuria are also inborn errors of metabolism but present with different clinical features and biochemical abnormalities, making them incorrect choices in this scenario.

Question 93: Correct Answer: C) Engaging in regular physical activity
Rationale: Engaging in regular physical activity postpartum helps promote bowel regularity and prevent constipation. It aids in stimulating bowel movements and maintaining overall bowel health. Avoiding fluid intake and limiting fiber-rich foods can exacerbate constipation. Ignoring the urge to defecate can lead to further complications such as hemorrhoids. Therefore, regular physical activity is crucial for postpartum mothers to maintain optimal bowel function.

Question 94: Correct Answer: B) Intravenous glucose infusion
Rationale: The recommended treatment for hypoglycemia in newborns is intravenous glucose infusion to rapidly increase blood glucose levels. Immediate feeding with formula can be used if intravenous access is not available. Skin-to-skin contact with the mother and observation without intervention are not appropriate treatments for hypoglycemia as they do not address the underlying issue of low blood glucose levels.

Question 95: Correct Answer: B) Dopamine
Rationale: Dopamine is a medication commonly used in newborn resuscitation due to its vasopressor effects, which help increase blood pressure and improve perfusion. Furosemide is a diuretic and not used for resuscitation purposes. Acetaminophen is an antipyretic and analgesic drug. Oxytocin is primarily used to induce or augment labor and control postpartum bleeding, not for resuscitation in newborns.

Question 96: Correct Answer: D) Rooting
Rationale: The correct answer is D) Rooting. When a newborn turns head side to side with mouth open and searches for the breast, it indicates the rooting reflex, a feeding cue. Hiccuping, spitting up, and burping are not feeding cues but rather normal physiological processes in newborns.

Question 97: Correct Answer: C) Breastfeeding should be established before introducing any supplementary feedings.
Rationale: It is crucial to establish breastfeeding before introducing any supplementary feedings to ensure that the newborn receives the full benefits of breastfeeding, including bonding with the mother, receiving essential nutrients, and stimulating milk production. Introducing supplementary feedings too early can interfere with the establishment of breastfeeding and may lead to nipple confusion or decreased milk supply. Therefore, it is recommended to wait until breastfeeding is well established before considering supplementary feedings.

Question 98: Correct Answer: A) The baby's respiratory

rate is within the normal range for a newborn.
Rationale: The normal respiratory rate for a newborn is between 30-60 breaths per minute. A rate of 60 breaths per minute falls within this range, indicating appropriate physiologic adaptation to extrauterine life. The heart rate of 140 beats per minute is also within the normal range for a newborn (120-160 bpm). The temperature of 36.8℃ is within the normal range (36.5-37.5℃) for a newborn. Pink skin color indicates good oxygenation, not hypoxia.

Question 99: Correct Answer: C) ABO incompatibility
Rationale: ABO incompatibility between the mother and baby can lead to the breakdown of red blood cells in the newborn, causing an increase in bilirubin levels and subsequent hyperbilirubinemia. Exclusive breastfeeding, term gestation, and maternal diabetes are not direct risk factors for hyperbilirubinemia. Term gestation is actually considered a protective factor against hyperbilirubinemia.

Question 100: Correct Answer: A) Dimming the lights and reducing noise levels
Rationale: Dimming the lights and reducing noise levels are essential comfort measures to create a soothing environment for newborns, promoting relaxation and sleep. Bright lights and loud noises can disrupt a newborn's sleep patterns and increase stress levels. Continuous loud white noise may also be overwhelming for the newborn. Strong scented candles for aromatherapy may not be recommended due to potential sensitivities in newborns.

Question 101: Correct Answer: B) Prepare for imminent delivery
Rationale: In a precipitous delivery scenario, where the fetal head is crowning, the priority nursing action is to prepare for imminent delivery to ensure a safe birth for both the mother and the baby. Instructing the patient to push without proper preparation or assessment can lead to complications. Performing a vaginal exam at this stage is unnecessary and may delay the delivery. Administering pain medication is not the priority when the baby is about to be born.

Question 102: Correct Answer: A) Previous preterm birth
Rationale: A history of previous preterm birth is a crucial antenatal risk factor as it increases the likelihood of experiencing another preterm birth. This history indicates a potential underlying risk factor that may predispose the mother to subsequent preterm deliveries. Maternal age over 35 years (option B) is a risk factor for certain pregnancy complications but not specifically related to obstetrical history. History of gestational diabetes (option C) and multiparity (option D) are important factors but do not directly correlate with antenatal risk factors for adverse pregnancy outcomes like previous preterm birth.

Question 103: Correct Answer: B) Hypokalemia
Rationale: Hypokalemia (Option B) is a potential complication of diuretic therapy, as these medications can lead to potassium loss. Decreased blood pressure (Option A) and increased urinary output (Option C) are expected effects of diuretics. Swelling in the lower extremities (Option D) would indicate inadequate response to diuretic therapy and may require further evaluation.

Question 104: Correct Answer: C) Anemia
Rationale: Anemia is a common hematologic complication in the postpartum period, often due to blood loss during delivery or inadequate iron intake. Symptoms include fatigue, weakness, and pallor. Thrombocytopenia (Option A) is a low platelet count, Polycythemia (Option B) is an excess of red blood cells, and Hemophilia (Option D) is a genetic disorder affecting clotting factors, none of which directly cause the characteristic decrease in red blood cells seen in anemia postpartum.

Question 105: Correct Answer: B) Notify the healthcare provider immediately.
Rationale: A blood pressure reading of 150/90 mmHg in the postpartum period is elevated and requires prompt notification of the healthcare provider for further evaluation and management. This reading is above the normal range and could indicate the development of postpartum preeclampsia, a serious condition that requires timely intervention. Options A, C, and D are incorrect as they do not address the urgency of the situation and the need for immediate medical attention.

Question 106: Correct Answer: A) Ultrasound
Rationale: Ultrasound is a non-invasive, safe, and effective method for assessing fetal growth, development, and well-being during pregnancy. It provides valuable information about the fetus, including size, position, and any potential abnormalities. Blood pressure measurement and urine analysis are essential for monitoring maternal health but do not directly assess fetal well-being. Weight measurement is important for tracking maternal weight gain but does not provide information about the fetus.

Question 107: Correct Answer: D) Gestational hypertension may progress to preeclampsia if proteinuria is detected.
Rationale: Gestational hypertension can progress to preeclampsia if proteinuria (?300 mg/24 hours) is detected, indicating the development of maternal organ dysfunction. Option A is incorrect as gestational hypertension usually resolves within 6 weeks postpartum. Option B is incorrect as gestational hypertension is defined as new-onset hypertension after 20 weeks gestation. Option C is incorrect as gestational hypertension is associated with an increased risk of adverse maternal outcomes, especially if it progresses to preeclampsia.

Question 108: Correct Answer: A) Zidovudine (AZT)
Rationale: Zidovudine (AZT) is a preferred antiretroviral medication during pregnancy as it has been shown to reduce the risk of vertical transmission of HIV. Efavirenz (EFV) is contraindicated in the first trimester due to potential teratogenic effects. Ritonavir (RTV) is often used as a booster in combination therapy, and Darunavir (DRV) is not typically a first-line option during pregnancy.

Question 109: Correct Answer: D) Electric breast pump
Rationale: An electric breast pump can help stimulate milk production by mimicking a baby's sucking pattern through adjustable suction levels and speed settings. Nipple shield, supplemental nursing system, and manual breast pump do not provide the same level of stimulation to increase milk supply effectively.

Question 110: Correct Answer: C) Prolonged second stage of labor
Rationale: Operative vaginal delivery using forceps or vacuum extraction may be indicated in cases of prolonged second stage of labor where maternal expulsive efforts are ineffective. Maternal exhaustion alone is not a primary indication for operative delivery. Fetal macrosomia may increase the risk of shoulder dystocia but is not a direct indication for operative

delivery. Maternal request for a quick delivery is not a sufficient medical indication for an operative vaginal delivery.

Question 111: Correct Answer: C) Weight gain of 1 kg in a week
Rationale: In a pregnant woman with a cardiac condition, sudden weight gain of 1 kg or more in a week can be indicative of cardiac decompensation, possibly due to fluid retention. This sign, along with symptoms such as increasing shortness of breath and fatigue, should raise concerns about worsening cardiac function. Leg cramps, decreased urinary frequency, and back pain are important to assess but are less specific indicators of cardiac decompensation compared to rapid weight gain in this context.

Question 112: Correct Answer: B) Keeping the cord stump clean and dry
Rationale: It is essential to keep the cord stump clean and dry to prevent infection. Cleaning with alcohol swabs can delay healing and increase infection risk. Applying powders and lotions can also introduce bacteria. Immersing the baby in water before the cord falls off can increase the risk of infection as well.

Question 113: Correct Answer: A) Every 2-3 hours
Rationale: In the early postpartum period, breastfeeding should occur every 2-3 hours to ensure the newborn receives adequate nutrition, stimulate milk production, and establish a strong bond between the mother and baby. Frequent breastfeeding also helps prevent engorgement and maintain milk supply. Options B, C, and D are incorrect as they suggest longer intervals between feedings, which can lead to decreased milk production, poor weight gain in the newborn, and potential breastfeeding difficulties.

Question 114: Correct Answer: C) Inadequate uterine contractions
Rationale: Prolonged labor is characterized by inadequate uterine contractions that impede cervical dilation and fetal descent. Options A and B suggest normal progress in labor, while option D is a consequence of prolonged labor rather than a defining feature. Inadequate uterine contractions can lead to maternal exhaustion and fatigue due to prolonged labor duration.

Question 115: Correct Answer: A) Hemoglobin
Rationale: Hemodilution during pregnancy leads to a decrease in hemoglobin levels, as the increase in plasma volume outpaces the increase in red blood cell production. This physiological adaptation is essential to support the increased oxygen demands of the mother and fetus. Platelet count, blood glucose levels, and serum creatinine are not typically affected by hemodilution during pregnancy, making options B, C, and D incorrect.

Question 116: Correct Answer: D) Nipple fissures
Rationale: Nipple fissures, or cracks in the skin of the nipple, can provide an entry point for bacteria, leading to mastitis. Nipple blanching, nipple blebs, and nipple vasospasm are associated with other nipple problems such as poor latch, milk stasis, and Raynaud's phenomenon, respectively. However, nipple fissures specifically increase the risk of developing mastitis due to the compromised skin barrier.

Question 117: Correct Answer: B) Hold the baby in a semi-upright position during feeding
Rationale: Holding the baby in a semi-upright position during bottle feeding helps prevent choking and allows for better digestion. Option A is incorrect as propping the bottle can lead to overfeeding and increases the risk of ear infections. Option C is incorrect as using a bottle nipple with a small hole can frustrate the baby and lead to feeding difficulties. Option D is incorrect as it is important to allow the baby to feed at their own pace, but the position during feeding should still be semi-upright for optimal safety and comfort.

Question 118: Correct Answer: B) Hand expression can help stimulate milk production and maintain milk supply
Rationale: Hand expression is a valuable skill that can aid in milk removal, especially in the early postpartum period. It can help stimulate milk production, maintain milk supply, and provide relief in case of engorgement. Option A is incorrect as hand expression can be as efficient as a breast pump. Option C is inaccurate as hand expression is beneficial for all mothers, not just those with inverted nipples. Option D is false as hand expression can actually help prevent engorgement when done appropriately.

Question 119: Correct Answer: C) Using a lanolin-based nipple cream after each feeding
Rationale: Cracked nipples can be painful and increase the risk of infection. Using a lanolin-based nipple cream after each feeding can help soothe the nipples, promote healing, and prevent further complications. Continuing to breastfeed on the affected side is important to maintain milk supply and promote healing. Applying soap to clean the nipples before each feeding can dry out the skin and worsen the condition. Switching to formula feeding temporarily is not necessary and can impact milk supply.

Question 120: Correct Answer: A) Oxytocin
Rationale: Oxytocin is a uterotonic agent frequently used in labor to prevent postpartum hemorrhage by stimulating uterine contractions. Magnesium sulfate (Option B) is primarily used for seizure prophylaxis in preeclampsia and eclampsia, not for promoting uterine contractions. Misoprostol (Option C) and Carboprost (Option D) are prostaglandin analogs used for postpartum hemorrhage treatment but are not the first-line agents for preventing hemorrhage during labor. Therefore, Oxytocin is the correct choice for promoting uterine contractions in labor.

Question 121: Correct Answer: C) Absence of a urethral meatus in a male newborn
Rationale: The absence of a urethral meatus in a male newborn is a critical finding that requires immediate intervention as it may indicate a genitourinary anomaly such as hypospadias. Hypospadias is a condition where the opening of the urethra is on the underside of the penis instead of at the tip. Surgical correction may be needed to prevent complications. Labial adhesions, presence of vernix caseosa, and physiologic jaundice are common findings in newborns that do not require immediate intervention related to the genitourinary system.

Question 122: Correct Answer: A) Pain relief during circumcision
Rationale: Oral sucrose is often used in newborn care to provide pain relief during procedures such as circumcision. It has been shown to have analgesic properties and can help reduce pain perception in infants undergoing minor painful procedures. Options B, C, and D are incorrect as oral sucrose is not indicated for the treatment of jaundice, prevention of hypoglycemia, or promotion of weight gain in newborns.

Question 123: Correct Answer: B) Tachypnea
Rationale: Tachypnea, or rapid breathing, is a common symptom of Cyanotic Heart Disease in newborns due to the body's compensatory mechanism to increase oxygenation. Option A is incorrect as hypertension is not a typical symptom of Cyanotic Heart Disease. Option C is incorrect as Cyanotic Heart Disease leads to hypoxemia, not hyperoxemia. Option D is incorrect as hypoglycemia is not directly associated with Cyanotic Heart Disease.

Question 124: Correct Answer: D) Foul-smelling vaginal discharge
Rationale: A foul-smelling vaginal discharge could indicate an infection, such as endometritis, which is a serious postpartum complication requiring immediate medical attention. Lochia rubra on day 2 postpartum is a normal finding. A firm and midline fundus at the level of the umbilicus indicates proper uterine involution. Perineal lacerations with minimal bleeding are common postpartum and may not require immediate intervention unless bleeding is excessive.

Question 125: Correct Answer: C) Epstein-Barr Virus (EBV)
Rationale: Epstein-Barr Virus (EBV) commonly presents with symptoms of fever, malaise, sore throat, and lymphadenopathy. Leukocytosis is often seen in EBV infection. While CMV, HSV, and Rubella can also cause similar symptoms, the presence of enlarged cervical lymph nodes and leukocytosis in this scenario points towards EBV as the most likely cause.

Question 126: Correct Answer: B) Using a properly secured infant car seat
Rationale: Ensuring newborn safety during transport within the healthcare facility is crucial. Placing the newborn in a prone position (Option A) is contraindicated due to the risk of sudden infant death syndrome (SIDS). Carrying the newborn in the nurse's arms (Option C) may pose a risk of accidental falls. Leaving the newborn unattended on a flat surface (Option D) is unsafe. Using a properly secured infant car seat (Option B) is the recommended method for safe transport, providing support and protection for the newborn during movement within the facility.

Question 127: Correct Answer: A) Group B Streptococcus (GBS)
Rationale: Group B Streptococcus (GBS) is a leading cause of early-onset neonatal sepsis, typically occurring within the first week of life. GBS can be transmitted from the mother to the newborn during childbirth. While Escherichia coli (E. coli), Listeria monocytogenes, and Staphylococcus aureus are also potential causes of neonatal infections, GBS is the most common pathogen associated with early-onset sepsis in newborns.

Question 128: Correct Answer: C) Assess for signs of infection and consult the healthcare provider.
Rationale: A moist cord stump with a foul odor may indicate infection. It is crucial to assess for other signs of infection such as redness, warmth, swelling, or discharge. Consulting the healthcare provider for further evaluation and treatment is necessary to prevent complications. Cleaning more frequently with soap and water, applying hydrogen peroxide, or covering with a gauze pad are not recommended actions and may worsen the condition if infection is present.

Question 129: Correct Answer: D) Eating a balanced diet rich in calories
Rationale: Breastfeeding mothers require additional calories to support milk production. Consuming a balanced diet rich in calories ensures an adequate milk supply for the infant. Limiting fluid intake can lead to dehydration and affect milk production. Caffeine should be consumed in moderation as excessive intake can be passed to the infant through breast milk. Carbohydrates are important for energy and should not be avoided as they provide essential nutrients for both the mother and the baby.

Question 130: Correct Answer: B) Tetralogy of Fallot (TOF)
Rationale: Tetralogy of Fallot (TOF) is a cyanotic heart defect characterized by four components: pulmonary stenosis, overriding aorta, ventricular septal defect, and right ventricular hypertrophy. The classic presentation includes cyanosis, tachypnea, poor feeding, and a loud single second heart sound (S2). While other defects like ASD, VSD, and PDA can also present with cyanosis, the specific combination of symptoms in Emily's case points towards TOF.

Question 131: Correct Answer: C) Nutramigen
Rationale: Nutramigen is a hypoallergenic formula specifically designed for infants with cow's milk protein allergy. It is extensively hydrolyzed, making it easier for infants to digest. Similac Advance, Enfamil Gentlease, and Gerber Good Start are not hypoallergenic formulas and may not be suitable for infants with cow's milk protein allergy. Nutramigen is the correct choice due to its specialized formulation for infants with this specific allergy.

Question 132: Correct Answer: A) Tummy time helps prevent flat spots on the baby's head.
Rationale: Tummy time is crucial for newborns to prevent flat spots on the baby's head and promote healthy development of neck and shoulder muscles. It is recommended to perform tummy time when the baby is awake and supervised, not immediately after feeding. Tummy time should be done on a firm, flat surface to ensure the baby's safety and prevent suffocation. Therefore, option A is the correct choice when educating parents about tummy time for newborns.

Question 133: Correct Answer: B) Fentanyl
Rationale: Fentanyl is a potent opioid analgesic commonly used in labor due to its rapid onset of action and short duration, making it suitable for pain relief during labor without significantly affecting the fetus. Morphine, although effective, has a longer duration of action and may cause respiratory depression in the newborn. Codeine and Tramadol are weaker opioids and are not typically used for labor pain relief.

Question 134: Correct Answer: D) Progestin-only pills
Rationale: Progestin-only pills, also known as the mini-pill, are the most suitable contraceptive method for breastfeeding mothers in the immediate postpartum period. This is because they do not affect milk supply and are safe to use while breastfeeding. Combined oral contraceptives containing estrogen are not recommended during this time as they can potentially decrease milk production. Intrauterine devices (IUDs) are generally safe but may be inserted after the uterus has involuted postpartum. Condoms are effective but may not be the most convenient option for long-term use in the postpartum period.

Question 135: Correct Answer: B) Erythromycin ointment
Rationale: Erythromycin ointment is the recommended

medication for eye prophylaxis in newborns to prevent ophthalmia neonatorum, which is caused by Neisseria gonorrhoeae and Chlamydia trachomatis. Tetracycline, Gentamicin, and Ciprofloxacin are not typically used for this purpose and may not provide adequate coverage against the pathogens causing ophthalmia neonatorum.

Question 136: Correct Answer: B) Notifying the healthcare provider
Rationale: When signs of infection are present in a postpartum mother with perineal edema and pain, the priority action is to notify the healthcare provider for further evaluation and initiation of appropriate antibiotic therapy. Increasing perineal care frequency and applying warm compresses may provide comfort but do not address the underlying infection. Antibiotic therapy should be prescribed by the healthcare provider after assessment and confirmation of infection.

Question 137: Correct Answer: B) Breastfeeding should be initiated within 1-2 hours after birth.
Rationale: Initiating breastfeeding within the first hour after birth is crucial for successful breastfeeding establishment. Colostrum, the first milk produced, is rich in nutrients and antibodies essential for the newborn's health. Delaying breastfeeding or supplementing with formula can interfere with establishing a good milk supply and may lead to breastfeeding difficulties. Nipple soreness is a common issue that can be addressed with proper latch techniques and support, and it is not a contraindication for breastfeeding.

Question 138: Correct Answer: B) Metoclopramide
Rationale: Metoclopramide is a GI motility drug commonly used to treat constipation by increasing muscle contractions in the upper digestive tract. Ondansetron is an antiemetic used for nausea and vomiting, Pantoprazole is a proton pump inhibitor for acid reflux, and Furosemide is a diuretic for fluid retention, making them incorrect options in this scenario.

Question 139: Correct Answer: C) Hormonal changes
Rationale: Hormonal changes, particularly fluctuations in estrogen and progesterone levels, play a significant role in causing sleep disturbances in postpartum women. These changes can disrupt the normal sleep-wake cycle, leading to difficulties in falling asleep or staying asleep. Options A, B, and D are incorrect as decreased anxiety levels, increased social support, and regular exercise are factors that can actually improve sleep quality rather than cause disturbances. Therefore, understanding the impact of hormonal changes is crucial in addressing sleep issues in postpartum women.

Question 140: Correct Answer: B) Oligohydramnios
Rationale: An AFI of 5 cm indicates oligohydramnios, which is a decreased volume of amniotic fluid and can be associated with fetal growth restriction, renal abnormalities, or placental insufficiency. Options A, C, and D are incorrect as they do not reflect the specific finding of oligohydramnios.

Question 141: Correct Answer: C) Teach the mother breast compression techniques to help stimulate milk flow.
Rationale: Breast compression techniques involve applying gentle pressure to the breast during breastfeeding to help the baby receive more milk efficiently. This can be particularly helpful for babies who exhibit weak sucking patterns or tend to fall asleep at the breast. Switching to bottle feeding (option A) may interfere with establishing a successful breastfeeding relationship. Nipple shields (option B) are not recommended unless there are specific latch issues. Limiting breastfeeding sessions (option D) can decrease milk supply and hinder the baby's ability to effectively nurse.

Question 142: Correct Answer: A) Encouraging frequent breastfeeding or pumping
Rationale: The most effective way to relieve breast engorgement is by encouraging frequent breastfeeding or pumping to empty the breasts and prevent milk stasis. This helps alleviate swelling and discomfort. Applying ice packs may reduce swelling temporarily but can also decrease milk supply. Avoiding breast stimulation can lead to further engorgement and potential issues like mastitis. Wearing tight-fitting bras can constrict milk flow and exacerbate the condition.

Question 143: Correct Answer: C) Blood glucose levels
Rationale: Monitoring blood glucose levels is crucial in pregnant women with a history of gestational diabetes to detect and manage any recurrence of the condition. While monitoring blood pressure, fetal movements, and maternal weight gain are important aspects of antenatal care, they may not be the priority in this scenario.

Question 144: Correct Answer: C) Arthrogryposis Multiplex Congenita
Rationale: The presentation of clenched fists and overlapping fingers is indicative of Arthrogryposis Multiplex Congenita, a condition characterized by multiple joint contractures at birth. Polydactyly is the presence of extra fingers or toes, Syndactyly is the fusion of digits, and Brachial Plexus Injury involves nerve damage leading to weakness or paralysis in the arm.

Question 145: Correct Answer: A) Normal
Rationale: The cord gas values fall within the normal range, indicating a normal acid-base status for the newborn. The pH is within the normal range of 7.35-7.45, pO2 and pCO2 values are also within normal limits, and the HCO3 level is within the expected range. These values suggest that the newborn did not experience significant acid-base disturbances during the delivery process.

Question 146: Correct Answer: D) Respect for persons
Rationale: Respect for persons is a fundamental ethical concept in maternal newborn nursing that requires healthcare providers to treat all individuals with dignity and respect, honoring their autonomy and worth. This principle is essential when addressing psychosocial and ethical issues, as it ensures that patients' beliefs and values are acknowledged and integrated into their care. While confidentiality, cultural competence, and informed consent are also crucial aspects of nursing practice, respect for persons specifically emphasizes the importance of upholding the dignity and autonomy of every individual, regardless of their background or beliefs.

Question 147: Correct Answer: D) Protein
Rationale: Protein is crucial for lactating mothers as it is the building block for breast milk production. While Vitamin C, Iron, and Calcium are essential nutrients for overall health, they do not directly impact milk supply. Protein-rich foods like lean meats, dairy, eggs, legumes, and nuts help in meeting the increased demands of breastfeeding.

Question 148: Correct Answer: A) Administering Rh immunoglobulin (RhIg) at 28 weeks gestation
Rationale: Rh incompatibility occurs when the mother is

Rh-negative and the fetus is Rh-positive. Administering RhIg at 28 weeks gestation helps prevent the mother from forming antibodies against the Rh-positive blood of the fetus, thus reducing the risk of hemolytic disease in the newborn. Delaying administration, monitoring without intervention, or administering RhIg only after birth are not recommended practices and can increase the risk of hemolytic disease.

Question 149: Correct Answer: D) Increased renal blood flow

Rationale: During pregnancy, there is an increase in plasma volume to support the growing fetus. This increase in plasma volume is facilitated by an increase in renal blood flow, allowing for enhanced filtration and excretion of waste products. Options A, B, and C are incorrect as pregnancy typically leads to an increased heart rate, increased red blood cell production to meet the demands of the growing fetus, and a relatively stable or slightly decreased blood pressure due to hormonal changes and increased blood volume.

Question 150: Correct Answer: B) Rh-negative mother with Rh-positive fetus

Rationale: Hemolytic disease of the newborn (HDN) occurs when a Rh-negative mother carries a Rh-positive fetus, leading to maternal antibodies attacking the fetal red blood cells. This mismatch in Rh factor can trigger an immune response in subsequent pregnancies, causing severe hemolysis in the newborn. Options A, C, and D are not directly associated with the development of HDN, making them incorrect choices. Maternal O positive blood type does not inherently predispose to HDN, maternal antibodies against fetal platelets are linked to a different condition (neonatal alloimmune thrombocytopenia), and premature birth, while posing other risks, is not a primary risk factor for HDN.

Made in the USA
Las Vegas, NV
22 April 2025